# Peptic Ulcer Disease

# Peptic Ulcer Disease

Edited by **Jessica Brown**

FOSTER
ACADEMICS

New Jersey

Published by Foster Academics,
61 Van Reypen Street,
Jersey City, NJ 07306, USA
www.fosteracademics.com

**Peptic Ulcer Disease**
Edited by Jessica Brown

International Standard Book Number: 978-1-63242-315-3 (Hardback)

Printed in the United States of America.

# Contents

# Preface

Peptic ulcer disease is one of the most common chronic infections amongst humans. In spite of centuries of study, this ailment still bothers a lot of people, especially those in third world countries. It can sometimes lead to serious complications like cancer or even, death. This book consists of the current information on peptic ulcer disease, contributed by distinguished researchers from various countries around the world. It discusses topics like the cause of the disease, pathophysiology and molecular-cellular mechanisms.

This book has been the outcome of endless efforts put in by authors and researchers on various issues and topics within the field. The book is a comprehensive collection of significant researches that are addressed in a variety of chapters. It will surely enhance the knowledge of the field among readers across the globe.

It is indeed an immense pleasure to thank our researchers and authors for their efforts to submit their piece of writing before the deadlines. Finally in the end, I would like to thank my family and colleagues who have been a great source of inspiration and support.

**Editor**

# Part 1

# Pathogenesis of Peptic Ulcer

# Gastric Ulcer Etiology

Maria Izabel Gomes Silva and
Francisca Cléa Florenço de Sousa
*Federal University of Ceará*
*Brazil*

## 1. Introduction

A gastric ulcer, also called stomach ulcer, is a break in the normal gastric mucosa integrity that extends through the muscularis mucosa into the submucosa or deeper. The incidence varies with the age, gender, geographical location and is associated with severe complications including hemorrhages, perforations, gastrointestinal obstruction, and malignancy. Thus, this clinical condition represents a worldwide health problem because of its high morbidity, mortality and economic loss (Brown & Wilson, 1999; Dimaline & Varro, 2007).

The normal stomach mucosa maintains a balance between protective and aggressive factors. Some of the main aggressive factors are gastric acid, abnormal motility, pepsin, bile salts, use of alcohol and nonsteroidal anti-inflammatory drugs (NSAID), as well as infection with microorganisms (*Helicobacter pylori* and others). On the other hand, mucus secretion, bicarbonate production, gastroprotective prostaglandin synthesis and normal tissue microcirculation protect against ulcer formation. Although in most cases the etiology of ulcer is unknown yet, it is generally accepted that gastric ulcers are multifactorial and develop when aggressive factors (endogenous, exogenous and/or infectious agents) overcome mucosal defense mechanisms (Allen & Garner, 1980; Wallace, 1992; Peskar & Marici, 1998; Tulassay & Herszényi, 2010).

In this context, the present chapter aims to address etiologies multiples of gastric ulcer development, clarifying how the imbalance between aggressive and defensive factors leads to this clinical condition. For this purpose, we review basic components of gastric mucosal defense and discuss conditions in which mucosal injury is directly related to impairment in mucosal defense.

## 2. Gastric protective factors

The stomach is lined by a complex epithelium that forms a selective barrier between the external environment (lumen) and the body, which is folded into several branching, tubular gastric glands that reach deep into the muscularis mucosa. The diverse range of functions performed by gastric epithelial cells is maintained in the face of a hostile luminal environment that can contain up to 150 mm HCl and aggressive proteases, which are capable of digesting tissue, as well as a variety of noxious pathogens (Dimaline &Varro, 2007). Despite continuous exposure to these injurious factors, under normal conditions a large number of defense mechanisms prevent local damage and maintain structural and functional mucosal integrity (Tulassay & Herszényi, 2010).

In general, gastric defense mechanisms consist of a gastric mucosal "barrier". It is a multilayer system, which include a preepithelial mucus-bicarbonate "barrier", an epithelial "barrier" (surface epithelial cells connected by tight junctions), and a subepithelial component including blood flow and nerves. (Henriksnäs et al., 2006; Dimaline & Varro, 2007; Nayeb-Hashemi & Kaunitz, 2009).

## 2.1 Gastric mucosal "barrier"
### 2.1.1 Preepithelial mucus-bicarbonate "barrier"

The regular exposure of the stomach to endogenously produced acid and degrading enzymes requires the presence of an efficient gastric mucosal "barrier". Since the first experimental evidence for the mucus bicarbonate barrier was reported about three decades ago (Allen, 1978; Allen & Garner, 1980), it has become firmly established as a key component of the gastroduodenal mucosal protective mechanisms against noxious agents (Allen & Flemström, 2005). This barrier constitutes the first line of mucosal defense and is formed by mucus gel, bicarbonate ($HCO_3^-$), and surfactant phospholipids, which cover the mucosal surface (Lichtenberger, 1999; Allen & Flemström, 2005).

The gastric mucus consists of a viscous, elastic, adherent and transparent gel secreted by apical expulsion from surface epithelial cells. It is formed by ~ 95% water and ~ 5% mucin glycoproteins that covers the entire gastrointestinal mucosa, and its luminal surface is coated with a film of surfactant phospholipids with strong hydrophobic properties. The $HCO_3^-$ is secreted by surface epithelial cells and its role is to neutralize acid diffusing into a stable, adherent mucus gel layer and to be quantitatively sufficient to maintain a near-neutral pH (~ 7.0) at the mucus-mucosal surface interface (Figure 1) (Hills et al., 1983; Lichtenberger 1999; Repetto & Llesuy, 2002; Tulassay & Herszényi, 2010).

In contrast to stomach acid, pepsin has received relatively little attention as the other endogenous aggressor in gastric juice. Pepsin damage is characterized by focal areas of discontinuity in the adherent mucus layer, localized hemorrhagic punctuate ulcers with bleeding into the lumen, and no evidence of reepithelialization or mucoid cap formation (Allen & Flemström, 2005). Thus, the unstirred mucus gel layer is also a physical barrier to luminal pepsin accessing the underlying mucosa. It retains $HCO_3^-$ secreted by surface epithelial cells, preventing penetration of pepsin and therefore proteolytic digestion of the surface epithelium (Tulassay & Herszényi, 2010). Therefore, a dissipation of the mucus gel and phospholipid layer by ulcerogenic substances (such as aspirin and bile salts) leads to both acid back-diffusion and mucosal injury. (Darling et al., 2004; Allen & Flemström , 2005). Moreover, if some oxygen radicals are generated in surface epithelium containing mucus, intracellular mucus could scavenge them, acting as an antioxidant and thus reducing mucosal damage mediated by oxygen free radicals. (Penissi & Piezzi, 1999; Repetto & Llesuy, 2002). Even when cells containing mucus are damaged by extracellular oxygen radicals, intracellular mucus may be released into the gastric tissue and prevent additional damage by scavenging them (Seno et al., 1995).

The efficacy of protective properties of the mucus barrier depends not only on the gel structure but also on the amount or thickness of the layer covering the mucosal surface (Penissi & Piezzi, 1999; Repetto & Llesuy, 2002). The thickness of this layer is the result of a dynamic balance between its secretion and its erosion mechanically by shear forces of the digestive process and by proteolytic degradation, particularly from luminal pepsin in stomach. Compared with other gastrointestinal secretions, the adherent mucus gel form is physically unique. Studies have shown that adherent mucus gels from stomach, duodenum, and colon are all well-defined viscoelastic gels that do not dissolve on dilution (Allen et al., 1976; Allen, 1989; Allen & Flemström, 2005). They flow over a relatively long time (30–120 min), reannealing when sectioned. Thus, mucus gels are known stable substances, and exposure of isolated gastric mucus gel to pH 1–8, hypertonic salt, or bile does not disperse or affect its rheological properties. In functional terms, these recognized properties contribute to the adherent mucus gel layer forming a continuous and effective protection over the mucosa (Allen & Flemström, 2005)

The mucus bicarbonate barrier is the only preepithelial barrier between epithelium and lumen. When it is overwhelmed or breaks down in different disease conditions, the next series of protective mechanisms come into play, including epithelial repair, and maintenance and distribution of mucosal blood flow (Tulassay & Herszényi, 2010).

## 2.1.2 Epithelial "barrier"

Subsequent to mucus-bicarbonate "barrier", the next line of mucosal protection is formed by a continuous layer of surface epithelial cells, which secrete mucus and bicarbonate and generate prostaglandins (PGs), heat shock proteins, trefoil factor family peptides (TFFs), and cathelicidins. This epithelial barrier serves to separate the digestive lumen from the internal compartments of the organism. Its main role is to maintain a selective exchange of different substances (secretions, nutrients, etc.) between these two compartments, and to assure the protection of the organism against the penetration of micro-organisms and other exogenous antigens, essentially contained in food. In this context, two crucial elements of the digestive epithelial barrier assure these functions: the epithelial cells and the intercellular junctions (tight junctions). Both structures provide two pathways for transepithelial transport: transcellular and paracellular routes, respectively (Figure 1). (Matysiak-Budnik, et al., 2003; Laine et al., 2008; Tulassay & Herszényi, 2010). Because of the presence of phospholipids on epithelial cells surfaces, these cells are hydrophobic and therefore repel acid- and water-soluble damaging agents (Lichtenberger et al., 1983).

The paracellular pathway seems to be the major route of transepithelial macromolecular permeation. This route is a complex array of structures that are mainly controlled by tight junctions between epithelial cells, which appear to be key regulators of gastrointestinal permeability to macromolecules such as endotoxin and other bacterial products. Also, interconnected by tight junctions, the surface epithelial cells form a "barrier" preventing back diffusion of acid and pepsin (Farhadi et al., 2003; Werther, 2000; Laine et al., 2008). The physiology of this tightly regulated conduit is not fully known. However, this dynamic gateway is able to change its size under various physiological and pathological conditions. For instance, an earlier study (Madara, 1983) showed that increases in guinea pig intestinal transepithelial resistance induced by osmotic loads were accompanied by alterations in absorptive-cell tight junction structure. This alteration in intestinal permeability after meal ingestion enhances the ability of the small intestine to harvest the maximal amount of nutrients, as well as also increase the risk of exposure to luminal proinflammatory compounds. Tight junctions are also composed of other structural proteins including actin anchoring protein (ZO-1) and occludin, which could be the target of oxidative or other toxin injury and result in disruption of gastrointestinal barrier integrity (Farhadi et al., 2003; Nusrat et al., 2001).

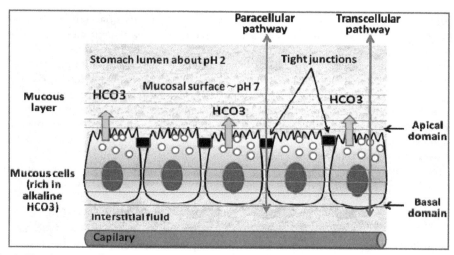

Fig. 1. Bicarbonate rich mucous secreted by surface epithelial cells.

Heat shock proteins generated by gastric epithelial cells are essential for the maintenance of cellular homeostasis during normal cell growth and for survival during various cellular stresses, such as increased temperature, oxidative stress, and cytotoxic agents, preventing protein denaturation and protecting cells against injury. Activation of heat shock protein response is one of the mucosal protective mechanisms of the antacid hydrotalcite. Also, cathelicidin and ß defensins are cationic peptides that play roles in the innate defensive system at mucosal surfaces preventing bacterial colonization. These elements have been demonstrated in gastric epithelial cells, and they accelerate ulcer healing (Tarnawski et al., 1999; Oyaka et al., 2006; Tanaka et al., 2007; Tulassay & Herszényi, 2010).

The trefoil factor family (TFFs) comprises a group of small peptides (6.5–12 kDa) secreted abundantly by surface epithelium, which has been demonstrated play an important role in mucosal integrity (Taupin & Podolsky, 2003). They regulate reepithelialization by stimulating cell migration and exert mucosal protective action from a broad range of toxic chemicals and drugs (Laine et al., 2008), as well as inhibiting apoptosis and inflammation, and augmenting the barrier function of mucus (Taupin & Podolsky, 2003; Hernández et al., 2009; Tulassay & Herszényi, 2010).

Maintenance of epithelial integrity requires a precise balance between cell proliferation and cell death. Thus, the epithelium is continually renewed by a well-coordinated and controlled proliferation of progenitor cells that enables replacement of damaged or aged surface epithelial cells. In this context, the gastric epithelium is populated by a variety of functionally-mature cells derived from proliferation of stem cells, such as mucous cells in the stomach, which show rapid turnover rates, and die within only a few days after their formation. Cell proliferation of progenitor cells is controlled by two peptides that have received attention for their potential role in barrier maintenance: epidermal growth factor (EGF), derived from salivary, esophageal and duodenal glands, and transforming growth factor alpha (TGF-alpha). Both peptides stimulate epithelial cell proliferation in case of injury as well as also enhance mucus secretion and inhibit acid production in the stomach (Murphy, 1998; Laine et al., 2008). However, after superficial injury, restitution of the surface epithelium occurs within minutes by migration of preserved epithelial cells located in the neck area of gastric glands. Such migration precedes and is independent of proliferation of progenitor cells, which occurs hours after injury (Lacy & Ito, 1984; Blikslager & Roberts, 1997; Laine et al., 2008).

Prostaglandins (PGs) are also synthesized by gastric mucosal epithelial cells from arachidonate metabolism through the action of cyclooxygenases (COX). The ability of exogenous PGs to attenuate or even completely prevent mucosal damage caused by corrosive substances such as absolute ethanol, concentrated bile or hiperosmolar solutions has been termed "cytoprotection" (Farhadi et al., 2003). Particularly prostaglandin E2 and prostacyclin have long been known to have "cytoprotective" effects on the gastrointestinal epithelium and therefore they can be crucial for the maintenance of the gastric integrity. In fact, it is well established that inhibition of their synthesis results in the reduction of gastric mucosal blood flow and gastric mucosal damage (Abdel Salam et al., 1997).

Thus, although the precise mechanism of cytoprotective action of prostaglandins remained unknown, it appears to result from a complex ability to stimulate mucosal mucus and bicarbonate secretion, to increase mucosal blood flow and sulfhydryl compounds and, particularly in the stomach, to limit back diffusion of acid into the epithelium (Tarnawski et al., 1985; Farhadi et al., 2003; Kato et al., 2005). Earlier studies confirm not only these finding but also document that certain growth factors, especially EGF, could be considered as gastroprotective because they were capable of reducing nonsteroidal anti-inflammatory drugs (NSAID)-induced gastric ulcerations in animals when endogenous PGs were completely inhibited by administration of these drugs (Konturek e a., 1981). Also, growth factors stimulated prostaglandin production in rat endometrial cells through a mechanism that involves an increase in cyclooxygenase activity (Bany & Kennedy, 1995). Moreover, previous studies (Matsuda et al. 2002; Sánchez et al. 2006), including that conducted by our group (Silva et al., 2009), reported that endogenous prostaglandins are involved in the protective effect of different natural or semi-synthetic terpenes.

In addition, other mediators such as nitric oxide (NO), calcitonin gene related peptide (CGRP) as well as some hormones including gastrin and cholecystokinin (CCK), ghrelin, leptin and gastrin-releasing peptide (GRP) have been also found to protect gastric mucosa against the damage induced by corrosive substances. This protective action has also been attributed in part to the release of PGs because it could be abolished by the pretreatment with indomethacin (a nonselective inhibitor of COX 1 and 2) and restored by the addition of exogenous PGE2 (Farhadi et al., 2003).

### 2.1.3 Subepithelial components (microcirculation and sensory innervations)

The modulation of the gastric mucosal microcirculation plays an essential role in the maintenance of gastric integrity, especially for delivering oxygen and nutrients and removing toxic substances. At the level of the muscularis mucosae, most gastric arteries branch into capillaries, which enter the lamina propria and travel upward in proximity to gastric glandular epithelial cells. At the base of surface epithelial cells, capillaries converge into collecting venules (Laine et al., 2008; Tulassay & Herszényi, 2010). Thus, blood flow is essential for many protective mechanisms. For instance, restitution, a process whereby denuded areas of the mucosa are covered by rapidly migrating cells from adjacent mucosa, depends to a large extent on adequate blood flow (Lacy & Ito, 1984; Guttu et al., 1994; Abdel-Salam et al., 2001). Also, exposure of the gastric mucosa to an irritant or acid back-diffusion occurrence leads to a marked increase in mucosal blood flow. This increase allows removal and/or dilution of the back-diffusing acid and/or noxious agents and seems to be essential for mucosal defense because its abolition through mechanical restriction of blood flow leads to hemorrhagic necrosis (Holzer, 2006, Laine et al., 2008).

The endothelial cells are also able to generate potent vasodilators agents such as nitric oxide (NO) and prostacyclin (PGI2). NO is produced from L-arginine in a reaction catalyzed by the enzyme nitric oxide synthase (NOS) (Bredt & Snyder, 1990). It is an important biological signaling molecule that influences circulation by regulating vascular smooth muscle tone and modulating systemic blood pressure. Therefore, it has been shown to exert positive effects on mucosal defense in the gastrointestinal system (Berg et al., 2004). Both NO and PGI2 oppose the mucosal damaging action of vasoconstrictors such as thromboxane A2, leukotriene C4, and endothelin. Consequently, these agents maintain viability of endothelial cells and prevent platelet and leukocyte adherence to the microvascular endothelial cells, preventing compromise of the microcirculation and thus protecting the gastric mucosa against injury (Laine et al., 2008). In addition to maintaining gastric blood flow, NO protects the gastrointestinal tract by inhibiting gastric acid secretion from parietal cells, stimulating mucus and bicarbonate secretion and by promotion angiogenesis in *vivo* and in *vitro* (Brown et al., 1993; Ma and Wallace, 2000).

Thus, for all its functions on gastric mucosal, NO has been shown to be beneficial in gastric ulcer healing. In fact, previous studies have demonstrated that NOS inhibition by N(G)-nitro- L-arginine (L-NNA) or N(G)-monomethyl-L-arginine (L-NMMA) significantly delayed ulcer healing, impaired angiogenesis in the granulation tissue and reduced gastric blood flow around the ulcer (Konturek et al., 1993). Also, NOS inhibitor N(G)-nitro-L-arginine methyl ester (L-NAME) has been showed to increase ethanol-induced gastric lesions in mice (Bulut et al., 1999; Silva et al., 2009). On the other hand, administration of an NO donor (glyceryl trinitrate) or L-arginine (the substrate of NOS) significantly reverses NOS inhibitor induced delayed healing and enhances healing (Elliott et al., 1995; Brzozowski et al., 1995; Moura Rocha et al.; 2010).

In addition to local mucosal protection factors, gastric mucosal defense is also regulated, at least in part, by the central nervous system and hormonal factors (Stroff et al., 1995; Peskar, 2001; Mózsik et al., 2001). Gastric mucosa and submucosal vessels are innervated by primary afferent sensory neurons and nerves forming a dense plexus at the mucosal base. Afferent neurons constitute an emergency system that is requested when the gastric mucosa is endangered by noxious agents. Thus, activation of these nerves in presence of gastric acid promotes releasing of neurotransmitters such as substance P and calcitonin gene-related peptide (CGRP), which relax the smooth muscle surrounding the arterioles, resulting in an elevation of mucosal blood flow, increase in mucus gel and surface cell intracellular pH in stomach. This mucosal protective action occurs most likely through vasodilatation of submucosal vessels mediated by NO generation. In this sense, interference with any aspect of the sensory innervations impairs the hyperemic response and therefore diminishes resistance of the gastric mucosa to injury (Tanaka et al., 1997; Holzer, 2007; Laine et al., 2008; Tulassay & Herszényi, 2010).

## 3. Etiologies multiples of gastric ulcer development

Despite its robust and multi-faceted nature, many factors directly related to impairment in mucosal defense can alter the epithelial barrier and encourage the formation of mucosal injury, the most important of which are acid secretion, bacteria and their products, nonsteroidal anti-inflammatory drugs, alcohol, reactive oxygen species, as well as different chemical compounds. Their effects on the gastric barrier represent important mechanisms of the pathogenesis of gastric ulcers, chronic gastritis and other gastric diseases, which are frequently generated through an imbalance between mucosal aggressive and defensive factors (Figure 2) (Wallace, 1992; Peskar & Marici, 1998; Tulassay & Herszényi, 2010).

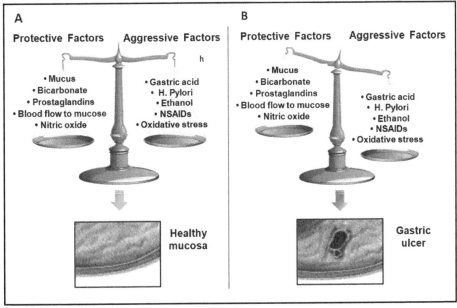

Fig. 2. (A) Healthy gastric mucosa: balance between mucosal aggressive and protective factors. (B) Gastric ulcer formation: imbalance between mucosal aggressive and protective factors.

## 3.1 Helicobacter Pylori

*Helicobacter pylori* is a common human pathogen and public health problem associated with the pathogenesis of gastritis and peptic ulcers. With a prevalence of up to 90% in developing populations, this microorganism is the second most common pathogen for human beings. It is a nonsporulating, gram-negative microaerophilic bacilli, spiral-shaped, having one to six polar-sheathed flagellae emerging from one of its rounded ends and a smooth surface (Dye et al.; 1989). This pathogen multiplies with great efficiency in the hostile environment within the stomach but survives poorly in the gastric lumen. It is mainly found under the mucous layer and in close proximity, or even attached, to gastric superficial epithelial cells, without substantial invasion of host tissue (Dubois, 1995).

*H. pylori* induces chronic gastritis of varying severity in infected subjects, which in around 10-15% progresses to peptic ulcer, while in 1-2% of subjects ultimately results in MALT lymphoma or gastric adenocarcinoma. The initial response to infection is an interaction of the host epithelial cells with the bacteria, however, the pathogenetic mechanisms of chronic infection with *H. pylori* and gastric ulcer are yet to be full determined (Parsonnet et al., 1991; Ernst & Gold, 2000; Calvino-Fernández & Parra-Cid, 2010).

A characteristics feature of this pathogen is the synthesis of urease, which was its first virulence factor studied. This enzyme may explain the extraordinary ability of bacteria to colonize the gastric mucosa and survive in an acid environment (Smoot, 1991). Because the ecologic niches of these bacteria are rich in urea, it catalyzes urea hydrolysis with the formation of ammonium (NH3), carbon dioxide and hydroxyl ions. By this mechanism, *H. pylori* neutralizes the surrounding gastric acid and protects itself from the strong acidity of the stomach (Smoot, 1991). On the other hand, although the neutralization of gastric acid benefits the bacteria, metabolites from urease activity are toxic to gastric epithelial cells (Figure 3). The formed ammonium reacts with OCl- produced by activated neutrophils to form highly toxic monochloramine (NH2Cl) in the stomach, a hallmark of *H. pylori* infection. In fact, inhibition of *H. pylori* urease has been showed significantly decrease this toxicity, suggesting that ammonia is at least partially responsible for the cytotoxicity found in association with this bacterium. Moreover, hydroxide ions are also considered toxic to gastric epithelial cells (Smoot, 1991; Handa et al., 2010).

Besides urease activity, further important virulence factors from *H. pylori* are their spiral shape and the motility of their flagellae, which render them resistant to peristaltic flushing of the gastric contents and enable them to persist in the mucous layer. Additionally, this pathogen produces other enzymes including catalase, oxidase, protease, and phospholipase, as well as it synthesizes specific adhesion proteins that enable them to adhere to mucous and epithelial cells (Boren et al., 1993; Dubois, 1995). In this context, although *H. pylori* typically colonizes the human stomach for many decades without adverse consequences, as referred above, the presence of this pathogen is associated with an increased risk of several diseases, including peptic ulcers, noncardia gastric adenocarcinoma, and gastric mucosa associated lymphoid tissue (MALT) lymphoma (Cover & Blaser, 2009).

The risks of developing gastric diseases are determined in part by the presence or absence of specific genotypes of the *H. pylori* strains with which an individual is colonized. For that reason, *H. pylori* pathogenicity may differ with respect to each of its virulence factors and this diversity is likely to contribute to variation in colonization or disease. (Dubois, 1995; Marshall & Windsor, 2005; Cover & Blaser, 2009). Thus, a number of *H pylori* strains can express multiple factors that interact with host tissue and therefore are associated with increased gastric mucosal inflammatory cell infiltration and increased gastric epithelial injury, whereas strains that lack these factors would be relatively noninteractive with the host. When virulent *H. pylori* strains are present, organisms adhere to the gastric epithelium, which disrupts membrane integrity and induces host cells to release toxic proteins, cytotoxins, platelet activating factor, , and lipopolysaccharides that all further damage the gastric mucosa. These changes would accelerate apoptosis and proliferation in the mucosal layer (Figure 3) (Crabtree, 1996; Kohda et al., 1999; Makola et al., 2007). However, it has been shown that this inflammation resolves after eradication of the infection, and presumably the concentrations of the pro-inflammatory and antisecretory cytokines also decrease. Thus, once the eradication of the bacterium is always followed by resolution of gastritis, the aim of treatment is eradication of the pathogen, defined as negative tests for the organism for one month after completion of the course of the antimicrobial (Pakodi et al., 2000; Kuipers et al., 2003; Brzozowski, et al., 2006).

Although much research and understanding have been gained in the last decades since the discovery of *H. pylori*, more questions have been raised than answered. The long road towards deciphering the fundamental mechanisms underlying the development of gastritis, intestinal metaplasia and gastric cancer has only just begun. Thus, currently it is apparent that infection with *H. pylori* negatively influences several of the important defense mechanisms in the gastric barrier, however, the exact mechanisms leading to the development of pathological changes by *H. pylori* remain to be further investigated.

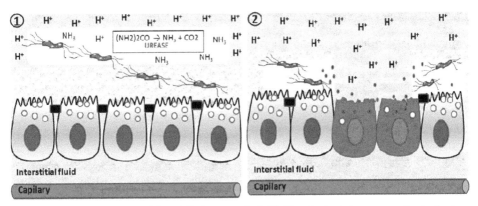

Fig. 3. Gastric ulcer formatted by *Helicobacter pylori*. (1) *H. pylori* catalyzes urea hydrolysis with the formation of ammonium (NH3) that neutralizes the surrounding gastric acid and protects itself from the strong acidity of the stomach. (2) *H. pylori* penetrates the mucus layer of stomach, adhere the surface of gastric mucosal epithelial cells, prolifirate and finally form the infectious focus. The gastric lesion is developed by destruction of mucosa, inflammation and mucosal cell death.

### 3.2 Non-steroidal anti-inflammatory drugs (NSAIDs)

Another important factor directly related to gastric injury initiated by impairment in mucosal defense is the prominent non-steroidal anti-inflammatory drugs (NSAIDs) use. As the prevalence of *H. pylori* infection has declined, because of continued efforts to eradicate the organism, the prevalence of NSAID-induced ulcers has risen and is taking on greater clinical importance. Studies show that NSAIDs are among the most commonly used drugs in the world. In United States, approximately 70 million prescriptions are written each year, while in Europe these medications represent more than 7.7% of all prescriptions (Graumlich, 2001; Jones, 2001). NSAIDs use is more frequent among women and increases with age, as does the incidence of rheumatic diseases. In fact, more than 90% of prescriptions for NSAIDs are made to patients aged >65 years. The major problem with the use of these drugs is that they induce predictable gastric mucosal injury, including complications in both upper and lower gastrointestinal tract (Laine et al., 2008; Sostres et al., 2010).

The major mechanism via which NSAIDs cause ulcers and gastrointestinal complications is thought to be by inhibition of cyclooxygenase (COX), a key enzyme in the biosynthesis of prostaglandins (PGs). There are two well identified isoforms of COX, COX 1 and COX 2 (Laine et al., 2008; Sostres et al., 2010). COX 1 isoform is expressed in most tissues, producing prostaglandins that play an essential protective role in the stomach by stimulating the synthesis and secretion of mucus and bicarbonate, increasing mucosal blood flow and promoting epithelial proliferation. So, the COX-1-mediated PG synthesis is mainly responsible for maintaining gastric mucosal integrity at baseline. On the other hand, COX2 has little or no expression in most tissues but is rapidly induced in response to inflammatory stimuli. Therefore, this isoform is the primary target for anti-inflammatory drugs.

In this context, the traditional NSAIDs nonselective inhibitors of both COX-1 and COX-2, such as indomethacin or ibuprofen, cause damage in the stomach with a marked decrease in the gastric mucosal PGE2 content. This effect occurs via COX 1 isoform inhibition, creating a gastric environment that is more susceptible to topical attack by endogenous and exogenous factors (Vane & Botting, 1995). Moreover, the inhibition of the COX 1 blocks platelet production of thromboxane, which increases bleeding when an active gastrointestinal bleeding site is present (Lanas & Scheiman, 2007; Sostres et al., 2010). This contention was further supported by the fact that COX-2 selective inhibitors, which do not inhibit COX-1 at therapeutic doses, do not affect the mucosal PGs production and do not produce gross gastric damage in experimental models (Laine et al., 2008).

Therefore, the development of NSAIDs which selectively inhibit COX-2 (Coxibs), while having little to no effect on COX-1, should result in effective pain relief with reduced adverse gastrointestinal effects. In fact, data from large gastrointestinal outcomes studies reveal that Coxibs significantly decrease gastroduodenal ulcers as compared with nonselective NSAIDs. Ulcer rates were significantly decreased with 5 tested Coxibs (celecoxib, valdecoxib, rofecoxib, lumiracoxib, etoricoxib) and when these drugs were tested against any of the most commonly used NSAIDs (diclofenac, naproxen or ibuprofen) (Rostom et al., 2007). Large randomized controlled outcome trials demonstrate a considerable reduction in upper gastrointestinal complications and overall upper gastrointestinal clinical events with Coxibs compared to traditional NSAIDs (Silverstein et al., 2000; Laine et al., 2007). Moreover, the results of another large outcomes study, celecoxib vs naproxen and diclofenac in osteoarthritis patients, confirmed the significantly better safety profile of celecoxib compared with traditional NSAIDs (Singh et al., 2006).

However, has been recognized that prostaglandins derived from COX-2 can be generated at the ulcer margin and appear to play an important role in ulcer healing through triggering the cell proliferation, promotion of angiogenesis and restoration of mucosal integrity (Konturek et al., 2005, Sostres et al., 2010). These observations indicate that, in contrast to the initial concept, COX-2 plays an important role in gastric mucosal defense. Accordingly to this, experimental studies have reported that inhibition of both COX-1 and COX-2 is required for NSAID-induced gastric injury (Wallace et al., 2000; Tanaka et al., 2001; Peskar et al., 2001) and therefore Coxibs markedly decrease but do not eliminate NSAIDs associated gastric and duodenal ulceration (Silverstein et al, 2000; Sostres et al., 2010). In fact, indomethacin and similar NSAIDs, which inhibit both isoforms of the COX enzyme, produce more severe damage in gastric tissue, even gastrointestinal bleeding, than more selective drugs (Delaney et al., 2007). Therefore, indomethacin became one of the first choice drugs to produce an experimental ulcer model (Sigthorsson et al., 2000; Suleyman et al., 2004). In this sense, the fact that nimesulide, which is considered to be less selective for COX-2 compared to Coxibs, is able to inhibit NSAID-induced gastric damage, while Coxibs agents (more selective for COX-2) are unable to inhibit these ulcers, indicates that it is impossible to attribute the gastrointestinal side effects of indomethacin and other NSAIDs to the inhibition of only the COX-1 enzyme (Suleyman et al., 2002).

In addition, studies have evidenced that NSAIDs may induce tissue and cell injury by mechanisms independent of prostaglandin inhibition, which include the inhibition of phosphorylating enzymes (kinases), inhibition of oxidative phosphorylation in mitochondria, and/or activation of apoptosis (Husain et al., 2001). These mechanisms, in combination with those related to prostaglandin suppression, lead to microvessel occlusion and subsequent hyperproduction of reactive oxygen metabolites. Such agents are then able to induce oxidative tissue injury that seems to play a prominent role in the development of mucosal ulceration caused by NSAIDs (Blandizzi et al., 2005). Furthermore, with the decrease in arachidonic acid metabolism via the COX pathway in NSAID users, arachidonic acid metabolism may be shifted to the alternative 5-lipoxygenase pathway, with a resultant increase in leukotriene production. In this way, a potential role for leukotrienes in NSAID induced gastric injury also has been postulated, since licofelone, an inhibitor of COX-1, COX-2, and 5-lipoxygenase, did not increase gastric mucosal injury (Bias et al., 2004).

Thus, because the prevalence and severity of NSAID-related gastrointestinal complications, recent efforts have been directed at the prevention of mucosal injury induced by these agents. In this sense, since NSAID and even Coxibs therapy delay the healing of active peptic ulcers, the best way to prevent mucosal injury is to avoid the use of NSAIDs or replace it with an agent less toxic to the gastroduodenal mucosa (Sostres et al., 2010).

### 3.3 Gastric acid secretion

For decades, surgeons were taught and believed that peptic ulcer disease was caused by acid, since the cure rate of peptic ulcer disease by acid-reduction operations (such as partial gastrectomies, gastroenterostomies or vagotomies) was substantial, impressive, and reported in the literature repeatedly, as described by Latarjet (1922) and Herrington et al. (1984). Thus, acid was meticulously measured in an attempt to better understand and treat peptic ulcer disease, the major clinical challenge at that time (Dotevall & Walan, 1971). In this sense, when pharmacologic means were developed such as histamine-2 blockers drugs (like cimetidine), which effectively eliminated acid and thus many patients found that their ulcer disease was healed, these observations validated the dictum "no acid, no ulcer"(Gustafson and Welling, 2010).

Over time, the prevalence as well as the management of these disorders has changed. With the advent of newer pharmacological therapy (potent antisecretory medications such as proton pump inhibitors) and the understanding of the role of *Helicobacter pylori* in the pathogenesis of peptic ulcer disease, more ulcers were successfully treated medically and the number of surgical cases drastically decreased (Lorentzon et al., 1987; Lindberg et al., 1990; Meyer-Rosberg et al., 1996; Fock et al., 2008; Schubert & Peura, 2008). As a result, the quantitative measurement of gastric acid secretion, for the most part, has become obsolete. Nevertheless, although there are multiple processes involved in the development of gastric lesions, the presence of acid hypersecretion continues to be a necessary condition for ulcer production and for a variety of common gastrointestinal disorders, since medical therapy for these illnesses involves both removing the injurious agent (eg, NSAIDs or *H. pilory*) and inhibiting acid secretion (Richardson et al., 1998; Schubert & Peura, 2008).

Parietal cells secrete hydrochloric acid at a concentration of approximately 160 mmol/L or pH 0.8. Acid facilitates the digestion of proteins and absorption of calcium, iron, and vitamin B-12, as well as it is the first line of mucosal defense to avoid microorganisms colonization thus preventing the bacterial overgrowth and consequent enteric infection (such as by *Helicobacter pylori*). However, when levels of acid (and pepsin) overwhelm mucosal defense mechanisms, common and potentially serious acid-related clinical conditions occur, including gastroesophageal reflux disease, Barrett's esophagus, where the usual squamous mucosal lining becomes replaced by columnar epithelial cells of putative specific aspect, peptic ulcer disease, and stress-related erosion/ulcer disease (Schubert & Peura, 2008; Schubert, 2008).

Acid is thought to gain access to the lumen by means of channels in the mucus layer created by the relatively high intraglandular hydrostatic pressures generated during secretion (approximately 17 mm Hg) (Johansson et al., 2001). Thus, luminal acid interferes with the process of restitution, resulting in the conversion of superficial injury to deeper mucosal lesion and inactivates the acid-labile growth factors important for maintenance of mucosal integrity and repair of superficial injury. A large amount of studies show that the rate of acid secretion by the human stomach changes little with aging unless there is coexisting disease of the oxyntic mucosa such as atrophic gastritis, infection with *H. pylori* or both (Trey et al., 1997; Schubert & Peura, 2008).

To prevent acid-induced mucosal damage, gastric acid must be precisely regulated through a highly coordinated interaction of neural, hormonal, and paracrine pathways (Schubert & Peura, 2008). In this sense, the principal stimulants of acid secretion include gastrin, histamine, gastrin-releasing peptide (GRP), orexin, ghrelin, and glucocorticoids, while the main inhibitor is somatostatin, released from oxyntic and pyloric D cells (paracrine). Gastrin, released from antral G cells into the blood stream during meals, stimulates acid secretion primarily by releasing histamine from histaminesecreting enterochromaffin-like (ECL) cells. GRP, released from antral nerve fibers in response to proteins, stimulates gastrin secretion. Ghrelin and orexin appear to stimulate acid secretion, although their physiologic roles in the stomach are not known. Glucocorticoids stimulate acid secretion acting via phosphoinositide 3 kinase, serum-inducible kinase and glucocorticoid-inducible kinase (Schubert, 2008). In addition, acetylcholine (Ach), released from postganglionic enteric neurons (neuronal stimulation), acts directly stimulating parietal cell acid secretion, as well as indirectly, by eliminating the inhibitory paracrine influence of somatostatin on parietal and ECL cells (Chuang et al., 1993; Schubert, 2008; Schubert & Peura, 2008).

Acid secretion by the parietal cell involves intracellular elevation of calcium, cyclic AMP, or both followed by a cascade that triggers the translocation of the proton pump, $H^+K^+$-ATPase, from cytoplasmic tubulovesicles to the apical plasma membrane. This pump is an integral membrane protein that transports hydronium ions from the cytoplasm into the canaliculus of the parietal cell in exchange for potassium. Most of the adult population chronically infected with *H. pylori* produce less than normal amounts of acid probably due to increased apoptosis via secreted mediators (such as VacA cytotoxin and lipopolysaccharide), induction of proinflammatory mediators (such as IL-1b), and inhibition of the $H^+K^+$-ATPase activity (Schubert, 2008). This condition may cause further reduction of acid production and, eventually, atrophy of the stomach lining, which may lead not only gastric ulcer but also increased risk for stomach cancer (Suerbaum & Michetti, 2002; Peek & Crabtree, 2006). Conversely, approximately 10% to 15% of patients chronically infected with this pathogen have antral predominant inflammation and are predisposed to duodenal ulcer. They produce increased amounts of acid as a result of reduced antral somatostatin content and elevated basal and stimulated gastrin secretion. Gastrin stimulates the parietal cells in the corpus to secrete even more acid into the stomach lumen and chronically may cause the number of parietal cells to also increase. The increased acid load ulcerations the duodenum (El-Omar, 2006; Schubert & Peura, 2008).

Thus, dosed before mealtime, proton pump inhibitors drugs are the most effective acid inhibitors currently available and are the most widely prescribed class of gastrointestinal medications. Not only can peptic ulcers be healed more rapidly with these agents, but refractory ulcers have all but disappeared. However, many clinical studies do support an accelerating effect of proton pump inhibitors on the development of atrophic gastritis in *H. pylori*-positive patients, while other evidences suggest that long-term acid suppression would result in relatively greater bacterial colonization in the corpus leading to diffuse or corpus-predominant gastritis or to acute gastroenteritis (Moayyedi et al., 2000; Rosh & Hassall, 2006; Schubert, 2008). Such observations have important implications given the extensive use of these drugs worldwide. Thus, continued progress in understanding of gastric acid secretion in health and disease is needed and this knowledge will be used to develop new more effective strategies to prevent and manage gastric disorders.

## 3.4 Alcohol

Throughout the world, alcohol has been used for centuries in social, medical, cultural, and religious settings. Currently, it is considered to be one of the most commonly abused drugs, related to a wide range of physical, mental, and social harms, and responsible for 3.8% of deaths and 4.6% of disability-adjusted life years lost worldwide. The World Health Organization (WHO) has estimated that there are about 2 billion people worldwide who consume alcoholic beverages and 76.3 million with diagnosable alcohol use disorders (Stermer, 2002; WHO, 2004, 2008; Rehm et al., 2009).

Among the various organ systems that mediate alcohol's effects on the human body and its health, the gastrointestinal tract plays a particularly important role. The alcohol absorption into the bloodstream occurs throughout the gastrointestinal tract and its direct contact with the mucosa can induce numerous metabolic and functional changes. These alterations may lead to marked mucosal damage, which can result in a broad spectrum of acute and chronic diseases, such as gastrointestinal bleeding and ulcers (Bode & Bode, 1997). In this context, pathogenesis of ethanol-induced gastric lesions is complex. Alcohol may interact directly with the gastric mucosa or it may act through a more general mechanism affecting the release of hormones and the regulation of nerve functions involved in acid secretion (Bode & Bode, 1997; Chari et al. 1993).

Intragastric application of absolute ethanol has long been used as a reproducible method to induce gastric mucosa lesions in experimental animals (Szabo et al., 1981; Arafa & Sayed-Ahmed, 2003). The effects of acute administration of absolute ethanol to rats and mice on the gastric mucosa are dose-dependent and the damage appears as early as 30 minutes after ingestion and reaches a peak at about 60 minutes. The ethanol-induced gastric musosal lesions and erosions are similar to those occurring in gastric ulcer (Stermer, 2002; Repetto & Llesuy, 2002). Thus, alcoholic gastritis leads to the impairment of the integrity of gastric mucosal barrier, contributing to acid reflux into the subluminal layers of the mucosa and submucosa (Oh et al., 2005).

Chari et al. (1993) relate that intravenous, oral, and intragastric alcohol at a concentration of up to 5% increases acid secretion principally by stimulating the secretion of gastrin and to a lesser extent by a direct effect on the parietal cells. On the other hand, an alcohol concentration of higher than 5% has no effect on gastric acid secretion (Stermer, 2002). Also, oxidative stress and depletion of non-protein sulfhydryls concentration, modulation of nitric oxide system and reduction of gastric mucosal blood flow frequently underlie the development of gastric lesions (Arafa & Sayed-Ahmed, 2003). According to Bode et al. (1996), the decreased formation of prostaglandins might also play a role in alcohol-induced mucosal injury, while other studies have indicated that an alcohol-dependent increase in the production of leukotrienes also might contribute to the development of alcohol-induced damage. It is important emphasize that changes induced by short-term exposure to alcoholic beverages are rapidly reversible while prolonged alcohol exposure leads to progressive structural mucosal damage (Bode & Bode, 1997).

Oxidative stress and depletion of anti-oxidants have been considered a crucial step in alcohol-induced mucosal damage and so they have been widely investigated in a number of studies (Hirokawa 1998; La Casa et al., 2000; Arafa & Sayed-Ahmed, 2003). Ethanol treatment induces intracellular oxidative stress and produces mitochondrial permeability transition and mitochondrial depolarization, which precede cell death in gastric mucosal cells. Thus, considering that ethanol is involved in the formation of oxidative stress generated extracellularly and/or intracellylary, the cytoprotective role of anti-oxidants in the prevention and healing of gastric lesions has also been widely investigated (Santos & Rao, 2001; Silva et al., 2009). In this sense, various studies point to intracellular antioxidants, such as glutathione (an endogenous sulfhydryl compound, as described below), as significant protective agents against ethanol in gastric mucosal cells (Repetto & Llesuy, 2002). Intragastric administration of superoxide dismutase was also able to protect the gastric mucosa against the damaging effect of ethanol (Terano et al., 1989). Also, ethanol-induced oxidative stress may account for the decreased NO release, because NO may be shunted toward scavenging free radicals. In this context, response to ethanol was prevented by increased production of nitric oxide and inducible NOS (Kato et al., 2000). In addition to ethanol-induced gastrointestinal tract alterations, alcohol consumption has been linked to increased risk of tumors in the pharynx, esophagus, stomach and colon (Stermer, 2002).

### 3.5 Oxidative stress

It is well documented in the literature that reactive oxygen species (ROS), such as superoxide anions, hydrogen peroxide, and hydroxyl radicals, are involved in the etiology and physiopathology of several human diseases including neurodegenerative disorders, viral infections, inflammation, autoimmune pathologies, as well as in digestive disturbances such as gastrointestinal inflammation and gastric ulcer (Repetto & Llesuy, 2002).

During gastric oxidative stress, the imbalance of aggressive and defensive factors in the stomach plays a pivotal role in gastric hemorrhage and ulcer formation (Hung, 2005). Overproduction of ROS has been concerned as one of the major pathogenic factors that directly results in oxidative damage, including lipid peroxidation, protein oxidation, and DNA damage, which can lead to cell death. Additionally, these agents are known to act as second messengers to activate diverse redox-sensitive signaling transduction cascades, including mitogen-activated protein kinases (MAPKs) and downstream transcription factors such as NF-kB and AP-1, which regulate the expression of several pro-inflammatory genes and, thereby, lead to the elaboration of chemical and humoral mediators of tissue inflammation and injury (Sun & Oberley, 1996; Ali & Harty, 2009). This is frequently evidenced by pro-ulcerative factors in the stomach and gut such as H pylori, use of NSAIDs, ethanol, smoking, psychological stress, corticosteroid use, and loss of sleep, while defensive factors involve glutathione (GSH), an important endogenous sulfhydryl compound, and mucus biosynthesis (Hung, 2005; Olaleye et al., 2007).

In the illness state, oxidative stress of the stomach may occur and result in an elevation of mucosal lipid peroxide that are generated from the reaction of oxyradicals and cellular polyunsaturated fatty acid, while GSH may act to prevent this aggressive action that can damage gastric mucosal cells. Malondialdehyde (MDA) is an end product resulting from peroxidation of polyunsaturated fatty acids and related esters within cell membranes, and the measurement of this substance represents a suitable index of oxidative tissue damage. On the other hand, sulfhydryl compounds such as GSH are involved in the maintenance of gastric integrity, particularly when reactive oxygen species are implicated in the pathophysiology of tissue injury (Blandizzi et al., 2005). Thus, the appearance of lipid free radicals and MDA in the blood and gastric juice could result from ROS-initiated chain reactions or initiated by indirect mechanisms that suppress the antioxidant capacity in both blood and gastric wall to scavenge ROS (Dotan et al., 2004; Tuorkey & Abdul-Aziz, 2011). In fact, numerous studies have demonstrated a decrease in GSH level in inflammatory and ulcerated gastric mucosa, as well as the protective effect of GSH on gastric damage induced by ethanol, nonsteroidal anti-inflammatory drugs, or lipopolysaccharide has been well documented (Hung, 2000; Hung, 2005; Silva et al., 2009; Al-Hashem, 2010).

On the other hand, a large body of research in both animal and human studies has examined the effect of psychological stress on the gastrointestinal tract. For instance, in accordance to Levenstein et al., (1999), susceptibility to gastric lesions is increased in rats by social stressors as premature separation of the rat pup from its mother (Ackerman et al., 1975). Also, subjects with psychological distress, self-described "stress or strain," or concrete life stressors at baseline have increased incidence of ulcer over 9 to 15 years (Levenstein et al., 1995; Levenstein et al., 1999). In this sense, according to Chang (2008), stressors can be acute or chronic and range from daily hassles to life-threatening situations like natural disasters and violence that trigger the "fight or flight" response. Over time, recurrent stress results in an increase demand on physiologic systems. Thus, several terms have been used to describe stress-related mucosal damage in critically ill patients, including stress ulcers, stress gastritis, stress erosions, hemorrhagic gastritis, erosive gastritis, and stress-related mucosal disease (Ali & Harty, 2009).

Stimulation of gastric acid secretion has historically been considered a mechanism by which physiological stress increases susceptibility to gastroduodenal ulceration. It is also known to modify gastric blood flow, which plays an important role in the gastric mucosal barrier, and to affect possible mediators such as cytokines, corticotropin-releasing hormone and thyrotropin- releasing hormone. Furthermore, stress seems to have different effects on gastric motility including delayed gastric emptying, which could increase the risk of gastric ulcer, while accelerated emptying could increase the net acid load delivered to the duodenum, enhancing the risk of duodenal ulcer. Psychological stress may also promote the growth of *H. pylori* in the duodenum if it increases duodenal acid load, since the *H. pylori*–inhibitory effects of bile seem to be reversed by acid (Levenstein et al., 1999).

## 4. Conclusion

Despite continuous exposure to several noxious factors, under normal conditions the gastric mucosa is able to maintain structural integrity and function. However, gastric mucosal injuries may occur when harmful factors overcome an intact mucosal defense or when the mucosal defensive mechanisms are impaired. Thus, much importance is attached to interactions and relationships among various ulcer-related factors, as well as to the individuality of the patients, including infections by *H. pylori*, alcohol and NSAIDs consume, and even smoking use, or stress-related disease.

Significant knowledge over the past three decades regarding gastric mucosal attack and defense mechanisms has led to the development of current and potential future therapies to reduce gastrointestinal injury and improve the quality of ulcer healing. Therefore, the incidence of gastric ulcers has declined, possibly as a result of the increasing use of proton pump inhibitors and decreasing rates of *Helicobacter pylori* infection. However, although there are many studies on gastroprotective therapies, their clinical effectiveness remains unclear. Thus, because gastric ulcer is a multifactorial disease, its medical management should not be based on a simple cause-effect relationship, instead a bio-psychosocial approach adjusted for the individual patient should be applied, with careful consideration of the association of this disease with many personal factors.

## 5. References

Abdel Salam, O.M.; Szolcsányi, J.; Mózsik. G. (1997). The indomethacin-induced gastric mucosal damage in rats. Effect of gastric acid, acid inhibition, capsaicin-type agents and prostacyclin. *Journal of Physiology – Paris, Vol.*91, No.1 (February), pp.7-19, ISSN 0928-4257.

Abdel-Salam, O.M.; Czimmer, J.; Debreceni, A.; Szolcsányi, J. & Mózsik, G. (2001). Gastric mucosal integrity: gastric mucosal blood flow and microcirculation. An overview. *Journal of Physiology (Paris)*, Vol.95, No.1-6 (January-December), pp.105-127, ISSN 0928-4257.

Ackerman, S.H.; Hofer, M.A. & Weiner, H. (1973). Age at maternal separation and gastric erosion susceptibility in the rat. *Psychosomatic Medicine*, Vol.37, No.2 (March-April), pp. 180-184, ISSN 0033-3174.

Al-Hashem, F.H. (2010). Gastroprotective effects of aqueous extract of *Chamomilla recutita* against ethanol-induced gastric ulcers. *Saudi Medical Journal.* Vol.31, No.11 (November), pp. 1211-1216, ISSN 0379-5284.

Ali, T. & Harty, R.F. (2009). Stress - Induced Ulcer Bleeding in Critically Ill Patients. *Gastroenterology Clinics of North America* 38, Vol.2 (June), pp. 245–265, ISSN 0889-8553.

Allen, A. & Flemström, G. (2005). Gastroduodenal mucus bicarbonate barrier: protection against acid and pepsin. *American Journal of Physiology - Cell Physiology*, Vol.288, No.1 (January), pp.C1–C19, ISSN: 1522-1563.

Allen, A. & Garner, A. (1980). Gastric mucus and bicarbonate secretion and their possible role in mucosal protection. *Gut*, Vol.21, No.3 (March), pp. 249–262, ISSN 0017-5749.

Allen, A. (1978). Structure of gastrointestinal mucus and the viscous and gel forming properties of mucus. *British Medical Bulletin*, Vol.34, No.1 (January), pp. 28–33, ISSN 0007-1420.

Allen, A. (1989). Gastrointestinal mucus, In: *Handbook of Physiology. Gastrointestinal Physiology. Salivary, Gastric, Pancreatic, and Hepatobiliary Secretion*, M.D. Bethesda, Am. Physiol. Soc. (Ed), sect. 6, vol. III, chapt. 19, pp. 359–382, ISBN-10: 0195208161, ISBN-13: 978-0195208160.

Allen, A.; Pain, R.H., & Robson, T. (1976). Model for the structure of gastric mucus gel. *Nature*, Vol.264 (November), p.88–89, ISSN 0028-0836.

Arafa, H.M. & Sayed-Ahmed, M.M. (2003). Protective role of carnitine esters against alcohol-induced gastric lesions in rats. *Pharmacological Research*, Vol.48, No.3 (September), pp. 285-90, ISSN 1043-6618.

Bany, B.M. & Kennedy, T.G. (1995). Regulation by epidermal growth factor of prostaglandin production and cyclooxygenase activity in sensitized rat endometrial stromal cells in vitro. *Journal of reproduction & fertility*, Vol.104, No.1 (May), pp. 57-62, ISSN 0022-4251.

Berg, A.; Redeen, S.; Ericson, A. & Sjöstrand, S.E. (2004). Nitric oxide-an endogenous inhibitor of gastric acid secretion in isolated human gastric glands. *BMC Gastroenterology*, Vol.6, (August), pp.4:16, ISSN 1471-230X.

Bias, P.; Buchner, A.; Klesser, B.; Laufer, S. (2004). The gastrointestinal tolerability of the LOX/COX inhibitor, licofelone, is similar to placebo and superior to naproxen therapy in healthy volunteers: results from a randomized, controlled trial. *American journal of gastroenterology*, Vol.99, No.4 (April), pp. 611–618, ISSN 0002-9270.

Blandizzi, C.; Fornai, M.; Colucci, R.; Natale, G.; Lubrano, V.; Vassalle, C.; Antonioli, L.; Lazzeri, G. & Del Tacca, M. (2005). Lansoprazole prevents experimental gastric injury induced by non-steroidal anti-inflammatory drugs through a reduction of mucosal oxidative damage. *World Journal of Gastroenterology*, Vol.14;11, No.26 (July), pp. 4052-4060, ISSN 1007-9327.

Blikslager, A.T. (1997). Roberts MC: Mechanisms of intestinal mucosal repair. *Journal of the American Veterinary Medical Association*,Vol.1;211, No.11 (December), pp.1437-1441, ISSN 0003-1488.

Bode, C. & Bode, J.C. (1997). Alcohol's role in gastrointestinal tract disorders. *Alcohol Health & Research World*, Vol.21, No.1, pp. 76-83, ISSN 0090-838X.

Bode, C.; Maute, G. & Bode, J.C. (1996). Prostaglandin E2 and prostaglandin F2 alpha biosynthesis in human gastric mucosa: Effect of chronic alcohol misuse. *Gut*, Vol.39, No.3 (September), pp. 348–352, ISSN 0017-5749.

Boren, T.; Falk, P.; Roth, K.A.; Larson, G. & Normark, S. (1993). Attachment of *Helicobacter pylori* to human gastric epithelium mediated by blood group antigens. *Science*, Vol.17;262, No.5141 (December), pp. 1892-1895, ISSN 0036-8075.

Bredt, D.S. & Snyder, S.H. (1990). Isolation of nitric oxide synthetase, a calmodulin-requiring enzyme. *Proceedings of the National Academy of Sciences of the United States of America*, Vol.87, No.2 (January), pp.682-685, ISSN 0027-8424.

Brown, J.F.; Kerates, A.C.; Hanson, P.J. & Whittle, B.J.R. (1993). Nitric oxide generators and cGMP stimulate mucus secretion by gastric mucosal cells. *American Journal of Physiology: Gastrointestinal and Liver Physiology*, Vol.265, No.3 (September), pp.G418–G422, ISSN 0193-1857.

Brown, L.F. & Wilson, D.E (1999). Gastroduodenal ulcers: causes, diagnosis, prevention and treatment. *Comprehensive Therapy*, Vol.25, No.1 (January), pp. 30-38, ISSN 0098-8243.

Brzozowski, T.; Konturek, S.J.; Drozdowicz, D.; Dembinski, A. & Stachura, J. (1995). Healing of chronic gastric ulcerations by L-arginine. Role of nitric oxide, prostaglandins, gastrin and polyamines. *Digestion* 56, No.6, pp. 463–471, ISSN 0012-2823.

Brzozowski,T.; Konturek, P.C.; Mierzwa, M.; Drozdowicz, D.; Bielanski, W.; Kwiecien, S.; Konturek, S.J.; Stachura, J.; Pawlik, W.W. & Hahn, E.G. (2006). Effect of probiotics and triple eradication therapy on the cyclooxygenase (COX)-2 expression, apoptosis, and functional gastric mucosal impairment in Helicobacter pylori-infected Mongolian gerbils. *Helicobacter*, Vol.11, No.1 (February), pp. 10-20, ISSN 1083-4389.

Bulut, R.; Unlucerci, Y; Bekpinar, S. & Kuntsal, L. (1999). Nitric Oxide-Mediated Regulation of Gastric H+, K+-ATPase and Alcohol Dehydrogenase Following Ethanol-Induced Injury in Rats. *Digestive diseases and sciences*, Vol.44, No.7 (July), pp. 1417-1422, ISSN 0163-2116.

Calvino-Fernández, M. & Parra-Cid, T. (2010). *H. pylori* and mitochondrial changes in epithelial cells. The role of oxidative stress. Revista Española de Enfermedades Digestivas (Madrid), Vol. 102, No 1 (January), pp. 41-50, ISSN 1130-0108.

Chang, L. (2008). The Role of Stress on Physiological Responses and Clinical Symptoms in Irritable Bowel Syndrome. *Current Molecular Medicine*, Vol.8, No.4, (June), pp. 299–312, ISSN 1566-5240.

Chari, S.; Teyssen, S.; and Singer, M.V. (1993). Alcohol and gastric acid secretion in humans. *Gut*, Vol.34, No.6 (June), pp. 843–847, ISSN 0017-5749.

Chuang, C.N.; Tanner, M.; Lloyd, K.C.K.; Wong, H.; Soll, A.H. (1993). Endogenous somatostatin inhibits histamine release from canine gastric mucosal cells in primary culture. *American Journal of Physiology: Gastrointestinal and Liver Physiology*, Vol.265, No.3 (September), pp.G521–G525, ISSN 0193-1857.

Cover, T.L. & Blaser, M.J. (2009). *Helicobacter pylori* in Health and Disease. *Gastroenterology*, Vol.136, No.6 (May), pp. 1863-1873, ISSN 0016-5085.

Crabtree,J.E. (1996). Immune and inflammatory responses to Helicobacter pylori infection. *Scandinavian Journal of Gastroenterology - Supplement*, Vol.215, pp. 3-10, ISSN 0085-5928.

Darling, R.L.; Romero, J.J.; Dial, E.J.; Akunda, J.K.; Langenbach, R. & Lichtenberger, L.M. (2004). The effects of aspirin on gastric mucosal integrity, surface hydrophobic, and prostaglandin metabolism in cyclooxygenase knockout mice. *Gastroenterology*, Vol.127, No.1 (July), pp.94–104, ISSN 0016-5085.

Delaney, J.A.; Opatrny, L.; Brophy, J.M. & Suissa, S. (2007). Drug drug interactions between antithrombotic medications and the risk of gastrointestinal bleeding. *Canadian Medical Association Journal*, Vol.14;177, No.4 (August), pp. 347–351, ISSN 0820-3946.

Dimaline, R. & Varro A. (2007). Attack and defence in the gastric epithelium - a delicate balance. *Experimental Physiology*, Vol.92, No.4 (July), pp.591-601, ISSN 0958-0670.

Dotan,Y.; Lichtenberg, D.; & Pinchuk, I. (2004). Lipid peroxidation cannot be used as a universal criterion of oxidative stress. *Progress in Lipid Research*, Vol.43, No.3 (May), pp. 200-227, ISSN 0163-7827.

Dotevall, G. & Walan, A. (1971). Clinical value of the gastric secretory test. *Nordisk medicin*, Vol. 11;86, No. 45 (November), pp. 1293-1297, ISSN 0029-1420.

Dubois, A. (1995). Spiral Bacteria in the Human Stomach: The Gastric Helicobacters. *Emerging Infectious Diseases*. Vol.1, No.3 (July-September), ISSN 1080-6059.

Dye, K.R.; Marshall, B.J.; Frierson, H.F.; Guerrant, R.L. & McCallum, R.W. (1989). Ultrastructure of another spiral organism associated with human gastritis.

*Digestive Diseases and Sciences*, Vol.34, No.11 (November), pp. 1787-1791, ISSN 0163-2116, 1573-2568.

Elliott, S.N.; McKnight, W.; Cirino, G. & Wallace, J.L. (1995). A nitric oxide-releasing nonsteroidal anti-inflammatory drug accelerates gastric ulcer healing in rats. *Gastroenterology*, Vol.109, No.2 (August), pp. 524–530, ISSN 0016-5085.

El-Omar, E.M. (2006). Mechanisms of increased acid secretion after eradication of *Helicobacter pylori* infection. *Gut*, Vol.55, No.2 (February), pp. 144–146, ISSN 0017-5749.

Ernst, P.B. & Gold, B.D. (2000). The disease spectrum of Helicobacter pylori: the immunopathogenesis of gastroduodenal ulcer and gastric cancer. *Annual Review of Microbiology*, Vol.54, pp. 615-640, ISSN 0066-4227.

Farhadi, A.; Banan, A. & Keshavarzian, A. (2003). Role of Cytoskeletal Structure in Modulation of Intestinal Permeability. *Archives of Iranian Medicine*, Vol.6, No.1 (January), pp. 49 – 53, ISSN 1029-2977.

Fock, K.M.; Ang, T.L.; Bee, L.C. & Lee, E.J.D. (2008). Proton pump inhibitors: do differences in pharmacokinetics translate into differences in clinical outcomes? *Clinical Pharmacokinetics*, Vol.47, No.1, pp.1–6, ISSN 0312-5963.

Graumlich, J.F. Preventing gastrointestinal complications of NSAIDs. *Postgraduate Medicine*, Vol.109, No.5 (May), pp.117-120, 123-128, ISSN 0032-5481.

Gustafson, J. & Welling, D. (2010). "No acid, no ulcer"--100 years later: a review of the history of peptic ulcer disease. *Journal of the American College of Surgeons*, Vol.210, No.1 (January), pp. 110-116, ISSN 1072-7515.

Guttu, K.; Sorbye, H.; Gislason, H.; Svanes, K. & Gronbech, J.E. (1994). Role of bicarbonate in blood flow-mediated protection and repair of damaged gastric mucosa in the cat. *Gastroenterology*, Vol.107, No.1 (July), pp. 149–159, ISSN 0016-5085.

Handa, O.; Naito, Y. & Yoshikawa, T. (2010). Helicobacter pylori: a ROS-inducing bacterial species in the stomach. *Inflammation Research*, Vol.59, No.12 (December), pp. 997–1003, ISSN 1023-3830.

Henriksnäs, J.; Phillipson, M.; Storm, M.; Engstrand, L.; Soleimani, M. & Holm, L. (2006). Impaired mucus-bicarbonate barrier in Helicobacter pylori-infected mice. *American Journal of Physiology: Gastrointestinal and Liver Physiology*, Vol.291, No.3 (September), pp.G396-G403, ISSN 0193-1857.

Hernández, C.; Santamatilde, E.; McCreath, K.J.; Cervera, A.M.; Díez, I.; Ortiz-Masiá, D.; Martínez, N.; Calatayud, S.; Esplugues, J.V. & Barrachina, M.D. (2009). Induction of trefoil factor (TFF)1, TFF2 and TFF3 by hypoxia is mediated by hypoxia inducible factor-1: implications for gastric mucosal healing. *British Journal of Pharmacology*, Vol.156, No.2 (January), pp.262–272, ISSN 0007-1188.

Hills, B.A.; Butler, B.D. & Lichtenberger, L.M. (1983). Gastric mucosal barrier: hydrophobic lining to the lumen of the stomach. *American Journal of Physiology*, Vol.244, No.5 (May), pp.G561–G568, *ISSN* 1522-1539.

Hirokawa, M.; Miura, S.; Yoshida, H.; Kurose, I.; Shigematsu, T.; Hokari, R.; Higuchi, H.; Watanabe, N.; Yokoyama, Y.; Kimura, H.; Kato, S; & Ishii, H. (1998). Oxidative stress and mitochondrial damage precedes gastric mucosal cell death induced by ethanol administration. *Alcoholism: Clinical and Experimental Research*, Vol.22, No.3 (May), pp. 111–114, ISSN 0145-6008.

Holzer, P. (2006). Neural regulation of gastrointestinal blood flow. In: *Physiology of the gastrointestinal tract*, L.R. Johnson, (4th Ed.), 817-839, Academic Press, ISBN 0120883945, New York, EUA.

Holzer, P. (2007). Role of visceral afferent neurons in mucosal inflammation and defense. *Current Opinion in Pharmacology*, Vol.7, No.6 (December), pp.563–569, ISSN1471-4892.

Hung, C. (2005). Effect of lysozyme chloride on betel quid chewing aggravated gastric oxidative stress and hemorrhagic ulcer in diabetic rats. *World Journal of Gastroenterology*, Vol.11, No.37 (October), pp. 5853-5858, ISSN 1007-9327.

Hung, C.R. (2000). Importance of histamine, glutathione and oxyradicals in modulating gastric hemorrhagic ulcer in septic rats. *Clinical and Experimental Pharmacology and Physiology* 2000; 27: 306-312, ISSN 1440-1681.

Husain, S.S.; Szabo, I.L.; Pai, R.; Soreghan, B.; Jones, M.K.; Tarnawski, A.S. (2001). MAP (ERK-2) kinase—a key target for NSAIDs-induced inhibition of gastric cancer cell proliferation and growth. *Life Sciences*, Vol.9;69, No.25-26 (November), pp. 3045-3054, ISSN 0730-9384.

Johansson, M.; Synnerstad, I. & Holm, L. (2001). Acid transport through channels in the mucous layer of rat stomach. *Gastroenterology*, Vol.119, No.5 (November), pp. 1297–1304, ISSN 0016-5085.

Jones, R. (2001). Nonsteroidal anti-inflammatory drug prescribing: past, present, and future. *American Journal of Medicine*, Vol.8;110, No.1A (January), pp. 4S-7S, ISSN 0002-9343.

Kato, S.; Aihara, E.; Yoshii, K.; Takeuchi K. (2005). Dual action of prostaglandin E2 on gastric acid secretion through different EP receptor subtypes in the rat. *American Journal of Physiology*, Vol.89, No.1 (July), pp. G64–G69, ISSN 1522-1539.

Kato, S.; Tanaka, A.; Kunikata, T.; Mizoguchi, H. & Takeuchi, K. (2000). The roles of nitric oxide and prostaglandins in alterations of ulcerogenic and healing responses in adjuvant- induced arthritic rat stomachs. *Alimentary Pharmacology and Therapeutics*, Vol.14, No.1 (April), pp. 18-25, ISSN 0269-2813.

Kohda,K.; Tanaka, K.; Aiba, Y.; Yasuda, M.; Miwa, T. & Koga, Y. (1999). Role of apoptosis induced by Helicobacter pylori infection in the development of duodenal ulcer. *Gut*, Vol.44, No.4 (April), pp. 456-462, ISSN 0017-5749.

Konturek, S.J.; Brzozowski, T.; Majka, J.; Pytko-Polonczyk, J. & Stachura, J. (1993). Inhibition of nitric oxide synthase delays healing of chronic gastric ulcers. *European Journal* of *Pharmacology*, Vol.2;239, No.1-3 (August), pp. 215–217, ISSN 0014-2999.

Konturek, S.J.; Konturek, P.C. & Brzozowski, T. (2005). Prostaglandins and ulcer healing. *Journal of Physiology and Pharmacology*, Vol.56, No.5 (september), pp.5–31, ISSN 0867-5910.

Konturek, S.J.; Piastucki, I.; Brzozowski, T.; Radecki, T.; Dembinska-Kiec, A.; Zmuda, A.; Gryglewski, R. (1981). Role of prostaglandins in the formation of aspirin induced gastric ulcers. *Gastroenterology*, Vol.80, No.1 (January), pp. 4-9, ISSN 0016-5085.

Kuipers, E.J.; Janssen, M.J. & Boer, W.A. (2003). Good bugs and bad bugs: indications and therapies for Helicobacter pylori eradication. *Current Opinion in Pharmacology*, Vol.3, No.5 (October, pp. 480-485, ISSN 1471- 4892.

La Casa, C.; Villegas, I.; Alarcon de La Lastra, C.; Motilva, V.; Martin Calero, M.J. (2000). Evidence for protective and antioxidant properties of rutin, a natural flavone, against ethanol induced gastric lesions. *Journal of Ethnopharmacology*, Vol.71, No.1/2 (July), pp. 45-53, ISSN 0378-8741.

Lacy, E.R. & Ito, R. (1984). Rapid epithelial restitution of the rat gastric mucosa after ethanol injury, *Laboratory Investigation*, Vol.51, No.5 (November), pp. 573-585, ISSN 0023-6837.

Laine, L.; Curtis, S.P.; Cryer, B.; Kaur, A.; Cannon, C.P. (2007). Assessment of upper gastrointestinal safety of etoricoxib and diclofenac in patients with osteoarthritis and rheumatoid arthritis in the Multinational Etoricoxib and Diclofenac Arthritis Long-term (MEDAL) programme: a randomised comparison. *Lancet*, Vol.10;369, No.9560 (February), pp. 465-473, ISSN 0140-6736.

Laine, L.; Takeuchi, K. & Tarnawski, A. (2008). Gastric mucosal defense and cytoprotection: bench to bedside. *Gastroenterology*, Vol.135, No.1 (July), pp. 41-60, ISSN 0016-5085.

Lanas, A. & Scheiman, J. (2007). Low-dose aspirin and upper gastrointestinal damage: epidemiology, prevention and treatment. *Current Medical Research and* Opinion, Vol.23, No.1 (January), pp.163-173, ISSN 0300-7995.

Latarjet A. (1922). Resection des nerfs de l'estomac Technique operatoire. Resultats Clin Bull Acad Med (Paris), Vol.67, pp. 661-691.

Levenstein, S.; Ackerman, S.; Kiecolt-Glaser, J.K.; Dubois, A. (1999). Stress and peptic ulcer disease. *Journal of the American Medical Association*, Vol.6;281, No.1 (January), pp.10-11, ISSN 00987484.

Levenstein, S.; Kaplan, G.A. & Smith, M. (1995). Sociodemographic characteristics, life stressors, and peptic ulcer: a prospective study. *Journal of Clinical Gastroenterology*, Vol.21, No.3 (October), pp. 185-192, ISSN 0192-0790.

Lichtenberger, L.; Graziani, L.A.; Dial, E.J.; Butler, B.D. & Hills, B.A. (1983). Role of surface active phospholipids in cytoprotection. *Science*, Vol.18;219, No.4590 (March), pp. 1327-1329, ISSN 0036-8075.

Lichtenberger, L.M. (1999). Gastroduodenal mucosal defense. *Current Opinion* in *Gastroenterology*, Vol.15, No.6 (November), pp.463-472, ISSN 0267-1379.

Lindberg, P.; Brändström, A.; Wallmark, B.; Mattsson, H.; Rikner, L. & Hoffmann, K.J. (1990). Omeprazole: the first proton pump inhibitor. *Medicinal Research Reviews*, Vol.10, No.1 (January-March), pp. 1-54, ISSN 0198-6325.

Ma, L. & Wallace, J.L. (2000). Endothelial nitric oxide synthase modulates gastric ulcer healing in rats. *American Journal* of *Physiology: Gastrointestinal and Liver Physiology*, Vol.279, No.2 (August), pp.G341-G6, ISSN 0193-1857.

Madara, J.L. (1983). Increases in guinea pig small intestinal transepithelial resistance induced by osmotic loads are accompanied by rapid alterations in absorptive-cell tightjunction structure. *Journal of Cell Biology*, Vol.97, No.1 (July), pp. 125 - 36, ISSN 0021-9525.

Makola, D.; Peura, D.A. (2007). Crowe SE. *Helicobacter pylori* infection and related gastrointestinal diseases. *Journal of Clinical Gastroenterology*, Vol.41, No.6 (July), pp. 548-558, ISSN 0192-0790, 1539-2031.

Marshall, B.J. & Windsor, H.M. (2005). The relation of Helicobacter pylori to gastric adenocarcinoma and lymphoma: pathophysiology, epidemiology, screening, clinical presentation, treatment, and prevention. *Medical Clinics of North America.*, Vol.89, No.2 (March), pp. 313–344, ISSN 00257125.

Matsuda, H.; Pongpiriyadacha, Y.; Morikawa, T.; Kashima, Y.; Nakano, K. & Yoshikawa, M. (2002) Protective effects of polygodial and related compounds on ethanol-induced gastric mucosal lesions in rats: structural requirements and mode of action. *Bioorganic & Medicinal Chemistry Letters*, Vol.11;12, No.3 (February), pp. 477–482, ISSN 0960-894X.

Matysiak-Budnik, T.; Heyman, M.; Mégraud, F. (2003). Review article: rebamipide and the digestive epithelial barrier. *Alimentary Pharmacology & Therapeutics*, Vol.18, No.1 (July), pp.55-62, ISSN 0269-2813.

Meyer-Rosberg, K.; Scott, D.R.; Rex, D.; Melchers, K.; Sachs, G. (1996). The effect of environmental pH on the proton motive force of *Helicobacter pylori*. *Gastroenterology*, Vol.111, No.4 (October), pp. 886–900, ISSN 0016-5085.

Moayyedi, P.; Wason, C.; Peacock, R.; Walan, A.; Bardhan, K.; Axon, A.T. & Dixon, M.F. (2000). Changing patterns of Helicobacter pylori gastritis in long-standing acid suppression. *Helicobacter*, Vol.5, no.4 (December), pp. 206-214, ISSN 1083-4389.

Moura Rocha, N.F.; Venâncio, E.T.; Moura, B.A.; Gomes Silva, M.I.; Aquino Neto, M.R.; Vasconcelos Rios, E.R.; de Sousa, D.P.; Mendes Vasconcelos, S.M.; de França Fonteles, M.M. & de Sousa, F.C. (2010). Gastroprotection of (-)-alpha-bisabolol on acute gastric mucosal lesions in mice: the possible involved pharmacological mechanisms. *Fundamental and Clinical Pharmacology*, Vol.24, No.1 (February), pp. 63-71, ISSN 0767-3981.

Mózsik, G.; Karádi, O.; Király, A.; Debreceni, A.; Figler, M.; Nagy, L.; Pár, A.; Pár, G.; Süto, G. & Vincze, A. (2001). The key-role of vagal nerve and adrenals in the cytoprotection and general gastric mucosal integrity. *Journal of Physiology (Paris)*, Vol.95, No. 1-6 (January-December), pp.229–237, ISSN 0928-4257.

Murphy, M.S. (1998). Growth factors and the gastrointestinal tract. *Nutrition*, Vol.14, No.10 (October), pp.771-774, ISSN 0899-9007 .

Nayeb-Hashemi, H. & Kaunitz, J.D. (2009). Gastroduodenal mucosal defense. *Current Opinion in Gastroenterology*, Vol.25, No.6 (November), pp. 537-543, ISSN 1531-7056.

Nusrat, A.; von Eichel-Streiber, C.; Turner, J.R. , Verkade, P.; Madara, J.L.; Parkos, C.A. (2001). Clostridium difficile toxins disrupt epithelial barrier function by altering membrane microdomain localization of tight junction proteins. *Infection and Immunity*, Vol.69, No.3 (March), pp. 1329 – 1336, ISSN 0019-9567.

Oh, T.Y.; Ahn, G.J.; Choi, S.M.; Ahn, B.O.; Kim, W.B. (2005). Increased susceptibility of ethanol-treated gastric mucosa to naproxen and its inhibition by DA-9601, an Artemisia asiatica extract. *World Journal of Gastroenterology*, Vol.11, No.47 (December), pp. 7450-7456, ISSN 1007-9327.

Olaleye, S.B.; Adaramoye, O.A.; Erigbali, P.P. & Adeniyi, O.S. (2007). Lead exposure increases oxidative stress in the gastric mucosa of HCl/ethanol-exposed rats. *World Journal of Gastroenterology*, Vol.14;13, No.38 (October), pp. 5121-5126, ISSN 1007-9327.

Oyaka, J. Otaka, M.; Matsuhashi, T.; Jin, M.; Odashima, M.; Komatsu, K.; Wada, I.; Horikawa, Y.; Ohba, R.; Hatakeyama, N.; Itoh, H. & Watanabe, S. (2006). Over-expression of 70-kDa heat shock protein confers protection against monochloramine- induced gastric mucosal cell injury. *Life Sciences*, Vol.79, No.3 (June), pp. 300–305, ISSN 0730-9384.

Pakodi,F.; Abdel-Salam, O.M.; Debreceni, A. & Mozsik, G. (2000). *Helicobacter pylori*. One bacterium and a broad spectrum of human disease! An overview. Journal of Physiology (Paris), Vol.94, No.2 (March-April), pp. 139-152, ISSN 0928-4257.

Parsonnet, J.; Friedman, G.D.; Vandersteen, D.P.; Chang, Y.; Vogelman, J.H.; Orentreich, N.; Sibley, R.K. (1991). Helicobacter pylori infection and the risk of gastric carcinoma. *New England Journal of Medicine*, Vol.325, No.16 (October), pp. 1127-1231, ISSN 0028-4793.

Peek, R.M. & Crabtree, J.E. (2006). *Helicobacter* infection and gastric neoplasia. *Journal of Pathology*, Vol.208, No.2 (January), pp. 233–248, ISSN 0022-3417.

Penissi, A. & Piezzi, R. (1999). Effect of dehydroleucodine on mucus production. A quantitative study. *Digestive Diseases and Sciences*, Vol.44, No.4 (April), pp. 708-712, ISSN 0163-2116.

Peskar, B.M. & Maricic, N. (1998). Role of prostaglandins in gastro protection. *Digestive Diseases and Sciences*, Vol. 43, No.9 (September), pp.23S-29S, ISSN 0163-2116.

Peskar, B.M. (2001). Neural aspects of prostaglandin involvement in gastric mucosal defense. *Journal of Physiology and Pharmacology*, Vol. 52, No.4 (December), pp.555–568, ISSN 0867-5910.

Peskar, B.M., Maricic, N.; Gretzera, B.; Schuligoi, R. & Schmassmann, A. (2001). Role of cyclooxygenase-2 in gastric mucosal defense. *Life Sciences*, Vol.9;69, No.25-26 (November), pp. 2993–3003, ISSN 0730-9384.

Rehm, J.; Mathers, C.; Popova, S.; Thavorncharoensap, M.; Teerawattananon, Y. & Patra, J. (2009). Global burden of disease and injury and economic cost attributable to alcohol use and alcohol-use disorders. *Lancet*. Vol.27;373, No.9682 (June), pp. 2223–2233, ISSN 0140-6736.

Repetto, M.G. & Llesuy, S.F. (2002). Antioxidant properties of natural compounds used in popular medicine for gastric ulcers. *Brazilian Journal of Medical and Biological Research*, Vol.35, No.5 (May), pp.523-534, ISSN: 0100-879X.

Richardson, P.; Hawkey, C.J.; & Stack, W.A. (1998). Proton pump inhibitors— pharmacology and rationale for use in gastrointestinal disorders. *Drugs*, Vol.56, No.3 (September), pp. 307–335, ISSN 0012-6667.

Rosh, J.R. & Hassall, E. (2006). Therapy with gastric acidity inhibitors increases the risk of acute gastroenteritis and community-acquired pneumonia in children. *Journal of Pediatric Gastroenterology & Nutrition*, Vol.43, No.4 (October), pp. 545, ISSN 0277-2116.

Rostom, A.; Muir, K.; Dube, C.; Jolicoeur, E.; Boucher, M.; Joyce, J.; Tugwell, P. & Wells, G.W. (2007). Gastrointestinal safety of cyclooxygenase-2 inhibitors: a Cochrane Collaboration Systematic Review. *Clinical Gastroenterology and Hepatology*, Vol.5, No.7 (Julho), pp. 818–828, ISSN 1542-3565.

Sánchez, M.; Theoduloz, C.; Schmeda-Hirschmann, G.; Razmilic, I.; Yáñez, T. & Rodríguez, J.A. (2006) Gastroprotective and ulcer-healing activity of oleanolic acid derivatives: in vitro–in vivo relationships. *Life Sciences*, Vol.79, No.14 (August), pp. 1349–1356, ISSN 0730-9384.

Santos, F.A. & Rao, V.S. (2001). 1,8-Cineol, a food-flavouring agent, prevents ethanol-induced gastric injury in rats. *Digestive Diseases and Sciences*, Vol.46, No.2 (February), pp. 331–337, ISSN 0163-2116.

Schubert, M.L. & Peura, D.A. (2008). Control of Gastric Acid Secretion in Health and Disease. *Gastroenterology*, Vol.134, No.7 (June), pp. 1842–1860, ISSN 0016-5085.

Schubert, M.L. (2008). Gastric secretion. *Current Opinion in Gastroenterology*, Vol.24, No.6 (November), pp. 659-664, ISSN: 0267-1379.

Seno, K.; Joh, T.; Yokoyama, Y. & Itoh, M. (1995). Role of mucus in gatric mucosal injury induced by local ischemia/reperfusion. *Journal of Laboratory and Clinical Medicine*, Vol.126, No.13), pp. 287-293, ISSN 0022-2143.

Sigthorsson, G.; Crane, R.; Simon, T.; Hoover, M. ; Quan, H.; Bolognese, J; Bjarnason, I. (2000). COX-2 inhibition with rofecoxib does not increase intestinal permeability in healthy subjects: a double blind crossover study comparing rofecoxib with placebo and indomethacin. *Gut*, Vol.47, No.4 (October), pp. 527–532, ISSN 0017-5749.

Silva, M.I.; Moura, B.A.; Neto, M.R.; Tomé, A.R.; Rocha, N.F.; de Carvalho, A.M.; Macêdo, D.S.; Vasconcelos, S.M.; de Sousa, D.P.; Viana, G.S. & de Sousa, F.C. (2009a). Gastroprotective activity of isopulegol on experimentally induced gastric lesions in mice: investigation of possible mechanisms of action. *Naunyn-Schmiedeberg's Archives of Pharmacology*, Vol.380, No.3 (September), pp. 233–245, ISSN 0028-1298.

Silverstein, F.E.; Faich, G.; Goldstein, J.L.; Simon, L.S.; Pincus, T.; Whelton, A.; Makuch, R.; Eisen, G.; Agrawal, N.M. & Stenson, W.F. (2000). Gastrointestinal toxicity with celecoxib vs nonsteroidal anti-inflammatory drugs for osteoarthritis and rheumatoid arthritis: the CLASS study: a randomized controlled trial. Celecoxib Long-term Arthritis Safety Study. *Journal of the American Medical Association*, Vol.13;284, No.10 (September), pp. 1247–1255, ISSN 0098-7484.

Singh, G.; Fort, J.G.; Goldstein, J.L.; Levy, R.A.; Hanrahan, P.S.; Bello, A.E.; Andrade-Ortega, L.; Wallemark, C.; Agrawal, N.M.; Eisen, G.M.; Stenson, W.F.; Triadafilopoulos, G. (2006). Celecoxib versus naproxen and diclofenac in osteoarthritis patients: SUCCESS-I Study. *American Journal of Medicine*, Vol.119, No.3 (March), pp. 255–66, ISSN 0002-9343.

Smoot, D.T.; Mobley, H.L.T.; Chippendaele, G.R.; Lewison, J.F. & Resau, J.H. (1991). *Helicobacter pylori* urease activity is toxic to human gastric epithelial cells. *Infection and Immunity*, Vol.59, No.6 (June), pp.1992-1994, ISSN 0019-9567.

Stermer, E. (2002). Alcohol Consumption and the Gastrointestinal Tract. *Israel Medical Association Journal.*, Vol.4, No.3 (March), pp. 200-202, ISSN 1565-1088.

Stroff, T.; Plate, S.; Respondek, M.; Müller, K.M. & Peskar, B.M. (1995). Protection by gastrin in the rat stomach involves afferent neurons, calcitonin gene-related peptide, and nitric oxide. *Gastroenterology*, Vol. 109, No.1 (July), pp.89–97, ISSN 0016-5085.

Suerbaum, S. & Michetti, P. (2002). *Helicobacter pylori* infection. *New England Journal of Medicine*, Vol.347, No.15 (October), pp. 1175–1186, ISSN 0028-4793.

Suleyman, H., Akcay, F.; & Altinkaynak, K. (2002). The effect of nimesulide on the indomethacin- and ethanol-induced gastric ulcer in rats. *Pharmacological Research* 45, No.2 (February), pp. 155–158, ISSN 1043-6618.

Suleyman, H.; Demirezer, L.O. & Kuruuzum-Uz, A. (2004). Effects of Rumex patientia root extract on indomethacine and ethanol induced gastric damage in rats. *Pharmazie*, Vol.59, No.2 (February), pp. 147–149, ISSN 0031-7144.

Szabo, S.; Trier, J.S. & Frankel, P.W. (1981). Sulfhydryl compounds may mediate gastric cytoprotection. *Science*, Vol.9;214, No. 4517 (October), pp. 200–202, ISSN 0036-8075.

Tanaka, A.; Araki, H.; Komoike, Y.; Hase, S. & Takeuchi, K. (2001). Inhibition of both COX-1 and COX-2 is required for development of gastric damage in response to nonsteroidal antiinflammatory drugs. *Journal of Physiology* (Paris), Vol.95, No.1-6 (January-December), p. 21–27, ISSN 0928-4257.

Tanaka, D.; Tsutsumi, S.; Arai, Y.; Hoshino, T.; Suzuki, K.; Takaki, E.; Ito, T.; Takeuchi, K.; Nakai, A. & Mizushima, T. (2007). Genetic evidence for a protective role of heat shock factor 1 against irritant-induced gastric lesions. *Molecular Pharmacology*, Vol.71, No.4, pp. 985–993, ISSN 0026-895X.

Tanaka, S.; Tache, Y.; Kaneko, H.; Guth, P.H. & Kaunitz, J.D. (1997). Central vagal activation increases mucous gel thickness and surface cell intracellular pH in rat stomach. *Gastroenterology*, Vol.122, No.2 (February), pp. 409–417, ISSN 0016-5085.

Tarnawski, A.; Hollander, D.; Stachura, J.; Krause, W.J.; Gergely, H. (1985). Prostaglandin protection of the gastric mucosa against alcohol injury — a dynamic time-related process. The role of mucosal proliferative zone. *Gastroenterology* Vol.88, No.1 (January), pp. 334–359, ISSN 0016-5085.

Tarnawski, A.; Wang, H.; Tomikawa. Talcid triggers induction of heat shock proteins HSP-70 in gastric mucosa: a key to its mucosal protective action? Gastroenterology, Vol.116, pp. A331, ISSN 0016-5085.

Taupin, D. & Podolsky, D.K. (2003). Trefoil factors initiators of mucosal healing. *Nature Reviews Molecular Cell Biology*, Vol.4, No.9 (October), 721-732, ISSN 1471-0072.

Terano, A.; Hiraishi, H.; Ota, S.; Shiga, J. & Sugimoto, T. (1989). Role of superoxide and hydroxyl radicals in rat gastric mucosal injury induced by ethanol. *Gastroenterologia Japonica*, Vol.24, No.5 (October), pp. 488-493, ISSN 0435-1339.

Trey, G.; Marks, I.N.; Louw, J.A.; Jaskiewicz, K.; Sipponen, P.; Novis, B.H.; Bank, S. & Tigler-Wybrandi, N.A. (1997). Changes in acid secretion over the years: a 30-year longitudinal study. *Journal of Clinical Gastroenterology*, Vol.25, No.6 (October), pp. 499–502, ISSN 0192-0790.

Tulassay, Z. & Herszényi, L. (2010). Gastric mucosal defense and cytoprotection. *Best Practice & Research Clinical Gastroenterology*, Vol.24, No. 2 (April), pp.99-108, ISSN 1521-6918.

Tuorkey, M.J. & Abdul-Aziz, K.K. (2011). Gastric Ulcer's Diseases Pathogenesis, Complications and Strategies for Prevention. *Webmedcentral*, Vol.2, No.3 (March), pp. 2–24, ISSN 2046-1690.

Vane, J.R. & Botting, R.M. (1995). A better understanding of anti-inflammatory drugs based on isoforms of cyclooxygenase (COX-1 and COX-2). *Advances in prostaglandin, thromboxane, and leukotriene research.* Vol.23, pp.41–48, ISSN 0732-8141.

Wallace, J.L. (1992). Prostaglandins, NSAIDs, and cytoprotection. *Gastroenterology Clinics of North America*, Vol.21, No.3 (September), pp. 631-641, ISSN 0889-8553.

Wallace, J.L.; McKnight, W.; Reuter, B.K. & Vergnolle N. (2000). NSAID-induced gastric damage in rats: requirement for inhibition of both cyclooxygenase 1 and 2. *Gastroenterology*, Vol.119, No.3 (September), pp. 706–714, ISSN 0016-5085.

Werther, J.L. (2000). The gastric mucosal barrier. *Mount Sinai journal of medicine*, Vol.67, No.1 (January), pp.41–53, ISSN 0027-2507.

*World Health Organization (WHO).* (2004). Global Status Report on Alcohol, In: *Webcite*, 11.11.2010, Available from http://www.who.int/substance_abuse/publications/global_status_report_2004_overview.pdf.

*World Health Organization (WHO).* (2008). Is harmful use of alcohol a public health problem?, In: *Webcite*, 11.11.2010, Available from http://www.who.int/features/qa/66/en/index.html

# Helicobacter Pylori Infection in Peptic Ulcer Disease

Tat-Kin Tsang[1] and Manish Prasad Shrestha[2]

*[1]University of Chicago,*
*[2]Saint Francis Hospital, University of Illinois*
*U.S.A*

## 1. Introduction

### 1.1 Background

Helicobacter pylori infection is one of the most common bacterial infections worldwide.[1,2] Nearly 50% of the world's population is affected.[3] Though the prevalence of this infection appears to be decreasing in many parts of the world, H. pylori remains an important factor linked to the development of peptic ulcer disease, gastric malignancy and dyspeptic symptoms.[4] Majority of H. pylori infected persons remain asymptomatic. Approximately 10-15% of the infected persons develop associated illnesses, 1 to 10% developing peptic ulcer disease, 0.1 to 3% developing gastric cancer and less than 0.01% developing gastric mucosa-associated lymphoid tissue (MALT) lymphoma.

There are several lines of evidence implicating H. Pylori in the development of gastric and duodenal ulcers.

1.  H. Pylori is found in most patients who have peptic ulcers in absence of NSAID use.
2.  Presence of H. Pylori is a risk factor for the development of ulcer.
3.  Eradication of H. Pylori significantly reduces the recurrence of gastric and duodenal ulcers.
4.  Treatment of H. Pylori infection leads to more rapid and reliable ulcer healing than does treatment with anti-secretory therapy alone.[15,21]

Early studies have estimated the rate of H. Pylori infection in patients with duodenal ulcer to be as high as 90% and in gastric ulcer to be as high as 70 to 90%.[5,6,7,29] Despite the decreasing prevalence of H. Pylori infection in developed countries, it is still an important factor in the aetiology of non-iatrogenic peptic ulcer disease. Up to 80% of duodenal ulcers and 70% of gastric ulcers are associated with H. Pylori infection. Several studies have shown that a pre- existing H. Pylori infection increases the risk for developing peptic ulcer disease.[8,9,10,11] In one study, 11% of patients with H. Pylori gastritis developed peptic ulcer disease compared to 1% of persons without gastritis.[10] Eradication of H. Pylori infection significantly reduces the recurrence of gastric and duodenal ulcers.[12,13,14,21] One study reviewed the relationship between H. Pylori eradication and reduced recurrence of duodenal and gastric ulcers. Ulcer recurrence was significantly less common among H. Pylori cured patients versus non-cured patients (6% versus 67% for patients with duodenal ulcers; 4% versus 59% for patients with gastric ulcers).[12]

H. Pylori has also been linked to the development of idiopathic thrombocytopenic purpura, ischemic heart disease and cerebrovascular accident. However, if confounding factors are taken into consideration, the strength of these associations is reduced.[16, 17, 221]

## 2. Bacteriology

Helicobacter pylori is a unipolar, multiflagellate, spiral shaped, microaerophilic, gram negative bacterium.[18] The bacterium was first isolated by Marshall and Warren in 1983 from gastroscopy biopsy specimens, which they described as a new species related to the genus Campylobacter.[18] The new genus Helicobacter was first published in October 1989. At least 22 species are now included in this genus, the majority of which colonise mammalian stomachs or intestines.

Helicobacter pylori is a slow growing bacterium. It can be cultured on non-selective agar media, such as blood agar, chocolate agar or on selective agar media, such as Skirrows media incubated in a humidified, micro-aerobic (5% oxygen) atmosphere at 35 to 37 degree centigrade for three to seven days.[19] Small, translucent circular colonies form and organisms are identified as Helicobacter pylori based on typical cellular morphology and positive results for oxidase, catalase and urease tests.

Under stress and nutritional deprivation, H. Pylori undergoes a morphological transformation from spiral bacilli to inactive coccoids.[19] H. Pylori cell wall enzyme Ami A, a peptidoglycan hydrolase, is involved in this morphologic transition.[20] Coccoid forms may be indicative of a dormant state. Coccoid forms may enable the organism to survive outside the human host in faeces or in water.

## 3. Epidemiology

Helicobacter pylori is one of the most common bacterial infections worldwide. At least 50% of the world's population is infected. The prevalence of H. Pylori infection in a community is related to three factors: 1. Rate of acquisition of infection, i.e. the incidence 2. the rate of loss of the infection 3. the prolonged prevalence of the bacterium in the gastro-duodenal mucosa between infection and eradication. [Prevalence is directly related to incidence and duration of illness].[2] Acute H. Pylori infection invariably passes undetected. Thus, the incidence of infection is determined indirectly from epidemiological studies. The incidence of H. Pylori infection is estimated to be approximately 0.5% per year in adults of developed countries. This incidence has been decreasing over time. However, the incidence of H. Pylori infection continues to be high in developing countries (3% to 10% per year).[25]

The infection is usually acquired in the first few years of life. Once acquired, infection persists indefinitely unless treated. In developing countries, the majority of children become infected during childhood and chronic infection continues during adulthood.[2,26] By age 1 year, approximately 20% are infected and by age 10 years, 50% are infected.[26] The prevalence of H. Pylori infection may be as high as 80% in adults.[30,31] However, in developed countries, such as, the United States, evidence of infection is rare before age 10, but increases to 10% between 18 and 30 years of age and to 50% in those older than age 60.[2] The higher prevalence in older age groups is thought to reflect a cohort effect related to poorer living conditions of children in previous decades. Within any age group, H. Pylori infection is more common in non-Hispanic blacks and Hispanics compared to the white population, which may be related to socioeconomic factors.[27, 28]

Important risk factors for H. Pylori infection are socioeconomic status and living conditions during childhood. Lower socioeconomic status and poor living conditions during childhood have been associated with higher risk of acquiring H. Pylori infection.[38,39,40,41] There may also be genetic susceptibility to H. Pylori infection.[42,43] Twin studies support hereditary susceptibility to infection, but this has not been proven. Individuals of certain ethnic groups including Hispanics and blacks have a higher rate of infection than Caucasians, which are not entirely explained by differences in socioeconomic status.[44]

## 4. Helicobacter pylori transmission

The mode of transmission of H. Pylori infection is poorly known.[1,45] Various modes of transmission have been suggested, such as person-to-person, water-borne, food-borne and zoonotic transmission.[45,46,47,48,49,50,51,52,53,54] The transmission of H. Pylori seems to be direct from person-to-person via faecal-oral or oral-oral routes.[45,46] Certain epidemiological studies have suggested water-borne and food-borne transmissions.[51,52,53,54] Zoonotic transmission has also been suggested based on isolation of H. Pylori from primates, domestic cats and sheep. [47,48,49]

Person-to person transmission is supported by the increased prevalence of infection among family members of patients with H. Pylori and among institutionalized patients. Isolation of genetically identical strains of H. Pylori from infected members of the same family and in patients in a chronic care facility further support this hypothesis.[32,33,34,35,36,37] Faecal-oral transmission is a possibility as H. Pylori has been cultured from faeces[54,55] and the organism seems to survive in water in non-culturable forms[50,51,52] (detected by PCR techniques). There is some indirect, but scarce evidence for oral-oral transmission.[45] H. Pylori has been identified in dental plaques[56], but it is unknown if this location can serve as a reservoir. Gastro-oral route of transmission through vomitus has also been suggested based on presence of bacteria in gastric secretions.[57,58]

Studies employing microbiological techniques have demonstrated that Helicobacter pylori is present in water and other environmental samples all over the world. Epidemiological studies have shown that water source and exposures related to water supply, including factors related to sewage disposal and exposure to animals, are risk factors for infection.[51] Children who swim in rivers, streams, pools, drink stream water or consume raw vegetables are more likely to be infected.[53] H. Pylori has also been detected in various food samples. So it has been hypothesised that food or water may be a reservoir in H. Pylori transmission. Iatrogenic transmission has also been documented after the use of inadequately disinfected endoscopes and endoscopic accessories.[58]

## 5. Patho-physiology

### 5.1 Patho-physiology of gastric ulcers

Up to 70% of gastric ulcers are associated with H. Pylori infection. Three types of gastric ulcers have been described. Type I ulcers occur in the body of the stomach and are not related to other gastro-duodenal disease. Type II ulcers also occur in the body of the stomach and are associated with a duodenal ulcer scar or active ulcer. Type III ulcers occur in the immediate pre-pyloric area. Type II and III ulcers are associated with higher levels of gastric acid secretion as seen in patients with duodenal ulcers, but type I ulcers tend to be associated with normal or low levels of gastric acid secretion. Role of H. Pylori in these different types of gastric ulcer is not known. Gastric acid secretion may not be the most important factor in the development of gastric ulcers as gastric ulcers have been seen in the presence of achlorhydria.[59] It has also been observed that basal and stimulated gastric acid secretion is within normal limits in groups of patients with gastric ulcers

## 5.2 Patho-physiology of duodenal ulcers

The mechanism by which Helicobacter pylori predisposes to duodenal ulcer is unclear. The pathogenesis of duodenal ulcer appears to be multi-factorial, involving an imbalance between "damaging" (e.g. acid, pepsin) and "protecting" (e.g. mucus, mucosal barrier, bicarbonate production, blood flow, cellular regeneration) factors.[60]The bacterium seems to affect different aspects of gastric and intestinal mucosal physiology that may contribute to development of ulcer disease. Disturbances in gastric acid secretion, gastric metaplasia, host inflammatory and immune response and down-regulation of various mucosal defence factors may contribute to ulcer formation. Various bacterial, host and environmental factors may also have a role in the pathogenesis of duodenal ulcer.

### 5.2.1 Disturbances in gastric acid secretion

Gastric acid secretion is elevated in patients with duodenal ulcers.[61,70] Helicobacter pylori infection can alter acid secretion in both directions. Acid secretion decreases temporarily during acute infection and may dwindle later if H. Pylori causes gastric atrophy.[63] In patients with duodenal ulcers, H. Pylori produces inflammation of non-acid secreting antral region of the stomach, whereas the more proximal acid-secreting fundic mucosa is relatively spared.[70,71] This may explain the increased gastric acid secretion in patients with duodenal ulcers. When compared to H. Pylori negative subjects, patients with duodenal ulcers have elevated basal acid output, peak acid output, fasting and meal-stimulated gastrin concentrations.[61,62,70]

H. Pylori infection is thought to change the physiological control of acid secretion. H. Pylori infection has been found to decrease the local expression of the inhibitory peptide somatostatin[63] and to increase the release of the acid-stimulating hormone, gastrin.[62,70] Hypergastrinemia, in addition to decreased inhibitory somatostatin, may be responsible for the increased gastric acid secretion. Hypergastrinemia may result from a decrease in the inhibitory peptide somatostatin.[64] Bacterial factors that inhibit somatostatin release have not been recognised, although TNF-alpha induced by H. Pylori infection may play a role in inhibiting somatostatin release.[65] In patients with H. Pylori infected duodenal ulcers, there is an exaggerate response to stimulation by gastrin.[61,70,71] This may be due to increased parietal cell mass in patients with duodenal ulcers[60,66,71] (Duodenal ulcer patients have approximately twice the normal parietal cell mass). But it is unclear whether or not this is due to H. Pylori infection.[67] Increased parietal cell mass may be due to trophic effects of hypergastrinemia over time or it may be related to host factors.

### 5.2.2 Gastric metaplasia

Elevated gastric acid secretion increases the duodenal acid load, which damages the duodenal mucosa, causing ulceration and gastric metaplasia. Gastric metaplasia occurs in the duodenum in response to acidic PH (when PH is less than 2.5).[68] Metaplastic gastric epithelium allows H. Pylori to colonise the duodenal mucosa, where it produces an acute inflammatory response. Colonization of these areas of gastric metaplasia by H. Pylori may significantly increase the risk of ulceration.[69]

However, gastric metaplasia is found in most, but not all patients with duodenal ulcers.[72,73,74] Gastric metaplasia can also be commonly found in the duodenum of healthy persons.[73,74,75] Studies have found a similar prevalence of gastric metaplasia among patients with duodenal ulcers and non ulcer dyspepsia.[76] Therefore, the role of gastric metaplasia in the pathogenesis of duodenal ulcer disease is unclear.

### 5.2.3 Host immune and inflammatory response

Host immune system responds to H. Pylori infection by production of inflammatory cytokines, such as interleukin(IL)-1, IL-6, tumor necrosis factor alpha, IL-8. These inflammatory cytokines may have a role in the development of duodenal ulcer.

### 5.2.4 Down-regulation of mucosal defence factors

i.  Mucus- Mucus is a protective coat overlying the intestinal mucosa. Helicobacter pylori produces proteolytic enzymes that degrade this mucus layer, thus exposing the underlying mucosa to damaging effects of acid.[77]

ii.  Bicarbonate- Most patients with duodenal ulcers have impaired proximal duodenal mucosal bicarbonate secretion. Impaired bicarbonate secretion in patients with duodenal ulcers could be caused by a cellular and/or physiological regulatory transport defect possibly related to H. Pylori infection as eradication of the infection normalises proximal mucosal bicarbonate secretion.[78]

iii.  Cellular regeneration- Epidermal growth factor (EGF) and transforming growth factor-alpha(TGF-alpha) are potent gastric acid inhibitors and stimuli of mucosal growth and protection. H. Pylori may contribute to ulcerogenesis by affecting these factors for cellular regeneration as eradication of H. Pylori infection has shown to increase mucosal content and expression of TGF-alpha, EGF and EGF receptor (EGFr).[79]

iv.  Blood flow- Thrombotic occlusion of surface capillaries is promoted by a bacterial platelet activating factor. Circulating platelet aggregates and activated platelets were detected in patients with H. Pylori infection. Platelet activation and aggregation may contribute to microvascular dysfunction.[84] This may play a role in producing mucosal damage and ulcer.

### 5.2.5 Other contributing factors

i.  Bacterial factors- Various bacterial factors, such as the bacterial strain may play role in the pathogenesis of duodenal ulcer. For example, Strains with the cytotoxin-associated gene A(cag A) are associated with duodenal ulcer. Approximately 95% of patients with duodenal ulcers have cag A+ strains compared to 65% of infected patients without ulcers.[80]

ii.  A specific Helicobacter pylori gene, duodenal ulcer promoting gene (dupA) is associated with an increased risk of duodenal ulcer. One study found that dup A was present in 42% of patients with duodenal ulcer versus 21% of patients with gastritis (adjusted odds ratio[OR]=3.1, 95% confidence interval; CI-1.7-5.7).[81] Its presence was also associated with more intense antral neutrophil infiltration and interleukin-8 levels and was a marker for protection against gastric atrophy, intestinal metaplasia, and gastric cancer.[81,82]

iii.  Host factors- Host factors may be important in the development of duodenal ulcer. For example, patients with Helicobacter pylori who develop duodenal ulcer have higher parietal cell mass or sensitivity to gastrin than Helicobacter pylori infected healthy persons.[60,66,71]

iv.  Environmental factors, such as NSAID use and smoking may also increase the risk of duodenal ulcer in patients with Helicobacter pylori infection.[83]

## 5.3 Pathogenesis of H. Pylori-induced peptic ulcer disease

H. pylori causes three major gastric morphologic changes.[87] The extent and distribution of H. Pylori-induced gastritis ultimately determine the clinical outcome. The commonest morphologic change is the "simple or benign gastritis", characterized by mild pangastritis with little disruption of gastric acid secretion. This form of gastritis is commonly seen in asymptomatic people with no serious gastrointestinal disease. Up to 15 % of infected subjects develop an antral-predominant gastritis with relative sparing of the acid producing corpus mucosa. Subjects with antral-predominant gastritis have high antral inflammatory scores, high gastrin levels, relatively healthy corpus mucosa and very high acid output.[70] These abnormalities lead to the development of peptic ulcers, particularly duodenal and a large proportion of pre-pyloric ulcers. Up to 1% of infected subjects develop a corpus predominant pattern of gastritis, gastric atrophy and hypo- or achlorhydria.[85] These abnormalities develop as a direct result of the chronic inflammation induced by the infection and increase the risk of gastric cancer.

It is believed that the complex interplay between the host and the bacterium determines the disease outcome. Various bacterial factors have been described which aid in the colonisation of the gastric mucosa and subsequent modulation of the host's immune response. Studies have investigated the impact of these bacterial factors on inflammation and disease outcome. Role of bacterial factors for disease outcome remains limited, with most "virulent" strains being found in asymptomatic subjects.[86] Therefore, the variation in the host's inflammatory and immune response to infection may play a key role in determining the disease outcome. Nonetheless, the bacterium is required to initiate the host's response.

### 5.3.1 Bacterial factors

i. Colonisation/ Bacterial attachment

H. pylori is very sensitive to acid and it dies rapidly in the acidic PH found in the gastric lumen. Bacterial motility, urease and its ability to adhere to gastric epithelium are the factors that allow it to survive in the acidic environment.[87]

Various changes are observed in H. Pylori expression of genes following exposure to low PH. There is an increase in the expression of genes encoding proteins involved in the motility apparatus as well as genes encoding urease and proteins associated with the optimal function of the urease.[88] These observations suggest that the bacterial genes are turned on in the gastric mucosa.

H. pylori is capable of swimming freely within the mucus gel by utilising its polar flagella. It seems that the bacterium is able to sense and respond to PH gradients by swimming away from the acidic PH.[89] This allows the bacterium to swim away from the acidic PH in the gastric lumen to the close proximity of gastric epithelium, where the PH is near normal. In this environment, it enjoys the same cytoprotective mechanism as the gastric epithelium.

Other remarkable feature of H. Pylori is its ability to produce large amounts of cytosolic and cell surface associated **urease**. The urease produced by H. Pylori functions optimally at 2 different PH values, 7.2 and 3.[91]Cell-surface associated urease hydrolyses gastric luminal urea to ammonia that helps neutralise gastric acid and form a protective cloud around the bacterium.[92] Within H. Pylori's urease gene cluster, there is a specific gene, Ure I, which encodes for a PH dependent urea channel.[22] The urea channel allows movement of urea from gastric lumen into the cytoplasm. The metabolism of urea by the cytosolic urease generates ammonia ions, which buffer hydrogen ions as they reach the cytoplasm of the organism.[93,94]

H. pylori infects gastric type epithelium to which it adheres closely. **Adherence of the bacterium to the gastric epithelium** is an important virulence factor and is necessary for the induction of pro-inflammatory responses. Adhesion to gastric epithelium may be beneficial to the bacterium in many ways. It may protect the bacterium against the mechanical clearance. Adhesion may promote invasion and persistence. The bacterium may use the cell surface as a site of replication. Increased inflammation and cellular damage caused by adhesion may release nutrients for H. Pylori. Adhesion also plays a major role in the delivery of toxins such as, Cag A and Vac A to host epithelial cell.[87]

Approximately 20% of H. Pylori in the stomach are found attached to the surfaces of mucus epithelial cells.[90] Adhesion is mediated by specific interactions between bacterial adhesin(s) and host receptor(s).[23,24] Over 30 genes in H. Pylori genomes are dedicated to the expression of outer membrane proteins (OMPs). Several of these OMPs have been classified as adhesins. Best described adhesins are BabA, Oip A and SabA. The leb-binding adhesin, BabA mediates binding to fucosylated Lewis b(Leb b) histo-blood group antigen on gastric epithelial cell.[95] Epidemiological studies also provide evidence in support of interaction between Leb and Bab A. For example, Strains of H. Pylori with BabA2 genotype are associated with inflammation, duodenal ulcer and gastric cancer.[96,97] Outer membrane protein (Oip A) coded by HPO638 gene may act as adhesins as well as promote inflammation by inducing IL-8 production.[98] However, their receptors have not yet been characterized. Sialic acid-binding adhesin (SabA) mediates binding to sialyl-dimeric-Lewix X glycosphingolipid in gastric epithelial cell.[99] Many strains of H. Pylori express a vacuolating cytotoxin Vac A, which may serve as a ligand for bacterial attachment. Although the majority of the Vac A is secreted, some may remain on the surface of the bacteria and serve as a ligand for bacterial attachment to epithelial cells, via an interaction with protein tyrosine phosphatases.[100] The Alp A and Alp B proteins have also been described as as adhesins in vitro.[101] However, there is a marked heterogeneity in H. Pylori adhesion system.[102] No individual adhesin is necessary for attachment to the gastric mucosa. Expression of adhesins is diverse between strains and variable within a single strain over time and these mechanisms of variability and adaptation are controlled at the genetic level by on/off switching of adhesin gene expression, gene inactivation or recombination.[87,102,103,104,105]

Le antigens expressed by host cells may serve as the major receptor for bacterial binding.[106,107] Bab A mediates binding to Leb receptor on host cell. However, there may be other host molecules besides Le antigens that can bind H. Pylori as it has been seen that the binding of H. Pylori to epithelial cells freshly isolated from human gastric biopsy specimens is unaffected by the expression of Le antigen[108] and individuals who do not express Leb can clearly be infected with H. Pylori.[109] One such host molecule may be class II major histocompatibility (MHC) molecule expressed on the surface of gastric epithelial cell.[110] H. Pylori can bind to class II MHC molecules on the surface of gastric epithelial cells and induce apoptosis.[111] A family of pathogen-associated molecular pattern receptors, the Toll-like receptors(TLRs) have also been examined for their role in binding of H. Pylori to the host epithelial cells. 11 TLRs have been described.[86] Each one appears to have a different specificity for various bacterial molecules.[112] These receptors may bind bacterial products and thereby, enhance both bacterial binding and signalling. For example, TLR5 binds bacterial flagellins[113], TLR4 binds bacterial lipopolysaccharide(LPS).[114,115] The gastric trefoil protein TFF1, predominantly expressed in the gastric mucosa and the gastric mucus may serve as another receptor for H. Pylori.[116] A host cell glycosylphosphatidylinositol( GPI)-anchored glycoprotein, DAF has also been described as a potential receptor for binding H. Pylori.[117]

ii. Virulence factors

H. pylori induced gastritis and damage to the gastric mucosa is probably secondary to immune recognition of the bacteria and damage from various bacterial products.[87] Various bacterial products have been described as "toxins" based on biological activity.

**Vac A**

Many strains of H. Pylori express a pore forming cytotoxin, Vac A.[118] Vac A has been shown to cause cell injury in vitro and gastric tissue damage in vivo.[23,120,121] However for Vac A to cause cell damage, it must be secreted from the bacteria and delivered in an active form to host cell membranes where it assembles into pores that allow the leakage of chloride ions.[122] The Vac A gene shows a considerable genetic diversity. The activities of different alleles of the toxin vary in their toxicity. For example, strains harbouring s1 types of Vac A are highly associated with ulcers and gastric cancer.[123] M1 types of Vac A are also associated with ulcers.[123] Although the majority of Vac A is secreted, some remain associated with the bacterial cell surface. The Vac A molecules that remain on the surface of the bacteria are functional and delivered to host cells by direct contact between adhered bacteria and the host cell membrane.[124] As described earlier, Vac A on the surface of the bacteria may also serve as a ligand for bacterial attachment via an interaction with protein tyrosine phosphatases.

Several toxigenic properties of Vac A have been described that may contribute to the development of the disease.[125,126] Vac A may lead to vacuolation of epithelial cells, probably through its effect on endosomal maturation.[87] Vac A also induces apoptosis of host cells, probably through the activation of pro-apoptotic signalling molecules[127] and pore formation in mitochondrial membranes.[128] Vac A may disrupt the barrier function of tight junctions, leading to the leakage of ions and small molecules, such as iron, sugars and amino acids.[129] Vac A was also found to be a powerful inhibitor of T-cell activation in vitro.[130]

**Cag A and the cag Pathogenicity island (Cag PAI)**

Cag A is an important virulence factor associated with H. Pylori. It was initially thought to be the most important virulence factor as patients with antibodies against this protein showed higher rates of peptic ulcer disease[119] and gastric cancer. [131,132,133] Cag A positive strains have also been associated with increased inflammation[134], cell proliferation[135] and gastric metaplasia.[136] However, 30 to 60% of patients infected with CagA + strains do not develop any significant disease.[80] Therefore, Cag A may not be the most important virulence factor.

Cag A is a 128 to 140 kd protein, that can activate a number of signalling mechanisms and thus, affect the structure, differentiation and behaviour of epithelial cells.[87] Cag A is translocated into the host cell by the type 4 secretion system( TFSS). Genes within the cag pathogenicity island(PAI) encode proteins for the type 4 secretion apparatus(TFSS), also referred to as Cag E.[125,137] These genes are co-transcribed and are genetically linked to Cag A.[120] TFSS allows bacterial macromolecules, such as Cag A, peptidoglycan to be translocated into the host cell.[125,137] The intact cag PAI of H. Pylori plays an important role in the pathogenesis of gastritis.[125,137,138] For example, Mutations of H. Pylori cag region were associated with decreased gastric mucosal inflammation in vivo and reduced activation of IL-8 or apoptosis in vitro.[139] It is believed that cag PAI results in the activation of nuclear factor(NF-kb) and AP-1, which in turn, regulate the expression of a wide variety of pro-inflammatory cytokines.[140,141] Cag PAI may collaborate with other bacterial factors, such as Oip A to enhance IL-8 production.[142] Bacterial peptidoglycan may also leak into the cell through the TFSS, resulting in the activation of Nod-1 mediated inflammatory response.[143]

Once inside the host cell, Cag A is tyrosine phosphorylated by host Src kinases.[144] Src kinases are normally involved in controlling basic cytoskeletal process, cell proliferation and differentiation. After its tyrosine phosphorylation, it interacts with a number of host proteins, triggering growth receptor-like signalling. Through these signal transduction events, Cag A affects the proliferative activities, adhesion and cytoskeletal organisation of epithelial cells.[87,145,146,147] Cag A also perturbs cell cycle control.[148] Cag A may also have a phosphorylation independent effect on gene transcription.[149] Independently of tyrosine phosphorylation, Cag A can form complexes with several junction proteins such as Zo-1, JAM and E-cadherin and can perturb the assembly and function of both the tight junction and the adherens junctions.[150,151] Phenotypically, this leads to the deregulation of epithelial cell-cell adhesion and loss of epithelial polarity.[152] Cag A, independent of cag TFSS, can activate the nuclear factor, NF-kb leading to activation of pro-inflammatory signal and IL-8 secretion.[140,141] Cag A may also induce DNA damage and apoptosis of gastric epithelial cells via oxidative stress.[171]

## Other virulence factors

Most persons infected with H. Pylori strains that produce Vac A and possess Cag A genotype nonetheless remain asymptomatic, suggesting that additional virulence factors are important in virulence. Several other H. Pylori virulence factors, such as ice A, Bab A2, Oip A have been described.[153,154,155,156,157] For example, "induced by contact with epithelium" ice A has been linked to peptic ulcers and increased mucosal concentrations of IL-8.[153,154,155] H. Pylori strains with "blood group antigen binding adhesin" Bab A2 genotype are associated with inflammation, duodenal ulcer and gastric cancer[156]. Oip A has been associated with duodenal ulcers.[157] However, the importance of these virulence factors in the life of H. Pylori is poorly understood.

## iii. Mechanism of persistence

In order to colonise the human stomach, H. Pylori must overcome the physical and chemical barriers as well as innate and adaptive immune responses that are triggered in the stomach by its presence.[87] H. Pylori urease functions mainly as a protective buffering enzyme against gastric acidity. Several bacterial factors including catalase and urease antagonise innate host immune responses.[158] H. Pylori may decrease the expression of the antibacterial molecule secretory leukocyte protease inhibitor.[159] H. Pylori produces an enzyme, arginase that inhibits nitric oxide production and may favour bacterial survival.[160] Virulent strains of H. Pylori may alter mucus production[161] and phagocytosis.[162] A number of H. Pylori factors may actually contribute to reduce inflammation or recognition by the immune system. Molecular mimicry may be an important mechanism employed by the bacterium to evade recognition by the host immune system. For example, H. Pylori flagellar proteins have evolved to avoid being recognised by toll-like receptors.[163] H. Pylori lipopolysaccharides mimic host molecules such as Lewis antigens.[164] H. Pylori virulence factors elicit both pro-inflammatory cytokines such as INF-gamma, TNF-alpha and anti-inflammatory cytokines, such as IL-4, !L-10 and transforming growth factor-beta. These anti-inflammatory cytokines may impair immune responses and may favour persistence.[86] However, these anti-inflammatory cytokines, IL-4, IL-10 and TGF-b are not expressed to the same levels as pro-inflammatory cytokines.[165,166,167,182] Hence, it has been hypothesized that H. Pylori induces a robust, but specific form of chronic inflammation that is ineffective in clearing the infection while avoiding forms of inflammation that would eliminate it.[87] This may be due to inappropriate T-cell responses or a lack of coordination in T-cell responses required for immunity.[86] A number of host polymorphisms may also lead to variations in the immune response.[87]

### 5.3.2 Role of host response in H. Pylori induced disease

As described earlier, the host response to H. Pylori infection is an important component in the pathogenesis of gastro-duodenal disease. H. Pylori induce chronic inflammation in the gastric mucosa, mediated by an array of pro- and anti-inflammatory cytokines. Heterogeneity in the regions of genome that control the magnitude of inflammation is thought to determine an individual's ultimate clinical outcome. For example, genetic polymorphisms in the regions controlling IL-1 beta were associated with an increased incidence of hypochlorhydria, gastric cancer and decreased occurrence of duodenal ulcer.[168,169] Il-1 beta has a profound pro-inflammatory effect and it is also a powerful acid inhibitor.[170] The pro-inflammatory genotypes of TNF-alpha, IL-8 and IL-10 were associated with the development of gastric cancer.[168]

i. Epithelial cell response to H. Pylori infection

The epithelial cell response to H. Pylori infection is determined by several variables: bacterial virulence factors, the signalling linked to specific receptors that recognise the bacterial components and the local effects of hormones, neurotransmitters, immune/inflammatory cytokines and stromal factors.[86] These responses include changes in epithelial cell morphology[175], increased epithelial cell proliferation[176], increased rates of epithelial cell death via apoptosis[177], disruption of the tight junctional complexes150, the production of inflammatory cytokines[137] and induction of numerous genes, most importantly genes involved in the regulation of the immune/inflammatory responses, epithelial cell turn over including apoptosis and proliferation and those affecting physiological properties in the stomach.[178,179,180,181] The expression of these genes in epithelial cells is modulated by transcription factors that are controlled by a series of signalling mechanisms. For example, nuclear factor kb(NF-kb) and AP-1 regulate the expression of pro-inflammatory cytokines and cellular adhesion molecules in response to infection.[182,183] These transcription factors are controlled by several signalling mechanisms including mitogen-activated protein kinases(MAPKs).[138,184] The MAPK cascades regulate several cell functions including proliferation, inflammatory responses and cell survival. ERK and P38 MAPK pathways regulate IL-8 production in gastric epithelial cells.[185,186] ERK and P38 also regulate the expression of other inflammatory response genes. Specific bacterial products as described earlier activate different transcription factors, which collaborate to enhance IL-8 production.[86] Interleukin-8 and related peptides in chemokine family secreted by gastric epithelial cells recruit and activate neutrophils and macrophages.

## ii. Host responses in the lamina propria

Although H. Pylori resides predominantly in the gastric lumen, it induces a robust inflammatory and immune response. The magnitude of the host inflammatory response cannot be explained solely based upon the host epithelial cell responses to the bacterium. Significant amounts of bacterial product may leak around epithelial cells and reach the lamina propria, where it can activate phagocytes, including macrophages and neutrophils.[86] Disruption of epithelial tight junctions may enhance bacterial antigen delivery to the lamina propria. Several studies have demonstrated the ability of H. Pylori to invade gastric epithelial cells in vitro and in vivo.[172,173] Transmission electron microscopy and immunogold detection have shown H. Pylori to be in direct contact with immune cells of the lamina propria in the majority of cases of gastritis.[174] Engulfment of H. Pylori infected epithelial cells by phagocytes may be one of the mechanisms by which H. Pylori can activate the host immune response.[187]

Several bacterial products have been shown to trigger immune response within the lamina propria. A broad array of cytokines is released in the lamina propria in response to intact bacteria or bacterial factors. One such bacterial factor is H. Pylori neutrophil-activating protein, a 150 kilodalton protein, which promotes neutrophil adhesion to endothelial cells and stimulates chemotaxis of monocytes and neutrophils.[188] Bacterial urease can induce he production of IL-6 and TNF-alpha by macrophages.[189] Heat shock protein 60 induces the production of IL-6.[190] Intact bacteria can induce the production of chemokines that recruit T-cells[191] as well as IL-12[192] and IL-18[193], that favour the selection of Th1 cell. Increased IL-1, IL-6, IL-8 and TNF-alpha in response to H. Pylori infection recruit and activate monocytes and neutrophils. Release of neutrophil mediators may in turn, disrupt epithelial cells and contribute to ulcer formation.

## iii. Gastric T-cell responses

Bacterial activation of epithelial cells, monocytes, macrophages and neutrophils leads to a T-helper cell type of adaptive response.[194,195] Different T-helper cell subsets emerge in response to infection with characteristic cytokine production. In H. Pylori infection, T-cell response is predominantly of T-helper cell 1(Th1) type.[138,196] Th1 cells promote cell-mediated immune responses, mainly through the production of INF-gamma and TNF-alpha while Th2 cells promote humoral immunity through the production of cytokines, such as IL-4, IL-5, IL-10 and IL-13. Previously, it was thought that the gastric mucosa is pre-conditioned to favour Th1 cell development.[165,192,197] One possible hypothesis is that H. Pylori selectively blocks Th2 development by interfering with STAT6 activation by IL-4.[198] IL-12 and IL-18 induced in response to infection may positively select for the Th1 response.[86] Activated Th1 cells produce INF-gamma and TNF-alpha which increase the expression of many pro-inflammatory genes in the epithelium including IL-8.[182] These cytokines also enhance bacterial binding[110] and may contribute to increased bacterial load.[199] Th1 cells may induce epithelial cell death through Fas-Fas L interactions.[200] In summary, Th1 activation may contribute to more severe inflammation and mucosal damage. However, Th1 type of T-cell response is a type of cell-mediated immunity against the control of intracellular pathogens.[196] It is unlikely to be effective against H. Pylori which is largely an extracellular pathogen. Hence, Th1 cell activation may produce inflammation, but not effective one which would clear the infection. In addition to Th1 cells, a subset of anti-inflammatory T-cells may be activated by H. Pylori infection. These cells may impair excessive inflammation which would otherwise lead to the clearance of the organism.[86]

iv. Gastric B-cell responses

Gastric T-cells can modulate B-cell responses, leading to the production of specific antibodies to a variety of H. Pylori antigens. During infection with H. Pylori, Ig G, Ig A and Ig M types of antibodies can be detected.[201,202] The role of these antibodies in the disease is poorly understood. Ig G class of antibody can activate complement and may contribute to immune-complex mediated inflammation.[203] In addition to producing antigen-specific antibodies, B-cells have also been shown to produce auto-reactive antibodies, that may be pathogenic.[204,205]

## 6. Indications for H. pylori testing

H. pylori is a common worldwide infection. The vast majority of patients with H. Pylori infection do not develop clinically significant gastroduodenal disease. Therefore, routine testing for H. Pylori is not recommended. When to test a patient for H. Pylori infection is an important question for a clinician. Guidelines from the American college of Gastroenterology [ACG] and the European Helicobacter study group [EHSG] have been published to assist clinicians in making this decision.

ACG recommendations[206]

Testing for H. Pylori should only be performed if the clinician plans to offer treatment for positive results.
Testing is indicated in patients with
1.    Active peptic ulcer disease( gastric or duodenal ulcer)
2.    Confirmed history of peptic ulcer disease( not previously treated for H. Pylori)
3.    Gastric MALT lymphoma( low grade)
4.    After endoscopic resection of early gastric cancer
5.    Uninvestigated dyspepsia( depending upon H. Pylori prevalence)
The test-and-treat strategy for H. Pylori infection is a proven management strategy for patients with uninvestigated dyspepsia who are under the age of 55 yr and have no "alarm features" ( bleeding, anaemia, early satiety, unexplained weight loss, progressive dysphagia, odynophagia, recurrent vomiting, family history of GI cancer, previous esophagogastric malignancy)
Deciding which test to use in which situation relies heavily upon whether a patient requires evaluation with upper endoscopy and an understanding of the strengths, weaknesses, and costs of the individual test.

EHSG recommendations[207]

Testing is indicated in patients with
1.    Gastroduodenal diseases such as peptic ulcer disease and low grade gastric MALT lymphoma
2.    Atrophic gastritis
3.    First degree relatives of patients with gastric cancer
4.    Unexplained iron deficiency anaemia
5.    Chronic Idiopathic thrombocytopenic purpura (ITP)
The test-and-treat strategy using a non-invasive test is recommended in adult patients with persistent dyspepsia under the age of 45 and no "alarm symptoms".
Testing is not recommended in GORD. However, testing should be considered in patients on long-term maintenance therapy with PPIs.

Testing should be considered in patients who are naive NSIADs users.

Testing should be considered in patients who are long-term aspirin users who bleed.

Children with recurrent abdominal pain, who have a positive family history of peptic ulcer and gastric cancer should be tested for H. Pylori after exclusion of other causes.

### Duodenal and gastric ulcer

Testing for H. Pylori is indicated in patients with confirmed gastric or duodenal ulcers. As described earlier, H. Pylori has been established as a major risk factor for both duodenal and gastric ulcers. H. Pylori eradication has also shown to reduce the recurrence of peptic ulcer disease. Therefore, both ACG and EHSG recommend testing patients with peptic ulcer disease for H. Pylori.

### Gastroduodenal bleeding

A meta-analysis performed by Sharma et al showed that H. Pylori treatment decreased recurrent ulcer bleeding by 17% and 4% compared with ulcer healing treatment alone ( bismuth, ranitidine or omeprazole) or ulcer healing treatment followed by maintenance therapy respectively.[208] Another study performed in Taiwanese patients with a history of ulcer bleeding showed that maintenance acid suppression was not routinely necessary to prevent ulcer recurrence after successful H. Pylori cure and ulcer healing.[209] Therefore, patients with a bleeding duodenal or gastric ulcer should be treated for H. Pylori.

### Uninvestigated dyspepsia

The Cochrane Systematic review confirmed that there is a small benefit of eradicating H. Pylori in patients with non-ulcer dyspepsia.[210] Eradication of H. Pylori may also reduce the incidence of peptic ulcer in patients with ulcer-like functional dyspepsia.[211] Therefore, the test-and-treat strategy is recommended in patients with uninvestigated dyspepsia who are under the age of 55 yrs or 45 yrs (depending upon the specific set of guidelines) and have no "alarm features". However, this strategy has been criticised. In a placebo-controlled trial of empirical treatment involving 294 patients with uninvestigated dyspepsia and a positive H. Pylori breath test, the 1-year rate of symptom resolution was 50% in those receiving H. Pylori eradication therapy, as compared with 36% of those receiving placebo ($p=0.02$)[212]; 7 patients would need to receive eradication therapy for 1 patient to have a benefit. This suggests that most patients treated with the test-and-treat strategy would incur the inconvenience, costs and potential side-effects of therapy without a benefit.

### Long-term maintenance therapy with PPIs

EHSG suggests H. Pylori testing in patients on long-term maintenance therapy with PPIs. Patients who are infected with H. Pylori and maintained on a PPI may be at risk for the development of atrophic gastritis.[213]However, the findings have not been confirmed in other studies.[214]

### Persons using NSAIDS or Aspirin

EHSG suggests H. Pylori testing in patients who are naive NSAIDs users. A meta-analysis of five studies including 939 patients showed that H. Pylori eradication was associated with a reduced incidence of peptic ulcer in patients taking NSAIDs(OR 0.43, 95% CI 0.20-0.93). Sub-analyses demonstrated that risk reduction was evident in NSAID-naive individuals, but not for those previously taking NSAIDs.[215,219]

### Iron-deficiency anaemia

EHSG recommends H. Pylori testing and eradication in patients with unexplained iron deficiency anaemia. There is emerging evidence to suggest that eradication of H. Pylori can improve iron deficiency anaemia[216,217], but the available data do not prove cause and effect.

### Chronic ITP

EHSG recommends H. Pylori testing and eradication in patients with chronic ITP. The available data support an association between H. Pylori infection and ITP.[218] Studies have also shown that there is a significant increase in platelet count in patients with ITP after H. Pylori eradication.[220,222,223,224]

### Prevention of gastric cancer

ACG recommends H. Pylori testing after endoscopic resection of early gastric cancer. EHSG recommends H. Pylori testing and eradication in first-degree relatives of patients with gastric cancer. Whether H. Pylori eradication reduces the risk of developing gastric cancer is unknown. H. Pylori eradication may protect against the progression of premalignant gastric lesions.[225,226] H. Pylori eradication may decrease the risk of developing cancer in individuals without precancerous lesions from high risk populations.[227] However, this may not apply to low-risk populations.

## 7. Diagnostic tests for H. pylori infection

Diagnostic tests for H. Pylori can be divided into endoscopic and non-endoscopic tests. Various diagnostic tests for H. Pylori infection are shown in Table 1-2. All the methods currently available for the detection of H. Pylori have their advantages and disadvantages regarding sensitivity, specificity, convenience, cost and immediacy. Choosing among these tests depends upon the clinical circumstance, the pre-test probability of infection, the accuracy of the tests, the availability and the relative costs.

### General recommendations from ACG

When endoscopy is indicated, the test of first choice is the rapid urease test (RUT) in patients who have not been on a PPI within 1-2 week or an antibiotic or bismuth within 4 week of endoscopy.

For patients who have been taking a PPI, antibiotics or bismuth, it is appropriate to obtain biopsies from the gastric body and antrum for histology with or without RUT or plan testing with Urea breath test(UBT) or faecal antigen test(FAT) at a later date after withholding the offending agents for an appropriate period of time.

Culture or PCR is not routinely recommended.

UBTs and faecal antigen tests provide reliable means of identifying active H. Pylori infection before antibiotic therapy.

In the setting of acute upper GI bleeding, a positive RUT indicates the presence of active H. Pylori infection, whereas a negative RUT and/or histology should be confirmed with another test. An antibody test provides a reasonably sensitive testing option. Alternatively, patient can undergo a UBT or FAT at a later date after withholding medications that can negatively affect the sensitivity of these tests for an appropriate period of time.

Antibody testing for H. Pylori is appropriate in patients with uninvestigated dyspepsia in regions where the prevalence of H. Pylori infection is high. In low prevalence populations (prevalence less than 20%), antibody tests should be avoided altogether or positive results should be confirmed with a test that identifies active infection, such as UBT or FAT prior to initiating eradication therapy.

| Tests | Advantages | Disadvantages |
|---|---|---|
| **Non- Endoscopic** | | |
| 1.Urea Breath Test (13$_C$ & 14$_C$) | • Rapid, inexpensive and identifies active infection.<br>• Excellent PPV regardless of H. Pylori prevalence.<br>• Useful after H. Pylori therapy. | • False negative results may be observed in patients who are taking PPIs, bismuth or antibiotics.<br>• May not be available consistently. |
| 2.Serological Test or Antibody Test | • Widely available.<br>• Least expensive test.<br>• Excellent NPV. | • The PPV is greatly influenced by the prevalence of H. pylori infection.<br>Not recommended for confirming eradication as positive results may reflect past rather than current infection. |
| 3. Fecal Antigen Test | • Identifies active H. pylori infection.<br>• High positive and negative predictive values.<br>• Useful before and after H. Pylori treatment. | • Collecting stool may be unpleasant to patients.<br>• False negative results may be observed in patients who are taking PPIs, bismuth or antibiotics.<br>• Polyclonal test less well validated. |
| **Endoscopic**<br>1.Rapid Urease Testing | • Rapid, inexpensive and accurate in properly selected patients. | • False negative results may be observed in patients who are taking PPIs, bismuth or antibiotics. |

| | | |
|---|---|---|
| 2.Histological assessment | • High sensitivity and specificity. | • Expensive.<br>• Requires trained personnel. |
| 3. Culture | • Excellent specificity.<br>• Allows determination of antibiotic sensitivities. | • Sensitivity variable.<br>• Requires infrastructure and trained personnel.<br>• Expensive, time consuming, difficult to perform and not widely available. |
| 4. Polymerase Chain Reaction | • High sensitivity and specificity.<br>• Provides opportunity to test for antibiotic sensitivity. | • False positive results may be due to contamination, homologous DNA sequences among various species, non-specific amplifications.<br>• False negative results may be due to reaction failure.<br>• Methodology not standardized across laboratories.<br>• Not widely available. |

Table 1.

| Test | Sensitivity | Specificity |
|---|---|---|
| **Non-Endoscopic Tests** | | |
| 1.Urea Breath Test | 90%-96% | 88%-98% |
| 2.Antibody Test | 88%-94% | 74%-88% |
| 3.Fecal Antigen Test | 86%-96% | 92%-97% |
| **Endoscopic Tests** | | |
| 1.Rapid Urease Test | 88%-95% | 95%-100% |
| 2.Histology | 93%-96% | 98%-99% |
| 3.Culture | 80%-98% | 100% |
| 4.Polymerase Chain Reaction | >95% | >95% |

Table 2.

Confirmation of eradication is indicated in any patients with an H. Pylori-associated ulcer, persistent dyspeptic symptoms despite the test-and-treat strategy, H. Pylori-associated MALT lymphoma and in individuals who have undergone resection of early gastric cancer. If testing to prove eradication were performed in the setting of endoscopy, histology or the combination of histology and RUT would be appropriate.

UBT is the most reliable non-endoscopic test to document eradication of H. Pylori infection. The monoclonal FAT provides another non-endoscopic means of establishing H. Pylori cure. Testing to prove H. Pylori cure appears to be most accurate if performed at least 4 wk after the completion of antibiotic therapy.

## 7.1 Endoscopic diagnostic tests
Currently available biopsy-based diagnostic methods for H. Pylori infection are the rapid urease test, histology, culture and polymerase chain reaction (PCR).

### 7.1.1 Rapid Urease test (RUT)
Rapid Urease tests depend on the activity of bacterial urease. Endoscopic biopsy specimens are placed into an agar gel or on a reaction strip containing urea, a buffering agent and a PH sensitive dye. If H. Pylori is present, its urease cleaves urea to liberate ammonia and bicarbonate, leading to an increase in the PH and change in the colour of the dye. CLO test, Hp Fast, HUT-test, Pyloritek and Pronto Dry are some of the commercially available RUT kits. The overall performance of these tests is comparable.[228,229]

Although RUTs are rapid, inexpensive and easy to perform, their sensitivity is reduced under certain circumstances. The tests may produce a false negative result in patients with active or recent bleeding from the upper gastrointestinal tract when gastric contents are contaminated with blood.[230,231,232] Furthermore, these tests may give a false negative result in patients who have recently been taking proton pump inhibitors (PPIs), H2-receptor antagonists (H2RAs), antibiotics, or bismuth containing compounds.[228]In these patients, the RUT is usually combined with other endoscopic or non-endoscopic tests to determine the presence or absence of the infection. It is also recommended to obtain biopsies from two sites, the body of the gastric angularis and greater curvature of the antrum.[233] This may increase the sensitivity of the test. An alternative is to withhold the offending agents, such as PPIs or antibiotics for an appropriate period of time prior to endoscopy. The duration of the deleterious effects of medications on the sensitivity of the RUT is unknown. However, based on data from UBT, it is probably reasonable to withhold a PPI for 1-2 weeks and bismuth and antibiotics for four weeks prior to the RUT.[234,235]

### 7.1.2 Histology
Histological testing of gastric biopsy specimens is another method of diagnosing H. Pylori infection. A significant advantage of histology over other diagnostic tests is the ability to evaluate for pathological changes associated with H. Pylori infection, such as gastritis, atrophy, intestinal metaplasia and malignancy.[236]The presence of type B chronic gastritis (non-atrophic diffuse antral gastritis or atrophic pangastritis) may be used as a surrogate marker for the infection when organisms are not detected whereas the absence of chronic gastritis may be used as a marker for the absence of infection. However, the sensitivity of histology is affected by several factors, such as the site, number and size of gastric biopsies, method of staining, level of training of the examining pathologist and use of medications, such as bismuth, antibiotics and PPIs. It is therefore recommended to obtain a minimum of three biopsies, one from the greater curvature of the corpus, one from the greater curvature of the antrum and one from the angularis to maximize the diagnostic yield of histology.[237]

### 7.1.3 Brush cytology
Brush cytology may be used as an alternative to histology for the diagnosis of H. Pylori infection, especially in patients who have an increased risk of bleeding following forces biopsy. Data with endoscopic brush cytology are encouraging, with reported sensitivity and specificity of more than 95%.[238]

### 7.1.4 Culture
Bacterial culture is highly specific method for detecting active H. Pylori infection. In addition to identifying infection, it permits testing for sensitivity to anti-microbial agents.[239] However, bacterial culture is relatively insensitive[240,241] and seldom performed in routine clinical practise. Not all hospital laboratories have necessary expertise or resources available to offer routine culturing. Furthermore, culturing H. Pylori is difficult, time consuming and expensive.

Culture and sensitivity testing may be useful in patients with refractory disease since the incidence of resistance is very high in this subgroup.

### 7.1.5 Polymerase chain reaction (PCR)
Detection of H. Pylori by PCR is based on the amplification of a target DNA sequence in the bacterial genome. The use of PCR for the detection of H. Pylori from environmental samples is well documented.[269,270] PCR can also be used to detect H. Pylori in biopsy specimens.[261,262,265] In fact, PCR may be more sensitive than other biopsy-based diagnostic techniques in diagnosing H. Pylori infection.[264,265] PCR testing may be more sensitive than other biopsy based tests in detecting H. Pylori infection in patients who are taking PPIs, H2 RAs, antibiotics or bismuth containing compounds.[263] The testing is also highly specific and allows testing for antibiotic sensitivities.[266,267,268]

Although PCR has many advantages, its clinical use is limited due to its tendency towards false positive and false negative results. False positives can result from clinical or laboratory contamination, carry over contaminations and most importantly, similarities between the primer binding regions of H. Pylori and other organisms especially at the 3' ends. False negatives can result from low number of target organisms, the presence of a specific PCR inhibitor, degenerated target DNA, and polymorphisms in the primer binding regions, especially at the 3' ends, that prevent the amplification of the target DNA. Furthermore, the test is not widely available and the methodology is not standardized across laboratories.

Newer PCR techniques, such as multiplex PCR assays may reduce false positive and false negative results and thereby improve the accuracy of the test. For example, TZAM HP multiplex PCR assay amplifies 10 DNA fragments from 5 DNA regions in the genome of H. Pylori at the same time. Amplifying more than one DNA region increases the sensitivity because the probability of amplifying several selected DNA regions is much higher than the chance of amplifying only one region. It also increases the specificity because probing different loci at the same time more accurately distinguishes one pathogen from another.[265]

### 7.2 Non-endoscopic diagnostic tests
Currently available non-endoscopic diagnostic tests for H. Pylori infection are urea breath test (UBT), antibody test and fecal antigen test (FAT).

### 7.2.1 Urea breat test (UBT)
The urea breath test, like the RUT, depends on the activity of bacterial urease. The test involves the ingestion of urea, labelled with either the non-radioactive isotope $^{13}$C or the radioactive isotope $^{14}$C, which is converted to labelled carbon dioxide by the bacterial urease. The labelled carbon dioxide can then be measured in expired air.[242,243,244] Although the dose of radiation exposure in $^{14}$C UBT is small, the $^{13}$C UBT is preferred in children and women of child bearing potential.[242,243]

The UBT has excellent sensitivity and specificity[242,243] therefore, it is considered to be the most reliable test to document H. Pylori infection. It can be used to screen for infection as well as to confirm eradication after H. Pylori treatment.[244,245,246,247] However, UBTs may produce a false negative result in patients who are taking PPIs, bismuth or antibiotics. It is currently recommended to withhold bismuth and antibiotics for at least 28 days and a PPI for 7-14 days prior to UBT to reduce false negative results.[234,235,248] It is unknown whether H2RAs affect the sensitivity of the UBT[249], although these drugs are generally stopped for 24-48 hours before the UBT.

A urease blood test, using a 13 C- bicarbonate assay also reliably detects active H. Pylori infection before and after treatment. In the presence of H. Pylori, the ingestion of a 13 C-urea rich meal results in the production of labelled bicarbonate, which can be measured in serum.[250,251]

## 7.2.2 Serological test or antibody test

Antibody testing is based upon the detection of H. Pylori specific Ig G antibodies in serum, whole blood or urine. Antibodies to H. Pylori can be quantitatively assessed using laboratory-based ELISA and latex agglutination techniques or qualitatively assessed using office-based serological kits.

Antibody testing is cheap, widely available and easy to perform. However, there are several factors limiting its usefulness in clinical practice. The test is less accurate when compared with other diagnostic tests.[252] The test has high sensitivity (88-94%), but variable specificity (74-88%) with accuracy ranging from 83 to 98%. In general, office based serological kits are less accurate than laboratory-based quantitative tests. The PPV of the test is greatly influenced by the prevalence of H. Pylori infection.[253] In a population with low prevalence of H. Pylori infection, a positive antibody test is more likely to be a false positive test. Finally, serological tests are unreliable indicators of H. pylori status in patients who have received treatment for the infection.[254] Although antibody titres fall in most patients after successful eradication, the rate and extent of the decline are highly variable and unpredictable.

## 7.2.3 Fecal antigen test (FAT)

H. pylori infection can be diagnosed by identifying H. Pylori specific antigens in the stool by enzyme immunoassay with the use of polyclonal or monoclonal anti-H. Pylori antibodies.[255,256] The FAT is a reliable test to diagnose H. Pylori infection as well as to confirm eradication after treatment and can be used interchangeably with the UBT. Both polyclonal and monoclonal tests have excellent sensitivity, specificity, positive and negative predictive values for diagnosing infection before treatment.[255] However, in the post-treatment setting, only the monoclonal test appears to have sensitivity, specificity and predictive values of greater than 90%. The polyclonal test appears to have less satisfactory sensitivity and positive predictive value.[255] Therefore, in the post-treatment setting, the monoclonal FAT is more reliable than the polyclonal test. The FAT may be effective in confirming eradication as early as 14 days after treatment[257] but, the general recommendation is to perform the test more than 4 weeks after treatment.[255]

The FAT has its own disadvantages. Like the UBT, the FAT may produce a false negative result in patients who are taking PPIs, antibiotics or bismuth.[258,259] To reduce false negative results, it is generally recommended to withhold bismuth and antibiotics for at least 4 weeks and a PPI for 2 weeks prior to the FAT. The FAT may produce a false positive result in patients with acute upper gastrointestinal bleeding.[231,260] This may be due to cross-reactivity with blood products. Furthermore, the process of stool collection may be unpleasant to patients.

## 8. References

[1] Cave DR. Transmission and epidemiology of Helicobacter pylori. Am J Med 1996;100:12S

[2] Pounder RE, Ng D. The prevalence of Helicobacter pylori infection in different countries. Aliment Pharmacol Ther 1995;9 Suppl 2:33

[3] Everhart JE. Recent developments in the epidemiology of Helicobacter pylori. Gastroenterol Clin North Am 2000;29:559-79

[4] Dooley CP, Cohen H. The clinical significance of Campylobacter pylori. Ann Intern Med 1988;108:70

[5] Hunt RH. The role of Helicobacter pylori in pathogenesis: the spectrum of clinical outcomes. Scand J Gastroenterol Suppl 1996; 220:3-9.

[6] Steer HW. The gastro-duodenal epithelium in peptic ulceration. J Pathol 1985;146:355

[7] Tytgat, G, Langenberg, W, Rauws, E, Rietra, P. Campylobacter-like organism(CLO) in the human stomach. Gastroenterology 1985; 88:1620

[8] Sipponen P, Varis K, Fraki O, et al. Cumulative 10-year risk of symptomatic duodenal and gastric ulcer in patients with or without chronic gastritis. A clinical follow-up study of 454 outpatients. Scand J Gastroentrol 1990; 25:966

[9] Nomura A, Stemmermann GN, Chyou PH, et al. Helicobacter pylori infection and the risk of duodenal and gastric ulceration. Ann Intern Med 1994; 120:977

[10] Cullen D, Collins B, Christiansen K, et al. Long term risk of peptic ulcer disease in people with H pylori infectin- A community based study. Gastroenterology 1993; 104(suppl):A60

[11] Leoci C, Ierardi E, Chiloiro M, et al. Incidence and risk factors of duodenal ulcer. A retrospective cohort study. J Clin Gastroenterol 1995; 20:104

[12] Hopkins RJ, Girardi LS, Turney EA. Relationship between Helicobacter pylori eradication and reduced duodenal and gastric ulcer recurrence: a review. Gastroenterology 1996; 110:1244.

[13] Graham DY, Lew Gm, Klein PD, et al. Effect of treatment of Helicobacter pylori infection on the long- term recurrence of gastric or duodenal ulcer: a randomized, controlled study. Ann Intern Med 1992; 116:705.

[14] Van der Hulst RWM, Rauws EAJ, Koycu B, et al. Prevention of ulcer recurrence after eradication of Helicobacter pylori: a prospective long-term follow up study. Gastroenterology 1997; 113:1082.

[15] Graham DY, Lew Gm, Evans DG, et al. Effect of triple therapy (antibiotics plus bismuth) on duodenal ulcer healing: a randomized controlled trial. Ann Intern Med 1991; 115:266.

[16] Byrne MF, Kerrigan SW, Corcoran PA, et al. Helicobacter pylori binds von Willebrand factor and interacts with GPIb to induce platelet aggregation. Gastroenterology 2003; 124:1846.

[17] Handlin RI. A hitchhiker's guide to the galaxy—an H. Pylori travel guides. Gastroenterology 2003; 124:1983.

[18] Marshall BJ, Warren JR. Unidentified curved bacilli in the stomach of patients with gastritis and peptic ulceration. Lancet 1984; 1:1311.

[19] Goodwin CS, Worsley BW. Microbiology of Helicobacter pylori. Gastroenterol Clin North Am 1993; 22:5.

[20] Chaput C, Ecobichon C, Cayet N, et al. Role of AmiA in the morphological transition of Helicobacter pylori and in the immune escape. PLoS pathog 2006; 2:e97.

[21] Hentschel E, Brandstatter G, Dragosics B, et al. Effect of ranitidine and amoxicillin plus metronidazole on the eradication of Helicobacter pylori and the recurrence of duodenal ulcer. N Engl J Med 1993; 328:308.

[22] Weeks DL, Eskandari S, Scott DR, Sachs G. A H+- gated urea channel: the link between Helicobacter pylori urease and gastric colonization. Science 2000; 287:482.

[23] Mobley HL. Defining Helicobacter pylori as a pathogen: strain heterogeneity and virulence. Am J Med 1996; 100:25.

[24] Logan RP. Adherence of Helicobacter pylori. Aliment Pharmacol Ther 1996; 10 Suppl 1:3.

[25] Parsonnet J. The incidence of Helicobacter pylori infection. Aliment Pharmacol Ther 1995; 9 Suppl 2:45.

[26] Torres J, Leal- Herrera Y, Perez G, et al. A Community-based seroepidemiologic study of Helicobacter pylori infection in Mexico. J Infect Dis 1998; 178:1089.

[27] Smoak BL, Kelley PW, Taylor DN. Seroprevalence of Helicobacter pylori infections in a cohort of US Army recruits. Am J Epidemiol 1994; 139:513.

[28] Everhart JE, Kruszon-Moran D, Perez GI, et al. Seroprevalence and ethnic differences in Helicobacter pylori infection among adults in the United States. J Infect Dis 2000; 181:1359.

[29] Graham DY, Klein PD, Opekun AR, et al. Effect of age on the frequency of active Campylobacter pylori infection diagnosed by the [13] C urea breath test in normal subjects and patients with peptic ulcer disease. J Infect Dis 1988;157:777

[30] Imai T, Kubo T, Watanabe H. Chronic gastritis in Japanese with reference to high incidence of gastric carcinoma. J Natl Cancer Inst 1971;47:179

[31] Dwyer B, Kaldor J, Tee W, et al. Antibody response to Campylobacter pylori in diverse ethnic groups. Scand J Infect Dis 1988;20:349

[32] Mitchell HM, Bohane TD, Berkowicz J, et al. Antibody to Campylobacetr pylori in families of index children with gastrointestinal illness due to C pylori [Letter]. Lancet 1987; 2:681.

[33] Drumm B, Perez-Perez GI, Blaster MJ, et al. Intrafamilial clustering of Helicobacter pylori infection. N Engl J Med 1990;322:359

[34] Malaty HM, Graham DY, Klein PD, et al. Transmission of Helicobacter pylori infection. Studies in families of healthy individuals. Scand J Gastroenterol 1991; 26:927.

[35] Perez-Perez GI, Taylor DN, Bodhidatta L, et al. Seroprevalence of Helicobacter pylori infections in Thialand. J Infect Dis 1990;161:1237

[36] Rauws EAJ, Langerberg W, Oudbier J, et al. Familial clustering of peptic ulcer disease colonized with C. Pylori of the same DNA composition [Abstract]. Gastroenterology 1989;96:409

[37] Kim F, Mobley HLT, Burken M, Morris JG. Molecular epidemiology of Campylobacter pylori infection in a chronic care facility [Abstract]. Gastroenterology 1989;96:256

[38] Hunt RH, Sumanac K, Huang JQ. Review article: should we kill or should we save Helicobacter pylori? Aliment Pharmacol Ther 2001; 15 Suppl 1:51-59.

[39] Webb PM, Knight T, Greaves S, et al. Relation between infection with Helicobacter pylori and living conditions in childhood: evidence for person to person transmission in early life. BMJ 1994; 308:750.

[40] Kivi M, Johansson AL, Reilly M, Tindberg Y. Helicobacter pylori status in family members as risk factors for infection in children. Epidemiol Infect 2005; 133:645.

[41] Mendall MA, Goggin PM, Molineaux N, et al. Childhood living conditions and Helicobacter pylori seropositivity in adult life. Lancet 1992;339:896

[42] Malaty HM, Engstrand L, Pedersen NL, Graham DY. Helicobacter pylori infection: genetic and environmental influences. A study of twins. Ann Intern Med 1994; 120:982.

[43] Riccardi VM, Rotter JI. Familial Helicobacter pylori infection. Societal factors, human genetics, and bacterial genetics. Ann Intern Med 1994; 120:1043.

[44] Graham DY, Malaty HM, Evans DG, et al. Epidemiology of Helicobacter pylori in an asymptomatic population in the United States. Effect of age, race, and socioeconomic status. Gastroenterology 1991; 100:1495.

[45] Mégraud F. Transmission of Helicobacter pylori: faecal-oral versus oral-oral route. Aliment Pharmacol Ther 1995; 9 Suppl 2:85.

[46] Perry S, de la Luz Sanchez M, Yang S, et al. Gastroenteritis and transmission of Helicobacter pylori infection in households. Emerg Infect Dis 2006; 12:1701.

[47] Fox JG. Non-human reservoirs of Helicobacter pylori. Aliment Pharmacol Ther 1995; 9 Suppl 2:93

[48] Handt LK, Fox JG, Dewhirst FE, et al. Helicobacter pylori isolated from the domestic cat: public health implications. Infect Immun 1994; 62:2367.

[49] Dore MP, Sepulveda AR, El-Zimaity H, et al. Isolation of Helicobacter pylori from sheep-implications for transmission to humans. Am J Gastroenterol 2001; 96:1396

[50] Hulten K, Han SW, Enroth H, et al. Helicobacter pylori in the drinking water in Peru. Gastroenterology 1996; 110:1031.

[51] Bellack NR, Koehoorn MW, MacNab YC, Morshed MG. A conceptual model of water's role as a reservoir in Helicobacter pylori transmission: a review of the evidence. Epidemiol Infect 2006; 134:439

[52] Queralt N, Bartolomé R, Araujo R. Detection of Helicobacter pylori DNA in human faeces and water with different levels of faecal pollution in the north-east of Spain. J Appl Microbiol 2005; 98:889.

[53] Goodman KJ, Correa P, Tenganá Aux HJ, et al. Helicobacter pylori infection in the Colombian Andes: a population-based study of transmission pathways. Am J Epidemiol 1996; 144:290.

[54] Thomas JE, Gibson GR, Darboe MK, et al. Isolation of Helicobacter pylori from human faeces. Lancet 1992; 340:1194.

[55] Kelly SM, Pitcher MC, Farmery SM, et al. Isolation of Helicobacter pylori from feces of patients with dyspepsia in the United Kingdom. Gastroenterology 1994;107:1671

[56] Hardo PG, Tugnait A, Hassan F, et al. Helicobacter pylori infection and dental care. Gut 1995; 37:44

[57] Axon AT. Review article: is Helicobacter pylori transmitted by the gastro-oral route? Aliment Pharmacol Ther 1995; 9:585

[58] Tytgat GN. Endoscopic transmission of Helicobacter pylori. Aliment Pharmacol Ther 1995; 9 Suppl 2:105.

[59] Reid J, Taylor TV, Holt S, et al. Benign gastric ulceration in pernicious anemia. Dig Dis Sci 1980;25:148

[60] Peura DA. Ulcerogenesis: integrating the roles of Helicobacter pylori and acid secretion in duodenal ulcer. Am J Gastroenterol 1997; 92:8S.

[61] el-Omar E, Penman I, Dorrian CA, et al. Eradicating Helicobacter pylori infection lowers gastrin mediated acid secretion by two thirds in patients with duodenal ulcer. Gut 1993; 34:1060.

[62] Peterson WL, Barnett CC, Evans DJ Jr, et al. Acid secretion and serum gastrin in normal subjects and patients with duodenal ulcer: the role of Helicobacter pylori. Am J Gastroenterol 1993; 88:2038.

[63] Calam, J. The somatostatin-gastrin link of Helicobacter pylori infection. Ann Med 1995; 27:569.

[64] Moss SF, Legon S, Bishop AE, et al. Effect of Helicobacter pylori on gastric somatostatin in duodenal ulcer disease. Lancet 1992; 340:930

[65] Beales I, Calam J, Post L, et al. Effect of tumor necrosis factor alpha and interleukin 8 on somatostatin release from canine fundic D cells. Gastroenterology 1997;112:136

[66] Graham, DY. Helicobacter pylori and perturbations in acid secretion: the end of the beginning. Gastroenterology 1996; 110:1647.

[67] Moss SF, Calam J. Acid secretion and sensitivity to gastrin in patients with duodenal ulcer: effect of eradication of Helicobacter pylori. Gut 1993; 34:888

[68] Wyatt JI, Rathbone BJ, Dixon MF, Heatley RV. Campylobacter pyloridis and acid induced gastric metaplasia in the pathogenesis of duodenitis. J Clin Pathol 1987; 40:841.

[69] Hamlet, A, Thoreson, AC, Nilsson, O, et al. Duodenal Helicobacter pylori infection differs in cagA genotype between asymptomatic subjects and patients with duodenal ulcers. Gastroenterology 1999; 116:259.

[70] el-Omar EM, Penman ID, Ardill JES, Chittajallu RS, Howie C, McColl KEL. Helicobacter pylori infection and abnormalities of acid secretion in patients with duodenal ulcer disease. Gastroenterology 1995;109:681-691

[71] Gillen D, el-Omar EM, Wirz AA, Ardill JES, McColl KEL. The acid response to gastrin distinguishes duodenal ulcer patients from Helicobacter pylori-infected healthy subjects. Gastroenterology 1998;114:50-57

[72] Borsch G, Schmidt G, Wegener M, et al. Campylobacter pylori: prospective analysis of clinical and histological factors associated with colonization of the upper gastrointestinal tract. Eur J Clin Invest 1988;18:133

[73] Fitzgibbons PL, Dooley CP, Cohen H, Appleman MD. Prevalence of gastric metaplasia, inflammation, and Campylobacter pylori in the duodenum of members of a normal population. Am J Clin Pathol 1988;90:711

[74] Hazell SL, Hennessy WB, Borody TJ, et al. Campylobacter pyloridis gastritis. II. Distribution of bacteria and associated inflammation in the gastroduodenal environment. Am J Gastroenterol 1987;82:297

[75] Kreuning J, Bosman FT, Kuiper G, et al. Gastric and duodenal mucosa in "healthy" individuals: an endoscopic and histopathological study of 50 volunteers. J Clin Pathol 1978; 31:69.

[76] Savarino V, Mela GS, Zentilin P, et al. 24 hour gastric PH and extent of duodenal gastric metaplasia in Helicobacter pylori-positive patients. Gastroenterology 1997; 113:741

[77] Isenberg J, McQuaid K, Laine L, Walsh J. Acid-Peptic Disorders. In: Textbook of Gastroenterology, Second Edition, Yamada, T (Ed), JP, Lippincott, Philadelphia 1995. p.1347.

[78] Hogan DL, Rapier RC, Dreilinger A, et al. Duodenal bicarbonate secretion: eradication of Helicobacter pylori and duodenal structure and function in humans. Gastroenterology 1996; 110:705.

[79] Konturek PC, Ernst H, Konturek SJ, et al. Mucosal expression and luminal release of epidermal and transforming growth factors in patients with duodenal ulcer before and after eradication of Helicobacter pylori. Gut 1997; 40:463.

[80] Weel JF, van der Hulst RW, Gerrits Y, et al. The interrelationship between cytotoxin-associated gene A, vacuolating cytotoxin, and Helicobacter pylori-related diseases. J Infect Dis 1996; 173:1171.

[81] Lu H, Hsu PI, Graham DY, Yamaoka Y. Duodenal ulcer promoting gene of Helicobacter pylori. Gastroenterology 2005; 128:833

[82] Yamaoka Y. Roles of the plasticity regions of Helicobacter pylori in gastroduodenal pathogenesis. J Med Microbiol 2008; 57:545.

[83] Kurata JH, Nogawa AN. Meta-analysis of risk factors for peptic ulcer: nonsteroidal anti-inflammatory drugs, Helicobacter pylori, and smoking. J Clin Gastroenterol 1997;24:2

[84] Elizalde JI, Gómez J, Panés J, et al. Platelet activation In mice and human Helicobacter pylori infection. J Clin Invest 1997; 100:996.

[85] El-Omar EM, Oien K, El Nujumi A, et al. Helicobacter pylori infection and chronic gastric acid hyposecretion. Gastroenterology 113 (1997), pp. 15–24.

[86] Ernst PB, Peura DA, Crowe SE. The translation of Helicobacter pylori basic research to patient care. Gastroenterology 2006; 130:188-199.

[87] Amieva MR, El-Omar EM. Host-Bacterial interactions in Helicobacter pylori infection. Gastroenterology 2008; 134:306-323

[88] Merrell DS, Goodrich ML, Otto G, Tompkins LS, Falkow S. pH-regulated gene expression of the gastric pathogen Helicobacter pylori. Infect Immun 71 (2003), pp. 3529–3539.

[89] Schreiber S, Konradt M, Groll C, et al. The spatial orientation of Helicobacter pylori in the gastric mucus. Proc Natl Acad Sci USA 101 (2004), pp. 5024–5029

[90] Hessey SJ, Spencer J, Wyatt JI, et al. Bacterial adhesion and disease activity in Helicobacter associated chronic gastritis. Gut 31 (1990), pp. 134–138.

[91] Mobley HL, Hu LT, Foxall PA. Helicobacter pylori urease: properties and role in pathogenesis. Scand J Gastroenterol 26 (1991) (Suppl 187), pp. 39–46.

[92] Phadnis SH, Parlow MH, Levy M, Ilver D, et al. Surface localization of a Helicobacter pylori urease and heat shock protein homolog requires bacterial lysis. Infect Immun 64 (1995), pp. 905–912.

[93] Scott DR, Weeks D, Hong C, Postius S, Melchers K, Sachs G. The role of internal urease in acid resistance of Helicobacter pylori. Gastroenterology 114 (1998), pp. 58–70

[94] Scott DR, Marcus EA, Weeks DL, Sachs G. Mechanisms of acid resistance due to the urease system of Helicobacter pylori. Gastroenterology 123 (2002), pp. 187–195.

[95] Ilver D, Arnqvist A, Ogren J, et al. Helicobacter pylori adhesin binding fucosylated histo-blood group antigens revealed by retagging. Science 1998; 279:373.

[96] Rad R, Gerhard M, Lang R, Schoniger M, et al. The Helicobacter pylori blood group antigen-binding adhesin facilitates bacterial colonization and augments a nonspecific immune response. J Immunol 168 (2002), pp. 3033–3041.

[97] Prinz C, Schoniger M, Rad R, et al. Key importance of the Helicobacter pylori adherence factor blood group antigen binding adhesin during chronic gastric inflammation. Cancer Res 61 (2001), pp. 1903–1909.

[98] Yamaoka Y, Kwon DH, Graham DY. A M(r) 34,000 proinflammatory outer membrane protein (oipA) of Helicobacter pylori. Proc Natl Acad Sci U S A 2000; 97:7533.

[99] Mahdavi J, Sondén B, Hurtig M, et al. Helicobacter pylori SabA adhesin in persistent infection and chronic inflammation. Science 2002; 297:573.

[100] Yahiro K, Wada A, Nakayama M, et al. Protein-tyrosine phosphatase alpha, RPTP alpha, is a Helicobacter pylori VacA receptor. J Biol Chem 278 (2003), pp. 19183–19189.

[101] de Jonge R, Durrani Z, Rijpkema SG, et al. Role of the Helicobacter pylori outer-membrane proteins AlpA and AlpB in colonization of the guinea pig stomach. J Med Microbiol 53 (2004), pp. 375–379.

[102] Aspholm-Hurtig M, Dailide G, Lahmann M, et al. Functional adaptation of BabA, the H pylori ABO blood group antigen binding adhesion. Science 305 (2004), pp. 519–522.

[103] Dossumbekova A, Prinz C, Mages J, et al. Helicobacter pylori HopH (OipA) and bacterial pathogenicity: genetic and functional genomic analysis of hopH gene polymorphisms. J Infect Dis 194 (2006), pp. 1346–1355.

[104] Solnick JV, Hansen LM, Salama NR, et al. Modification of Helicobacter pylori outer membrane protein expression during experimental infection of rhesus macaques. Proc Natl Acad Sci U S A 101 (2004), pp. 2106–2111

[105] de Jonge R, Pot RG, Loffeld RJ, et al. The functional status of the Helicobacter pylori sabB adhesin gene as a putative marker for disease outcome. Helicobacter 9 (2004), pp. 158–164.

[106] Boren T, Falk P, Roth KA, Larson G, Normark S. Attachment of Helicobacter pylori to human gastric epithelium mediated by blood group antigens. Science 262 (1993), pp. 1892–1895.

[107] Falk P, Roth KA, Boren T, et al. An in vitro adherence assay reveals that Helicobacter pylori exhibits cell lineage-specific tropism in the human gastric epithelium. Proc Natl Acad Sci U S A 90 (1993), pp. 2035–2039.

[108] Clyne M, Drumm B. Absence of effect of Lewis A and Lewis B expression on adherence of Helicobacter pylori to human gastric cells. Gastroenterology 113 (1997), pp. 72–80.

[109] Niv Y, Fraser G, Delpre G, et al. Helicobacter pylori infection and blood groups. Am J Gastroenterol 91 (1996), pp. 101–104.

[110] Fan XJ, Crowe SE, Behar S, et al. The effect of class II MHC expression on adherence of Helicobacter pylori and induction of apoptosis in gastric epithelial cells: a mechanism for Th1 cell-mediated damage. J Exp Med 187 (1998), pp. 1659–1669.

[111] Fan X, Gunasena H, Cheng Z, et al. Helicobacter pylori urease binds to class II MHC on gastric epithelial cells and induces their apoptosis. J Immunol 165 (2000), pp. 1918–1924.

[112] Medzhitov R. Toll-like receptors and innate immunity. Nat Rev Immunol 1 (2001), pp. 135–145.

[113] Smith MF Jr, Mitchell A, Li G, et al. TLR2 and TLR5, but not TLR4, are required for Helicobacter pylori-induced NF-kappa B activation and chemokine expression by epithelial cells. J Biol Chem 278 (2003), pp. 32552–32560.

[114] Su B, Ceponis PJ, Lebel S, Huynh H, Sherman P.M. Helicobacter pylori activates Toll-like receptor 4 expression in gastrointestinal epithelial cells. Infect Immun 71 (2003), pp. 3496–3502.

[115] Ishihara S, Rumi MA, Kadowaki Y, et al. Essential role of MD-2 in TLR4-dependent signaling during Helicobacter pylori-associated gastritis. J Immunol 173 (2004), pp. 1406–1416.

[116] Clyne M, Dillon P, Daly S, et al. Helicobacter pylori interacts with the human single-domain trefoil protein TFF1. Proc Natl Acad Sci U S A 101 (2004), pp. 7409–7414.

[117] O'Brien DP, Israel DA, Krishna U, et al. The role of decay-accelerating factor as a receptor for Helicobacter pylori and a mediator of gastric inflammation. J Biol Chem 281 (2006), pp. 13317–13323.

[118] Leunk RD, Johnson PT, David BC, et al. Cytotoxic activity in broth-culture filtrates of Campylobacter pylori. J Med Microbiol 26 (1988), pp. 93–99.

[119] Nomura AM, Perez-Perez GI, Lee J, et al. Relation between Helicobacter pylori cagA status and risk of peptic ulcer disease. Am J Epidemiol 2002; 155:1054-1059.

[120] Blaser MJ. Role of vacA and the cagA locus of Helicobacter pylori in human disease. Aliment Pharmacol Ther 1996; 10 Suppl 1:73.

[121] Figura N. Helicobacter pylori exotoxins and gastroduodenal diseases associated with cytotoxic strain infection. Aliment Pharmacol Ther 1996; 10 Suppl 1:79.

[122] Iwamoto H, Czajkowsky DM, Cover TL, et al. VacA from Helicobacter pylori: a hexameric chloride channel. FEBS Lett 450 (1999), pp. 101–104.

[123] Atherton JC, Cao P, Peek RM Jr. Mosaicism in vacuolating cytotoxin alleles of Helicobacter pylori: Association of specific vacA types with cytotoxin production and peptic ulceration. J Biol Chem 270 (1995), pp. 17771-17777.

[124] Ilver D, Barone S, Mercati D, et al. Helicobacter pylori toxin VacA is transferred to host cells via a novel contact-dependent mechanism. Cell Microbiol 6 (2004), pp. 167-174.

[125] Blaser MJ, Atherton JC. Helicobacter pylori persistence: biology and disease. J Clin Invest 113 (2004), pp. 321-333.

[126] Cover TL. The vacuolating cytotoxin of Helicobacter pylori. Mol Microbiol 20 (1996), pp. 241-246.

[127] Yamasaki E, Wada A, Kumatori A, et al. Helicobacter pylori vacuolating cytotoxin induces activation of the proapoptotic proteins Bax and Bak, leading to cytochrome c release and cell death, independent of vacuolation. J Biol Chem 281 (2006), pp. 11250-11259.

[128] Willhite DC, Blanke SR. Helicobacter pylori vacuolating cytotoxin enters cells, localizes to the mitochondria, and induces mitochondrial membrane permeability changes correlated to toxin channel activity. Cell Microbiol 6 (2004), pp. 143-154.

[129] Papini E, Satin B, Norais N, et al. Selective increase of the permeability of polarized epithelial cell monolayers by Helicobacter pylori vacuolating toxin. J Clin Invest 102 (1998), pp. 813-820.

[130] Gebert B, Fischer W, Weiss E, et al. Helicobacter pylori vacuolating cytotoxin inhibits T lymphocyte activation. Science 301 (2003), pp. 1099-1102.

[131] Blaser MJ, Perez-Perez GI, Kleanthous H, et al. Infection with Helicobacter pylori strains possessing cagA is associated with an increased risk of developing adenocarcinoma of the stomach. Cancer Res 55 (1995), pp. 2111-2115.

[132] Wu AH, Crabtree JE, Bernstein L, et al. Role of Helicobacter pylori CagA+ strains and risk of adenocarcinoma of the stomach and esophagus. Int J Cancer 103 (2003), pp. 815-821.

[133] Huang JQ, Zheng GF, Sumanac K, et al. Meta-analysis of the relationship between cagA seropositivity and gastric cancer. Gastroenterology 125 (2003), pp. 1636-1644.

[134] Peek RM Jr, Miller GG, Tham KT, et al. Heightened inflammatory response and cytokine expression in vivo to cagA+ Helicobacter pylori strains. Lab Invest 73 (1995), pp. 760-770.

[135] Peek RM Jr, Moss SF, Tham KT, et al. Helicobacter pylori cagA+ strains and dissociation of gastric epithelial cell proliferation from apoptosis. J Natl Cancer Inst 89 (1997), pp. 863-868.

[136] Figura N, Vindigni C, Covacci A, et al. cagA positive and negative Helicobacter pylori strains are simultaneously present in the stomach of most patients with non-ulcer dyspepsia: relevance to histological damage. Gut 42 (1998), pp. 772-778.

[137] Naumann M, Crabtree JE. Helicobacter pylori-induced epithelial cell signalling in gastric carcinogenesis. Trends Microbiol 12 (2004), pp. 29-36.

[138] Elliott SN, Ernst PB, Kelly CP. The year in Helicobacter pylori 2001: molecular inflammation. Curr Opin Gastroenterol 17 (2002), pp. s12-s18.

[139] Israel DA, Salama N, Arnold CN, Moss SF, et al. Helicobacter pylori strain-specific differences in genetic content, identified by microarray, influence host inflammatory responses. J Clin Invest 107 (2001), pp. 611–620.

[140] Brandt S, Kwok T, Hartig R, et al. NF-κB activation and potentiation of proinflammatory responses by the Helicobacter pylori CagA protein. Proc Natl Acad Sci U S A 102 (2005), pp. 9300–9305.

[141] Kim SY, Lee YC, Kim HK, et al. Helicobacter pylori CagA transfection of gastric epithelial cells induces interleukin-8. Cell Microbiol 8 (2006), pp. 97–106.

[142] Yamaoka Y, Kudo T, Lu H, Casola A, Braiser AR, Graham DY. Role of interferon-stimulated responsive element-like element in interleukin-8 promoter in Helicobacter pylori infection. Gastroenterology 2004; 126:1030-1043.

[143] Viala J, Chaput C, Boneca IG, Cardona A, et al. Nod1 responds to peptidoglycan delivered by the Helicobacter pylori cag pathogenicity island. Nat Immunol 2004; 5:1166-1174.

[144] Stein M, Bagnoli F, Halenbeck R, et al. c-Src/Lyn kinases activate Helicobacter pylori CagA through tyrosine phosphorylation of the EPIYA motifs. Mol Microbiol 43 (2002), pp. 971–980

[145] Stein M, Rappuoli R, Covacci A. Tyrosine phosphorylation of the Helicobacter pylori CagA antigen after cag-driven host cell translocation. Proc Natl Acad Sci U S A 97 (2000), pp. 1263–1268.

[146] Selbach M, Moese S, Hauck CR, Meyer TF, Backert S. Src is the kinase of the Helicobacter pylori CagA protein in vitro and in vivo. J Biol Chem 277 (2002), pp. 6775–6778.

[147] Tsutsumi R, Higashi H, Higuchi M, Okada M, Hatakeyama M. Attenuation of Helicobacter pylori CagA x SHP-2 signaling by interaction between CagA and C-terminal Src kinase. J Biol Chem 278 (2003), pp. 3664–3670.

[148] Chang YJ,Wu MS, Lin JT et al. Mechanisms for Helicobacter pylori CagA-induced cyclin D1 expression that affect cell cycle. Cell Microbiol 8 (2006), pp. 1740-1752.

[149] Hirata Y, Maeda S, Mitsuno Y, et al. Helicobacter pylori CagA protein activates serum response element-driven transcription independently of tyrosine phosphorylation. Gastroenterology 123 (2002), pp. 1962–1971.

[150] Amieva MR, Vogelmann R, Covacci A, et al. Disruption of the epithelial apical-junctional complex by Helicobacter pylori CagA. Science 300 (2003), pp. 1430–1434.

[151] Murata-Kamiya N, Kurashima Y, Teishikata Y, et al. Helicobacter pylori CagA interacts with E-cadherin and deregulates the β-catenin signal that promotes intestinal transdifferentiation in gastric epithelial cells. Oncogene 26 (2007), pp. 4617–4626.

[152] Bagnoli F, Buti L, Tompkins L, et al. Helicobacter pylori CagA induces a transition from polarized to invasive phenotypes in MDCK cells. Proc Natl Acad Sci U S A 102 (2005), pp. 16339-16344.

[153] van Doorn LJ, Figueiredo C, Sanna R, et al. Clinical relevance of the cagA, vacA, and iceA status of Helicobacter pylori. Gastroenterology 1998; 115:58

[154] Peek RM Jr, Thompson SA, Donahue JP, et al. Adherence to gastric epithelial cells induces expression of a Helicobacter pylori gene, iceA, that is associated with clinical outcome. Proc Assoc Am Physicians 1998; 110:531.

[155] Nogueira C, Figueiredo C, Carneiro F, et al. Helicobacter pylori genotypes may determine gastric histopathology. Am J Pathol 2001; 158:647.

[156] Gerhard M, Lehn N, Neumayer N, et al. Clinical relevance of the Helicobacter pylori gene for blood-group antigen-binding adhesin. Proc Natl Acad Sci U S A 1999; 96:12778.

[157] Yamaoka Y, Kikuchi S, el-Zimaity HM, et al. Importance of Helicobacter pylori oipA in clinical presentation, gastric inflammation, and mucosal interleukin 8 production. Gastroenterology 2002; 123:414.

[158] Nilius M, Malfertheiner P. Helicobacter pylori enzymes. Aliment Pharmacol Ther 1996; 10 Suppl 1:65.

[159] Wex T, Treiber G, Nilius M, Vieth M, Roessner A, Malfertheiner P. Helicobacter pylori-mediated gastritis induces local downregulation of secretory leukocyte protease inhibitor in the antrum. Infect Immun 72 (2004), pp. 2383–2385.

[160] Gobert AP, McGee DJ, Akhtar M, Mendz GL, Newton JC, Cheng Y, Mobley HL, Wilson KT. Helicobacter pylori arginase inhibits nitric oxide production by eukaryotic cells: a strategy for bacterial survival. Proc Natl Acad Sci U S A 98 (2001), pp. 13844–13849.

[161] Byrd JC, Yunker CK, Xu QS, Sternberg L.R, Bresalier RS. Inhibition of gastric mucin synthesis by Helicobacter pylori. Gastroenterology 118 (2000), pp. 1072–1079.

[162] Allen LA, Schlesinger LS, Kang B. Virulent strains of Helicobacter pylori demonstrate delayed phagocytosis and stimulate homotypic phagosome fusion in macrophages. J Exp Med 191 (2000), pp. 115–128.

[163] Gewirtz AT, Yu Y, Krishna US, et al., Helicobacter pylori flagellin evades toll-like receptor 5-mediated innate immunity. J Infect Dis 189 (2004), pp. 1914–1920.

[164] Moran AP, Knirel YA, Senchenkova SN, et al. Phenotypic variation in molecular mimicry between Helicobacter pylori lipopolysaccharides and human gastric epithelial cell surface glycoforms: Acid-induced phase variation in Lewis(x) and Lewis(y) expression by H pylori lipopolysaccharides. J Biol Chem 277 (2002), pp. 5785–5795.

[165] Karttunen R, Karttunen T, Ekre HP, MacDonald TT. Interferon gamma and interleukin 4 secreting cells in the gastric antrum in Helicobacter pylori positive and negative gastritis. Gut 36 (1995), pp. 341–345.

[166] Lindholm C, Quiding-Jarbrink M, Lonroth H, Hamlet A, Svennerholm AM. Local cytokine response in Helicobacter pylori-infected subjects. Infect Immun 66 (1998), pp. 5964–5971.

[167] D'Elios MM, Manghetti M, Almerigogna F, Amedei A, et al. Different cytokine profile and antigen-specificity repertoire in Helicobacter pylori-specific T cell clones from the antrum of chronic gastritis patients with or without peptic ulcer. Eur J Immunol 27 (1997), pp. 1751–1755.

[168] El-Omar EM, Rabkin CS, Gammon MD et al. Increased risk of noncardia gastric cancer associated with proinflammatory cytokine gene polymorphisms. Gastroenterology 124 (2003), pp. 1193–1201.

[169] El-Omar EM, Carrington M, Chow WH et al., Interleukin-1 polymorphisms associated with increased risk of gastric cancer. Nature 404 (2000), pp. 398–402.

[170] El-Omar EM, The importance of interleukin 1β in Helicobacter pylori associated disease. Gut 48 (2001), pp. 743–747.

[171] Chaturvedi R, Asim M, Bussiere FI, Singh K, Casero RAJ, Peek RM, et al. Spermine oxidase as the link between H pylori cagA and gastric carcinogenesis. Gastroenterology. 2006;130:A60

[172] Amieva MR, Salama NR, Tompkins LS, Falkow S. Helicobacter pylori enter and survive within multivesicular vacuoles of epithelial cells. Cell Microbiol. 2002;4:677–690

[173] Semino-Mora C, Doi SQ, Marty A, Simko V, Carlstedt I, Dubois A. Intracellular and interstitial expression of Helicobacter pylori virulence genes in gastric precancerous intestinal metaplasia and adenocarcinoma. J Infect Dis. 2003;187:1165–1177

[174] Necchi V, Candusso ME, Tava F, Luinetti O, Ventura U, Fiocca R, et al. Intracellular, intercellular, and stromal invasion of gastric mucosa, preneoplastic lesions, and cancer by Helicobacter pylori. Gastroenterology. 2007;132:1009-1023.

[175] Segal ED , Cha J , Lo J , Falkow S , Tompkins LS . Altered states (involvement of phosphorylated CagA in the induction of host cellular growth changes by Helicobacter pylori). Proc Natl Acad Sci U S A . 1999;96:14559–14564

[176] Peek RM . IV. Helicobacter pylori strain-specific activation of signal transduction cascades related to gastric inflammation. Am J Physiol Gastrointest Liver Physiol . 2001;280:G525–G530

[177] Moss SF, Sordillo EM, Abdalla AM, Makarov V, Hanzely Z, Perez-Perez GI, et al. Increased gastric epithelial cell apoptosis associated with colonization with cagA + Helicobacter pylori strains. Cancer Res 2001;61:1406–1411

[178] Chiou CC , Chan CC , Sheu DL , Chen KT , Li YS , Chan EC . Helicobacter pylori infection induced alteration of gene expression in human gastric cells. Gut 2001;48:598-604.

[179] Cox JM , Clayton CL , Tomita T , Wallace DM , Robinson PA , Crabtree JE . cDNA array analysis of cag pathogenicity island-associated Helicobacter pylori epithelial cell response genes. Infect Immun 2001;69:6970–6980

[180] Guillemin K, Salama NR , Tompkins LS , Falkow S . Cag pathogenicity island-specific responses of gastric epithelial cells to Helicobacter pylori infection. Proc Natl Acad Sci U S A . 2002;99:15136–15141

[181] Sepulveda AR , Tao H , Carloni E , Sepulveda J , Graham DY , Peterson LE . Screening of gene expression profiles in gastric epithelial cells induced by Helicobacter pylori using microarray analysis. Aliment Pharmacol Ther. 2002;16(Suppl 2):145–157

[182] Yasumoto K , Okamoto S , Mukaida N , Murakami S , Mai M , Matsushima K . Tumor necrosis factor α and interferon γ synergistically induce interleukin 8 production in a human gastric cancer cell line through acting concurrently on AP-1 and NF-

kappaB-like binding sites of the interleukin 8 gene . J Biol Chem. 1992;267:22506–22511

[183] Aihara M, Tsuchimoto D, Takizawa H, Azuma A, Wakebe H, Ohmoto Y, et al. Mechanisms involved in Helicobacter pylori-induced interleukin-8 production by a gastric cancer cell line, MKN45 . Infect Immun. 1997;65:3218–3224

[184] Maeda S, Yoshida H, Ogura K, Mitsuno Y, Hirata Y, Yamaji Y, et al. H. pylori activates NF-kappaB through a signaling pathway involving IkappaB kinases, NF-kappaB-inducing kinase, TRAF2, and TRAF6 in gastric cancer cells . Gastroenterology 2000;119:97–108

[185] Keates S , Keates AC , Warny M , Peek RM , Murray PG , Kelly CP . Differential activation of mitogen-activated protein kinases in AGS gastric epithelial cells by cag+ and cag- Helicobacter pylori. J Immunol.1999;163:5552–5559

[186] Naumann M, Wessler S, Bartsch C, Wieland B, Covacci A, Haas R, et al. Activation of activator protein 1 and stress response kinases in epithelial cells colonized by Helicobacter pylori encoding the cag pathogenicity island . J Biol Chem. 1999;274:31655–31662

[187] Hawley AT, Ryan KA, Ravichandran KS, Ernst PB. Complement-mediated phagocytosis of Helicobacter pylori-infected gastric epithelial cells: a novel mechanism for sensing luminal bacterial infection. Gastroenterology (in press).

[188] Satin B, Del Giudice G, Della Bianca V, Dusi S, Laudanna C, Tonello F, et al. The neutrophil-activating protein (HP-NAP) of Helicobacter pylori is a protective antigen and a major virulence factor. J Exp Med. 2000;191:1467–1476

[189] Harris PR , Mobley HLT , Perez-Perez GI , Blaser MJ , Smith PD . Helicobacter pylori urease is a potent stimulus of mononuclear phagocyte activation and inflammatory cytokine production. Gastroenterology. 1996;111:419–425

[190] Gobert AP, Bambou JC, Werts C, Balloy V, Chignard M, Moran AP, et al. Helicobacter pylori heat shock protein 60 mediates interleukin-6 production by macrophages via a toll-like receptor (TLR)-2-, TLR-4-, and myeloid differentiation factor 88-independent mechanism . J Biol Chem . 2004;279:245–250

[191] Eck M, Schmausser B, Scheller K, Toksoy A, Kraus M, Menzel T, et al. CXC chemokines Gro(alpha)/IL-8 and IP-10/MIG in Helicobacter pylori gastritis . Clin Exp Immunol. 2000;122:192–199

[192] Haeberle HA, Kubin M, Bamford KB, Garofalo R, Graham DY, El Zaatari F, et al. Differential stimulation of interleukin-12 (IL-12) and IL-10 by live and killed Helicobacter pylori in vitro and association of IL-12 production with gamma interferon-producing T cells in the human gastric mucosa. Infect Immun. 1997;65:4229–4235

[193] Tomita T, Jackson AM, Hida N, Hayat M, Dixon MF, Shimoyama T, et al. Expression of interleukin-18, a Th1 cytokine, in human gastric mucosa is increased in Helicobacter pylori infection . J Infect Dis. 2001;183:620–627

[194] Ernst PB, Jin Y, Reyes VE, Crowe SE. The role of the local immune response in the pathogenesis of peptic ulcer formation. Scand J Gastroenterol Suppl 1994; 205:22.

[195] Di Tommaso A, Xiang Z, Bugnoli M, et al. Helicobacter pylori-specific CD4+ T-cell clones from peripheral blood and gastric biopsies. Infect Immun 1995; 63:1102.

[196] Bamford K.B,Fan X and. Crowe S.E et al., Lymphocytes in the human gastric mucosa during Helicobacter pylori have a T helper cell 1 phenotype. Gastroenterology 114 (1998), pp. 482–492.

[197] Hida N, Shimoyama T, Neville P, Dixon MF, Axon AT, Shimoyama T, et al. Increased expression of IL-10 and IL-12 (p40) mRNA in Helicobacter pylori infected gastric mucosa (relation to bacterial cag status and peptic ulceration). J Clin Pathol 1999;52:658–664

[198] Ceponis PJ, McKay DM , Menaker RJ , Galindo-Mata E , Jones NL . Helicobacter pylori infection interferes with epithelial Stat6-mediated interleukin-4 signal transduction independent of cagA, cagE, or VacA. J Immunol. 2003;171:2035–2041

[199] Lehmann FS, Terracciano L, Carena I, Baeriswyl C, Drewe J, Tornillo L, et al. In situ correlation of cytokine secretion and apoptosis in Helicobacter pylori-associated gastritis. Am J Physiol Gastrointest Liver Physiol . 2002;283:G481–G488

[200] Wang J, Fan XJ, Lindholm C, Bennet M, O'Connell J, Shanahan F, et al. Helicobacter pylori modulates lymphoepithelial cell interactions leading to epithelial cell damage through Fas/Fas Ligand interactions. Infect Immun. 2000;68:4303–4311

[201] Valnes K , Brandtzaeg P , Elgjo K , Stave R . Quantitative distribution of immunoglobulin-producing cells in gastric mucosa (relation to chronic gastritis and glandular atrophy). Gut 1986;27:505–514

[202] Kosunen, TU. Antibody titres in Helicobacter pylori infection: implications in the follow-up of antimicrobial therapy. Ann Med 1995; 27:605.

[203] Berstad AE , Brandtzaeg P , Stave R , Halstensen TS . Epithelium related deposition of activated complement in Helicobacter pylori associated gastritis. Gut 1997;40:196–203

[204] Negrini R, Lisato L, Zanella I, Cavazzini L, Gullini S, Villanacci V, et al. Helicobacter pylori infection induces antibodies cross-reacting with human gastric mucosa . Gastroenterology 1991;101:437–445

[205] Appelmelk BJ, Simoons-Smit I, Negrini R, Moran AP, Aspinall GO, Forte JG, et al. Potential role of molecular mimicry between Helicobacter pylori lipopolysaccharide and host Lewis blood group antigens in autoimmunity . Infect Immun 1996;64:2031–2040

[206] Chey, WD, Wong, BC, Practice Parameters Committee of the American College of Gastroenterology. American College of Gastroenterology guideline on the management of Helicobacter pylori infection. Am J Gastroenterol 2007; 102:1808-1816.

[207] Malfertheiner, P, Megraud, F, O'Morain, C, et al. Current concepts in the management of Helicobacter pylori infection: the Maastricht III Consensus Report. Gut 2007; 56:772

[208] Sharma VK, Sahai AV, Corder FA, et al. Helicobacter pylori eradication is superior to ulcer healing with or without maintenance therapy to prevent further ulcer haemorrhage. Aliment Pharmacol Ther 2001; 15:1939-47

[209] Liu CC, Lee CL, Chan CC, et al. Maintenance treatment is not necessary after Helicobacter pylori eradication and healing of bleeding peptic ulcer. Arch Intern Med 2003; 163:2020-4

[210] Moayyedi P, Deeks J, Talley NJ, et al. An update of the Cochrane systematic review of Helicobacter eradication therapy in nonulcer dyspepsia: Resolving the discrepancy between systematic reviews. Am J Gastroenterol 2003; 98:2621-6.

[211] Hsu PI, Lai KH, Tseng HH, et al. Eradication of Helicobacter pylori prevents ulcer development in patients with ulcer-like functional dyspepsia. Aliment Pharmacol ther 2001; 15:195-201.

[212] Chiba N, Van Zanten SJO, Sinclair P, Ferguson RA, Escobedo S, Grace E. Treating Helicobacter pylori infection in primary care patients with uninvestigated dyspepsia: the Canadian adult dyspepsia empiric treatment-Helicobacter pylori positive (CADET-Hp) randomised controlled trial. BMJ 2002;324:1012-1016.

[213] Kuipers, EJ, Lundell, L, Klinkenberg-Knol, EC, et al. Atrophic gastritis and Helicobacter pylori infection in patients with reflux esophagitis treated with omeprazole or fundoplication. N Engl J Med 1996; 334:1018.

[214] Lundell L, Miettinen P, Myrvold HE, et al. Lack of effect of acid suppression therapy on gastric atrophy. Nordic Gerd Study Group. Gastroenterology 1999; 117:319.

[215] Schaeverbeke T, Broutet N, Zerbib F, et al. Should we eradicate Helicobacter pylori before prescribing an NSAID? Results of a placebo-controlled study. Am J Gastroenterol 2005; 100:2637-43.

[216] Annibale B, Marignani M, Monarca B, et al. Reversal of iron deficiency anaemia after Helicobacter pylori eradication in patients with asymptomatic gastritis. Ann Inten Med 1999; 131:668-72.

[217] Hacihanefioglu A, Edebali F, Celebi A, et al. Improvement of complete blood count in patients with iron deficiency anemia and Helicobacter pylori infection after the eradication of Helicobacter pylori. Hepatogastroenterology 2004; 51:313-5.

[218] Gasbarrini A, Franceschi F, Armuzzi A, Ojetti V, Candelli M, Torre ES, De Lorenzo A, Anti M, Pretolani S, Gasbarrini G. Extradigestive manifestations of Helicobacter pylori gastric infection. Gut. 1999 Jul;45 Suppl 1:I9-I12.

[219] Chan FK, Sung JY, Chan SC, et al. Randomized trial of eradication of Helicobacter pylori before non-steroidal anti-inflammatory drug therapy to prevent peptic ulcers. Lancet 1997; 350: 975-9.

[220] Gasbarrini A, Franceschi F, Taraglione R, et al. Regression of autoimmune thrombocytopenia after eradication of Helicobacter pylori. Lancet 1998; 352:878.

[221] Franchini M, Veneri D. Helicobacter pylori infection and immune thrombocytopenic purpura: an uptodate. Helicobacter 2004; 9:342-6.

[222] Fujimura K, Kuwana M, Kurata Y, et al. Is eradication therapy useful as the first line of treatment in H. pylori-positive idiopathic thrombocytopenic purpura? Analysis of 207 eradicated chronic ITP cases in Japan. Int J Hematol 2005; 81:162-8.

[223] Franchini M, Veneri D, Helicobacter pylori-associated immune thrombocytopenia. Platelets 2006; 17:712-17.

[224] Tsutsumi Y, Kanamori H, Yamato H, et al. Randomized study of H. pylori eradication therapy and proton pump inhibitor monotherapy for idiopathic thrombocytopenic purpura. Ann Hematol 2005; 84:807-11.

[225] Leung WK, Lin SR, ching JY, et al. Factors predicting progression of gastric intestinal metaplasia: Results of a randomized trial on Helicobacter pylori eradication. Gut 2004; 53:1244-9.

[226] Mera R, Fontham ETH, Bravo LE, et al. Long term follow up of patients treated for Helicobacter pylori infection. Gut 2005; 54:1536-40.

[227] Wong BCY, Lam SK, Wong WM, et al. Helicobacter pylori eradication to prevent gastric cancer in a high risk region of China. JAMA 2004; 29:187-94.

[228] Midolo P, Marshall BJ. Accurate diagnosis of Helicobacter pylori. Urease tests. Gastroenterol Clin N Am 2000; 29:871-8.

[229] Perna F, Ricci C, Gatta L, et al. Diagnostic accuracy of a new rapid urease test (Pronto Dry), before and after treatment of Helicobacter pylori infection. Minerva Gastroenterol Dietol 2005; 51:247-54.

[230] Lee JM, Breslin NP, Fallon C, et al. Rapid urease tests lack sensitivity in Helicobacter pylori diagnosis when peptic ulcer disease presents with bleeding. Am J Gastroenterol 2000; 95:1166-70.

[231] Grino P, Pascual S, Such J, et al. Comparison of stool antigen immunoassay with standard methods for detection of Helicobacter pylori infection in patients with upper gastrointestinal bleeding of peptic origin. Eur J Gastroenterol Hepatol 2003; 15:525-9.

[232] Gisbert JP, Abraira V. Accuracy of Helicobacter pylori diagnostic tests in patients with bleeding peptic ulcer: A systematic review and meta-analysis. Am J Gastroenterol 2006; 101:848-63.

[233] Woo JS, el-Zimaity HM, Genta RM, et al. The best gastric site for obtaining a positive rapid urease test. Helicobacter 1996; 1:256-9.

[234] Chey WD, Woods M, Sheiman JM, et al. Lansoprazole and ranitidine affect the accuracy of the 14 C-urea breath test by a PH-dependent mechanism. Am J Gastroenterol 1997; 92:446-50.

[235] Laine L, Esrada R, Trujillo M, et al. Effect of proton-pump inhibitor therapy on diagnostic testing for Helicobacter pylori. Ann Intern Med 1998; 129:547-50.

[236] Dixon MF, Genta RM, Yardley JH, et al. Classification and grading of gastritis. The updated Sydney system. International workshop on the histopathology of gastritis, Houston 1994. Am J Surg Pathol 1996; 20:1161-81.

[237] El-Zimaity HM. Accurate diagnosis of Helicobacter pylori with biopsy. Gastroenterol Clin N Am 2000; 29:863-9.

[238] Huang MS, Wang WM, Wu DC, et al. Utility of brushing cytology in the diagnosis of Helicobacter pylori infection. Acta Cytol 1996; 40:714.

[239] Perez-Perez GI. Accurate diagnosis of Helicobacter pylori. Culture, including transport. Gastroenterol Clin N Am 2000; 29:879-84.

[240] Makristathis A, Hirschl AM, Lehourst P, et al. Diagnosis of Helicobacter pylori infection. Helicobacter 2004; 9:7-14.

[241] Lehours P, Ruskone-Fourmestraux A, Lavergne A, et al. Which test to use to detect Helicobacter pylori infection in patients with low grade gastric mucosa-associated lymphoid tissue lymphoma? Am J Gastroenterol 2003; 98: 291-5.

[242] Gisbert JP, Pajares JM. Review article: 13 C-urea breath test in the diagnosis of Helicobacter pylori infection- a critical review. Aliment Pharmacol Ther 2004; 20:1001-17.

[243] Chey WD, Accurate diagnosis of Helicobacter pylori. 14-C urea breath test. Gastroenterol Clin N Am 2000; 29:895-902.

[244] Leodolter A, Domingues-Munoz JE, von Arnim U, et al. Validity of a modified 13-C-urea breath test for pre- and post-treatment diagnosis of Helicobacter pylori infection in the routine clinical setting. Am J Gastroenterol 1999; 94:2100-4.

[245] Chey WD, Metz DC, Shaw S, et al. Appropriate timing of the 14 C-urea breath test to establish eradication of Helicobacter pylori infection. Am J Gastroenterol 2000; 95:1171-4.

[246] Perri F, Giampiero M, Neri M, et al. Helicobacter pylori antigen stool test and 13 C-urea breath test in patients after eradication treatments. Am J Gastroenterol 2002; 97:2756-62.

[247] Gatta L, Ricci C, Tampieri A, et al. Accuracy of breath tests using low doses of 13 C-urea to diagnose Helicobacter pylori infection. Gut 2006; 55:457-62.

[248] Graham DY, Opekun AR, Hammoud F, et al. Studies regarding the mechanism of false negative urea breath tests with proton pump inhibitors. Am J Gastroenterol 2003; 98:1005-9.

[249] Savarino V, Tracci D, Dulbecco P, et al. Negative effect of ranitidine on the results of urea breath test for the diagnosis of Helicobacter pylori. Am J Gastroenterol 2001; 96:348-52.

[250] Chey WD, Murthy U, Toskes P, et al. The 13 C-urea blood test accurately detects active Helicobacter pylori infection. Am J Gastroenterol 1999; 94: 1522-4.

[251] Ahmed F, Chey WD, Murthy U, et al. Evaluation of the Ez-HBT Helicobacter blood test to establish eradication. Aliment Pharmacol Ther 2005; 22:875-80.

[252] Loy CT, Irwig LM, Katelaris PH, et al. Do commercial serological kits for Helicobacter pylori infection differ in accuracy? A meta-analysis. Am J Gastroenterol 1996; 91:1138-44.

[253] Nurgalieva ZZ, Graham DY. Pearls and pitfalls of assessing Helicobacter pylori status. Dig Liver Dis 2003; 35:375-7.

[254] Ho B, Marshall BJ. Accurate diagnosis of Helicobacter pylori. Serological testing. Gastroenterol Clin N Am 2000; 29:853-62.

[255] Gisbert JP, Pajares JM, Stool antigen test for the diagnosis of Helicobacter pylori: A systematic review. Helicobacter 2004; 9:347-68.

[256] Gisbert JP, de la Morena F, Abraira V. Accuracy of monoclonal stool antigen test for the diagnosis of H. pylori infection: A systematic review and meta-analysis. Am J Gastroenterol 2006; 101:1921-30.

[257] Odaka T, Yamaguchi T, Koyama H, et al. Evaluation of the Helicobacter pylori stool antigen test for monitoring eradication therapy. Am J Gastroenterol 2002; 97:594-9.

[258] Bravo LE, Realpe JL, Campo C, et al. Effects of acid suppression and bismuth medications on the performance of diagnostic tests for Helicobacter pylori infection. . Am J Gastroenterol 1999; 94:2380-3.

[259] Manes G, Balzano A, Iaquinto G, et al. Accuracy of the stool antigen test in the diagnosis of Helicobacter pylori infection before treatment and in patients on omeprazole therapy. Aliment Pharmacol Ther 2001; 15:73-9.

[260] Van Leerdam ME, van Der Ende A, ten Kate FJW, et al. Lack of accuracy of the non-invasive Helicobacter pylori stool antigen test in patients with gastroduodenal ulcer bleeding. Am J Gastroenterol 2003; 98: 798-801.

[261] Pacheco N, Mago V, Gomez I, et al. Comparison of PCR and common clinical tests for the diagnosis of H. pylori in dyspeptic patients. Diagn Microbiol Infect Dis. 2001; 39:207-210.

[262] He Q, Wang JP, Osato M, et al. Real-time quantitative PCR for detection of Helicobacter pylori. J Clin Microbiol. 2002; 40:3720-3728.

[263] Meng XW, Scheer MA, Zhang HJ, Tsang TK: Detection of H. pylori from patients with PPIs treatment. ACG 2008[Poster presentation].

[264] Zsikla V, Hailemariam S, Baumann M, et al. Increased rate of Helicobacter pylori infection detected by PCR in biopsies with chronic gastritis. Am J Surg Pathol 2006; 30:242-8.

[265] Weiss J, Tsang TK, Meng X, Zhang H, Kilner E, Wang E, Watkin W. Correlation with inflammation scores and immunohistochemical and CLO test findings. Am J Clin Pathol 2008; 129:89-96.

[266] Lawson AJ, Elviss NC, Owen RJ. Real-time PCR detection and frequency of 16 S rDNA mutations associated with resistance and reduced susceptibility to tetracycline in Helicobacter pylori from England and Wales, Antimicrob Chemother 2005; 56:282-6.

[267] Rimbara E, Noguchi N, Yamaguchi T, et al. Development of a highly sensitive method for detection of clarithromycin-resistant Helicobacter pylori from human feces. Current Microbiol 2005; 51:1-5.

[268] De Francesco V, Maargiotta M, Zullo M, et al. Primary clarithromycin resistance in Italy assessed on Helicobacter pylori DNA sequences by TaqMan real-time polymerase chain reaction. Aliment Pharmacol Ther 2006; 23:429-35.

[269] Kabir S. Detection of Helicobacter pylori in feces by culture, PCR and enzyme immunoassay. J Med Microbiol. 2001;50:1021-1029.

[270] Meng X, Zhang H, Law J, Tsang R, Tsang T. Detection of Helicobacter pylori from food sources by a novel multiplex PCR assay. J of food safety 2008; 28:609-619.

# 3

# NSAIDs and Peptic Ulcer Disease

Iván Ferraz-Amaro and Federico Díaz-González
*Rheumatology Service*
*Hospital Universitario de Canarias*
*Santa Cruz de Tenerife*
*Spain*

## 1. Introduction

In 1897 Felix Hoffman, a 29-year-old scientist working for the Bayer Company patented a chemical procedure that enabled the acetylation of salicylic acid with the enough purity to be used commercially (Wallace, 1997). The new product was evaluated by Dreser Heinrich, head of marketing at Bayer, who - despite some initial misgivings - gave his approval for marketing acetylsalicylic acid under the name "Aspirin" in 1899. The new compound was commercialized by Bayer as an effective therapy for fever and aches, one that, unlike its source molecule (salicylic acid), had no gastric side effects. For over six decades aspirin remained the mainstay of non-narcotic analgesic treatment and nonsteroidal anti-inflammatory drug (NSAIDs) therapy. Beginning with the sale of indomethacin in 1963, used for the treatment of rheumatoid arthritis, at least twenty other NSAIDs with aspirin-like actions have been developed over the past half-century. Although aspirin's preeminence as an over-the-counter analgesic has been progressively displaced by new NSAIDs, new studies exploring its antiplatelet effect led to aspirin's development as a major antithrombotic agent (Patrono et al., 2005). Today, NSAIDs are popular because of their versatile effectiveness as analgesics, antipyretics, and as anti-inflammatory agents, and they remain among the most frequently prescribed medications worldwide.

The long-standing confidence in the gastric safety of aspirin went unchallenged for 40 years until 1938 when two researchers at Guy's Hospital in London, Douthwaite and Lintott, showed unquestionably that it had a major gastro-erosive activity (Douthwaite & Lintott 1938). Unfortunately, most of the NSAIDs currently available on the market can injure the gastric and duodenal mucosa (Cryer & Feldman, 1992; Soll et al., 1991), much like aspirin, with considerable rates of morbidity and mortality. The standard evolution of peptic ulcers resulting from NSAIDs ranges from resolution without intervention to the development of complications, such as bleeding and perforation. To variable degrees aspirin and NSAIDs inhibit the cyclooxygenase (COX) enzymes COX-1 and COX-2, which synthesize the inflammatory mediators known as prostaglandins and thromboxane. Prostaglandin inhibition plays a critical role in the pathogenesis of NSAIDs-induced gastric injury. Beginning ten years ago new specific inhibitors of COX-2 became available, compounds that have significantly reduced gastrointestinal (GI) side effects compared with COX-1 inhibitors (Bombardier et al., 2000; Laine et al., 2007; Silverstein et al., 2000).

Peptic ulcers are defects in the GI mucosa that extend throughout the muscularis mucosae, and which are often associated with *Helicobacter pylori* (*H. pylori*) infection or with consumption of *NSAIDs*. As the prevalence of *H. pylori* infection has declined in Western countries, gastric ulcers have increasingly been linked to *NSAID* use, with acetylsalicylic acid (Yuan et al., 2006) being an important cause of morbidity and rising health care costs related to work loss, hospitalization, and outpatient care (Ramakrishnan & Salinas, 2007). Management of peptic ulcer disease has improved radically during the past few decades, culminating in the widespread use of proton pump inhibitor (PPI)-based triple therapy for *H. pylori* eradication. However, prescriptions for drugs such as aspirin and *NSAIDs* have also increased over this same time period and adherence to gastroprotection protocols to prevent *NSAID*-induced peptic ulcer disease still seem to be far from optimal (Jones, 2001).

## 2. Epidemiology

### 2.1 Ulcers and NSAIDs. Incidence and prevalence

In the United States alone sales of over-the-counter analgesics approach 3 billion dollars annually, with *NSAIDs* accounting for about 60% of sales (the other 40% is attributed to acetaminophen) (Laine, 2001). An estimated 14 million patients use *NSAIDs* for the relief of symptoms associated with arthritis alone (Wolfe, 1996), and among patients older that 65, as many as 70% take NSAIDs at least once a week, with at least 34% of this population taking a *NSAID* tablet daily (Talley et al., 1995).

A systematic review of the worldwide literature estimated that the annual incidence of peptic ulcer disease ranged from 0.1 to 0.19 percent for physician-diagnosed and 0.01 to 0.17 percent when based upon hospitalized patients (Sung et al., 2009). Upper GI symptoms, such as dyspepsia, occur in 15% to 60% of NSAID users, twice as often as in individuals not taking NSAIDs. The prevalence of gastric or duodenal ulcers in patients taking NSAIDs regularly is approximately 15% to 30%. The annual incidence of NSAID-related clinical upper GI events (complicated and symptomatic ulcers) is approximately 2.5% to 4.5%, with the annual incidence of serious complications (severe bleeding, perforation, and obstruction) running about 1% to 1.5% (Laine, 2002).

### 2.2 Trends

The epidemiology of peptic ulcer disease largely reflects environmental factors, primarily *H. pylori* infection, but also *NSAID* use and smoking. The incidence of *H. pylori* below age 50 is falling dramatically in developed countries due, in part, to improved hygiene and socioeconomic conditions; however, the prevalence of *H. pylori* infection remains high for older individuals and in certain predisposed subpopulations. The epidemiology of peptic ulcer disease has changed in the past decade due to the enormous efforts made to eradicate *H. pylori* infection, which is the single largest cause of peptic ulcers. As the prevalence of *H. pylori* infection has declined, the proportion (and actual numbers) of patients with *H. pylori*-negative idiopathic ulcers, and with ulcers attributed to the use of NSAIDs, has risen (Chow & Sung, 2007). A prospective cohort study in Hong Kong (Chan et al., 2001; Hung et al., 2005) demonstrated that the number and proportion of *H. pylori*-associated ulcers decreased from 50.3% in 1997–1998 and to 33.4% in 2000–2001. This study also showed that there was a 4.5-fold increase in the absolute number of idiopathic ulcers, from 4.1% to 18.8% during that same time period. By contrast, the relative proportion of *NSAID*-associated ulcers remained constant (45.5% in 1997–1998 versus 47.8% in 2000–2001). On the basis of these data, the incidence of non-*H. pylori*, non-*NSAID* peptic ulcer bleeding is thought to be on the rise in Asia. Similar prospective studies are awaited in the West; however, it is clear that the global prevalence of idiopathic ulcers is on increasing. Although *H. pylori* is the predominant cause of peptic ulcer disease worldwide, it appears that there are regional differences in prevalence that cannot be explained by this infection per se. Patterns of *NSAID* use and smoking are likely to be important, too.

At a minimum, smoking clearly exacerbates *H. pylori*-associated ulcer disease. The decline in smoking in younger individuals, particularly in males, and the concomitant increase in women, may be a factor in the declining male/female ratio of ulcer disease. Smoking does not appear to be a factor in the ulcerative complications found in older women or in *NSAID*-related ulcers. It should also be borne in mind that *NSAID* use increases as a function of age and is an independent risk factor for ulcers. In addition, older subjects are more likely not only to develop complications from *NSAID*-related ulcers, but also to suffer increased morbidity and mortality from these complications because of co-morbidities.

## 3. Mechanisms of therapeutic action of NSAIDs

Based on their chemical structure, there are now at least 20 different *NSAIDs* from six major groups available for use in humans (Table 1). All of them are absorbed completely, have negligible first-pass hepatic metabolism, are tightly bound to albumin, and have small volumes of distribution. The half-lives of *NSAIDs* vary, though in general can be divided into "short" (less than six hours) and "long" (more than six hours) lasting drugs. These compounds differ in their doses, interaction with other drugs, and some specific side effects. The inhibition of prostaglandin synthesis via the blockade of cyclooxygenase (COX) has been widely accepted as the main mechanism of action and toxicity utilized by these compounds (Moncada et al., 1973). However, during the last decade, many groups have described a number of non-prostaglandin-mediated anti-inflammatory effects from NSAIDs, suggesting that COX inhibition is not the only explanation for either the anti-inflammatory action or the gastric toxicity observed with this group of therapeutic agents (Abramson & Weissmann, 1989; Amin et al., 1995; Kopp & Ghosh, 1994; Mahmud et al., 1996).

---

**Non-selective nonsteroidal anti-inflammatory (NSAID) agents**
    Salicylate (acetylated): Aspirin
    Salicylates (non-acetylated): Diflunisal, Choline magnesium trisalicylate, Salsalate
    Propionic acids: Ibuprofen, Naproxen, Ketoprofen, Flurbiprofen, Oxaprozin
    Acetic acids: Diclofenac, Etodolac, Tolmetin, Sulindac, Ketorolac, Indomethacin
    Oxicams (enolic acids): Meloxicam, Piroxicam
    Fenamates (anthranilic acids): Meclofenamic acid, Mefenamic acid
    Non-acidic (naphthylalkanone): Nabumetone

**Selective COX-2 inhibitors:**
    Celecoxib, Eterocoxib, Parecoxib

---

Table 1. NSAID families

### 3.1 COX inhibition

As stated above, NSAIDs target COX, and hence the synthesis of prostaglandins, particularly prostaglandin E2 (PGE2). This inflammatory molecule lowers pain thresholds, and the primary goal of NSAIDs is to reduce pain. Tissue prostaglandins are produced from membrane arachidonic acid via two pathways: cyclooxygenase-1 (COX-1) and COX-2. The COX-1 pathway is the predominant constitutive pathway; prostaglandins derived from this enzyme mediate many effects, most notably they facilitate gastroduodenal cytoprotection, renal perfusion, and platelet activity. In contrast, the COX-2 pathway is inducible by inflammatory stimuli and mediates effects through prostaglandins, which results in inflammation, pain, and fever. COX-2 induces at least two orders of magnitude more PGE2 than COX-1. Specific inhibitors of COX-2 represent a major advance in the treatment of pain, particularly in patients with osteoarthritis or rheumatoid arthritis. For the most part, COX-2 inhibitors have significantly reduced gastrointestinal side effects compared with COX-1 inhibitors (Rostom et al., 2007).

All of the non-salicylate, non-COX-2 selective *NSAIDs* including aspirin can interfere with platelet aggregation and secretion (McQueen et al., 1986; O'Brien, 1968) through the inactivation of platelet COX-1. In platelets, this enzyme is a rate-limiting step in the transformation of arachidonic acid into thromboxane A2, a potent platelet-aggregating agent. However, aspirin inhibits platelet COX-1 in an irreversible manner and thus has proven beneficial in reducing the risk of secondary thrombotic cardiovascular events (Berger et al., 2008). These properties may be important enough to warrant its continued use in those patients also needing common *NSAIDs*. Thus, if needed, such patients can be continued on low dose aspirin. Administration of some *NSAIDs* may interfere with the desirable antiplatelet effects of aspirin (Catella-Lawson et al., 2001).

### 3.2 Nonprostaglandin-mediated effects

Although *NSAIDs'* degree of potency as inhibitors of prostaglandin synthesis *in vitro* tends to reflect their anti-inflammatory potency *in vivo*, several experimental and clinical studies suggest that prostaglandin inhibition is only part of the story. The necessary dose of any given *NSAID*, notably aspirin, which is essential for suppressing inflammation, may well exceed that required to substantially inhibit prostaglandin synthesis, at least in plasma. In this regard, salicylate, which is a weak inhibitor of COX activity, appears to be as effective as aspirin, a potent inhibitor of COX activity, in controlling inflammation in patients with rheumatoid arthritis (Brooks & Day, 1991). These and other data have led to the suggestion that these drugs are driven by prostaglandin-independent mechanistic actions, particularly in terms of their anti-inflammatory properties.

Therefore, several non-prostaglandin-mediated *NSAID*-induced mechanisms of action may also be important. These mechanisms are generally related to the ability of *NSAIDs* to insert themselves into biological membranes and disrupt a wide range of cell functions and cell-cell interactions. For example, *NSAIDs* might interfere with neutrophil-endothelial cell adherence by decreasing the availability of L-selectins in the membranes of neutrophils, thereby removing a critical step in the migration of granulocytes to sites of inflammation (Diaz-Gonzalez et al., 1995). *NSAIDs* also inhibit nuclear factor *kappa B (NF-kB)*-dependent transcription *in vitro*, resulting in a decrease in available nitric oxide synthetase (Amin et al., 1995). This enzyme produces nitric oxide in large amounts, thereby causing vasodilation, cytotoxicity, and increased vascular permeability (Hawkey, 1995). The anti-nociceptive actions of some *NSAIDs*, though not all, appear to involve L-arginine-NO-cyclic GMP-potassium channel pathways (Ortiz et al., 2003).

The role and importance of these non-prostaglandin-mediated processes in clinical inflammation remains unclear. Also unknown is whether any of these potential mechanisms of action might explain the great variability in individual patient response to *NSAIDs*.

## 4. Mechanisms underlying NSAID-induced gastrointestinal toxicity

*NSAIDs* damage gastrointestinal mucosa by causing both local injuries and by systemically inhibiting prostaglandin production. However, current consensus on the pathogenesis of symptomatic peptic ulcer disease resulting from exposure to *NSAIDs* holds that it is mainly a consequence of systemic (post-absorptive) inhibition of GI mucosal COX activity rather than a local effect (van Oijen et al., 2008).

### 4.1 COX inhibition
NSAIDs induce gastrointestinal cytotoxicity through the inhibition of COX enzyme activity, a correlation which has been well established (Warner et al., 1999). In addition, while it is now known that certain prostaglandins such as *PGE2* reduce gastric acid secretion, the onset of hypochlorhydria does not entirely explain the mucosal protection observed with PGE2. This has led to the notion that prostaglandins have antisecretory-independent effects that have been collectively referred to as "cytoprotection". Some of the cytoprotective mechanisms employed by prostaglandins include stimulation of glycoprotein (mucin), bicarbonate and phospholipid production by epithelial cells, enhancement of mucosal blood flow and oxygen delivery to epithelial cells via local vasodilation, increased epithelial cell migration towards the luminal surface (restitution), and enhanced epithelial cell proliferation (Robert et al., 1979). Inhibition of the COX-1 pathway blocks production of prostaglandins in epithelial cells and, consequently, these compounds impair any protective capabilities, resulting in a gastric environment that is more susceptible to topical attack by endogenous factors, such as acid, pepsin, and bile salts. Many *NSAIDs* block COX-1 and COX-2 more or less equally (i.e., are non-selective) and thus they may impair gastric prostaglandin production even at low concentrations. Since prostaglandins are essential to both the maintenance of intact GI defenses and normal platelet function, *NSAIDs* promote ulcer formation as well as bleeding. Drugs that more selectively inhibit COX-2 than COX-1 have less suppressive effects on gastric prostaglandin synthesis. As a result, selective inhibitors of COX-2 preserve prostaglandin-mediated GI mucosal protection. However, COX-2 selective inhibitors may still block COX-1 at clinically recommended doses, and thus have the potential to also block COX-1 in the stomach and duodenum and thereby cause damage.

### 4.2 Nonprostaglandin-mediated effects
Most *NSAIDs* are carboxylic acid derivatives. As a result, they are not ionized at the acidic pH levels found in the gastric lumen and can thus be absorbed across the gastric mucosa. Once the drug moves from the acidic environment of the gastric lumen into the pH–neutral mucosa, the drug ionizes and is trapped temporarily in epithelial cells where it may inflict damage.

The ability to uncouple mitochondrial oxidative phosphorylation is a common characteristic of NSAIDs containing an ionizable group. NSAIDs are able to interfere with mitochondrial oxidative phosphorylation (Krause et al., 2003), reducing intracellular ATP synthesis *in vivo* (Mingatto et al., 1996), an effect that has been postulated as representing an early pathogenic event in NSAID-mediated enteropathy (Mahmud et al., 1996; Rainsford, 1980). Recently, novel pathways, independent of COX inhibition, have been identified for some NSAIDs, as has their ability to bind and disrupt cell membranes. *In vitro* exposure of gastric epithelial cells to different concentrations of NSAIDs can result in altered cell-membrane permeability. This can lead to profound and rapid changes in cell morphology, suggesting that the cytotoxicity and biological actions of NSAIDs are mediated by the cell membrane and are not dependent upon COX (Zhou et al.).

### 4.3 Role of Helicobacter pylori infection

Until recently, data analysis on the role of *H. pylori* infection as a risk factor for GI bleeding in *NSAID* users was complicated by a failure, in many studies, to account for the variable influence of multiple, co-existing risk factors. Not surprisingly, therefore, these studies have yielded conflicting results (Graham et al., 1992).

A comprehensive meta-analysis of 16 case–controlled studies demonstrated that the risk of peptic ulcer bleeding was increased by a factor of 1.79 with *H. pylori* infection, by 4.85 with *NSAID* usage, and by 6.13 in the presence of both *NSAID* use and *H. pylori* infection, strongly suggesting the possibility of an additive effect (Huang et al., 2002). Further evidence of *H. pylori* infection's additive role in the context of *NSAID* use comes from trials measuring the impact of *H. pylori* eradication. Indeed, the eradication of *H. pylori* in high-risk patients prior to the initiation of *NSAID* therapy has been shown to significantly reduce the risk of subsequent ulceration (Bazzoli et al., 2001; Malfertheiner et al., 2002). Two systematic reviews have clearly shown that eradication of *H. pylori* is superior to placebo therapy in the primary prevention of peptic ulcers among *NSAID* users (risk ratio (95 % CI) 0.35 (0.20 – 0.61)) (Leontiadis et al., 2007). Using a Markov model, Leontiadis *et al.* (Leontiadis et al., 2007) showed that the most cost-effective strategy for primary prevention of *NSAID*-associated ulcers was *H. pylori* eradication in patients over age 50. Interestingly, sensitivity analysis showed that eradication therapy remained cost-effective even when the *H. pylori* prevalence was as low as 5%. However, eradication seems less effective than treatment with a maintenance PPI for preventing non-steroidal anti-inflammatory drug-associated ulcers (Vergara et al., 2005).

It must be added that many patients take *NSAIDs* intermittently and often for only short periods at a time. Whether a "test-and-treat" strategy would be cost effective for such a large population group is unknown. Furthermore, it has also been noted that eradication of *H. pylori* infection alone is not sufficient for the secondary prevention of peptic ulcer bleeding in chronic *NSAID* users (Vergara et al., 2005).

### 5. Risk of GI complications in patients taking different NSAIDs

Recent studies suggest that the risk of GI complications may be lower with the use of some *NSAIDs*, including ibuprofen, nabumetone, meloxicam, and etodolac, but higher with others such as sulindac, piroxicam, and ketorolac (de Abajo & Garcia Rodriguez, 2001; Garcia Rodriguez & Hernandez-Diaz, 2001; Hernandez-Diaz & Rodriguez, 2000). In the case of ibuprofen, this may be due to the use, in general, of lower analgesic doses, especially in relation to ibuprofen preparations that are available over-the-counter. Nabumetone, meloxicam, and etodolac may possess some degree of COX-2 selectivity, whereas sulindac, piroxicam, and ketorolac may owe their increased toxicity to the presence of relatively long plasma half-lives, which would thereby result in more prolonged mucosal exposure (Simon & Mills, 1980). With respect to aspirin, its use at low doses alone, in the absence of other risk factors, is also associated with an increased risk for both GI bleeding and death from GI complications. Numerous studies in patients taking low-dose aspirin alone have shown a relative risk of 2–4 for GI bleeding (Lanas et al., 2005). Furthermore, a large percentage of patients on low-dose aspirin are elderly, have multiple co-morbidities, and cardiovascular disease, in particular, and are likely to be concurrently taking anticoagulants, *NSAIDs* and corticosteroids, any one of which will elevate their relative risk for GI events to several times that of low-dose aspirin alone. It is important to emphasize that physicians are often unaware that patients are self-medicating with low-dose aspirin when they prescribe *NSAIDs* for pain relief or anti-inflammatory effects.

In regards to COX-2 inhibitors, there have been several large randomized, controlled, outcome trials comparing COX-2 inhibitors to traditional NSAIDs. The CLASS study (Silverstein et al., 2000) compared celecoxib 400 mg b.i.d. with ibuprofen 800 mg t.i.d., or diclofenac 75 mg b.i.d., in osteoarthritis or rheumatoid arthritis patients. A non-significant 50% reduction in ulcer complications was observed in the celecoxib group compared with those who received the conventional *NSAID* after 6 months of therapy. After 1 year, however, there was little or no difference between the three groups. Another large trial, the VIGOR study (Bombardier et al., 2000), compared outcomes in rheumatoid arthritis patients taking either 500 mg of naproxen b.i.d. or 50 mg of rofecoxib daily. At 6 months, rofecoxib was associated with a significantly lower incidence of GI events (2.1 *vs.* 4.5%, $P < 0.001$), and GI complications (0.6 *vs.* 1.42 %, $P = 0.005$). The TARGET study (Schnitzer et al., 2004) compared lumiracoxib with traditional *NSAIDs* in patients with osteoarthritis. After 1 year, a significant reduction in ulcer complication rates was noted for lumiracoxib among the entire study population (0.3 *vs.* 0.9%), as well as among those who were not taking aspirin (0.2 *vs.* 0.9%), but not in those taking aspirin. In a report summarizing the results of eterocoxib, based on three prospective randomized, double-blind trials (Laine et al., 2007), 34,701 arthritic patients were treated with 60 or 90 mg of etoricoxib or 150 mg of diclofenac daily. This study included patients on low-dose aspirin and/or PPI therapy. It was found that the overall incidence of uncomplicated GI events was significantly less with etoricoxib than with diclofenac (Hazard ratio 0.69, 95 % CI; 0.57 – 0.83) ($P < 0.001$). There were no differences between the groups for complicated events (bleeding, perforation, and/or obstruction).

A Cochrane systematic review of GI safety revealed that COX-2 inhibitors produced significantly fewer gastroduodenal ulcers (relative risk, 0.26; 95 % confidence interval, 0.23 – 0.30) and ulcer complications (relative risk, 0.39; 95 % confidence interval, 0.31–0.50), as well as fewer withdrawals caused by GI symptoms when compared with nonselective *NSAIDs* (Rostom et al., 2007).

## 6. Clinical spectrum of gastroduodenal mucosal injury by NSAIDs

NSAIDs are valuable agents in the treatment of arthritis and many other musculoskeletal disorders, and as analgesics in a wide variety of clinical scenarios. However, as stated above, their use has been limited mainly by their association with mucosal injury to the upper gastrointestinal tract, including the development of peptic ulcer disease and its complications, most notably upper gastrointestinal hemorrhage and perforation (Cryer & Feldman, 1992; Soll et al., 1991).

### 6.1 Gastric damage
Upper GI symptoms, such as dyspepsia, occur in 15% to 60% of *NSAID* users, twice as often as in individuals not taking *NSAIDs*. Dyspepsia occurs in three common patterns: ulcer-like

or acid dyspepsia (e.g., burning, epigastric hunger pain with food, antacid, and antisecretory agent relief); indigestion (also called functional dyspepsia or dysmotility-like dyspepsia, with postprandial belching, bloating, epigastric fullness, anorexia, early satiety, nausea, and occasional vomiting); and reflux-like dyspepsia. These patterns overlap considerably. Although poorly correlated with endoscopic lesions and clinical events, dyspepsia and other GI symptoms limit the use of *NSAIDs*, affect quality of life, and frequently require medical co-therapy with H2-receptor antagonists or PPIs. For example, it has been estimated that 5% to 15% of patients with rheumatoid arthritis can expect to discontinue *NSAID* therapy because of dyspepsia (Singh & Triadafilopoulos, 1999).

Endoscopically visible lesions associated with *NSAID* use include subepithelial hemorrhages, erosions, and ulcers. Subepithelial hemorrhages appear as bright red areas without any clear break in the mucosa. Microscopically, they appear as large numbers of red blood cells in the superficial portion of the mucosa, beneath the epithelium. Erosions are breaks in the mucosa that remain confined therein. Subepithelial hemorrhages occur in virtually 100% of people within 15 to 30 minutes after ingestion of a single 650-mg dose of aspirin. Repeated dosing of aspirin (650 mg 4 times daily) leads to development of gastric erosions within 24 hours in virtually all patients (Laine, 1996). With longer-term therapy, adaptation may occur, although gastric erosions are still found in approximately 40% to 60% of patients taking regular doses of *NSAIDs*.

An ulcer is defined histologically as a break that extends into the submucosa or deeper, and endoscopically as a break in the mucosa of >3 mm in diameter with unequivocal depth. For this reason, only ulcers can cause serious GI complications, such as bleeding, perforation, and obstruction. Subepithelial hemorrhages and erosions do not cause major GI bleeding because they are confined to the mucosal layer, where there are no blood vessels of significant size. Furthermore, they cannot cause the most dreaded of GI complications, perforation, since perforation requires an extension of the break in the mucosa through all 4 layers of the GI tract (mucosa, submucosa, musclaris propria, and serosa) (Laine, 2002). Ulcers may be formed in healthy subjects within 1 week of regular *NSAID* use. The prevalence of ulcers in patients taking *NSAIDs* regularly is approximately 15% to 30% (Laine, 1996; Larkai et al., 1987). The cumulative incidence of *NSAID*-associated ulcers in recent double-blind trials has been as high as 45% after 6 months. Most ulcers do not cause clinically important GI events. In fact, large outcome studies of arthritis patients indicate that the annual incidence of *NSAID*-related clinical upper GI events (complicated and symptomatic ulcers) is approximately 2.5% to 4.5%, while the annual incidence of serious complications (severe bleeding, perforation, and obstruction) is about 1% to 1.5%(Bombardier et al., 2000; Silverstein et al., 2000). Although these percentages are relatively small, the consumption of *NSAIDs* is so extensive that a large number of GI events are caused by *NSAIDs*, making GI complications the most important concern limiting use of *NSAIDs*.

### 6.2 Duodenal damage

In contrast to the stomach, damage to the duodenal mucosa by aspirin and *NSAIDs* seems to largely depend upon gastric acid. The "classic" symptoms of a duodenal ulcer occur when acid is secreted in the absence of a food buffer. Food is usually well emptied by two to three hours after meals, although food-stimulated acid secretion can persist for three to five hours; thus, classic duodenal ulcer symptoms occur two to five hours after meals or on an empty stomach. Symptoms also occur at night when the circadian stimulation of acid secretion is maximal. The ability of alkali, food, and antisecretory agents to produce relief suggests that acid plays a role in this process. Thus, "acid dyspepsia" is a fitting term. Symptomatic periods lasting a few weeks, followed by symptom-free periods of weeks or months, is a pattern characteristic of classic duodenal ulcers.

Numerous findings suggest that *NSAIDs* represent the most relevant factor in duodenal ulcers not associated with *H. pylori* infection. The history of *NSAID* use is more common in duodenal ulcer patients who have a normal, non-infected stomach than in those in whom the ulcer is associated with *H. pylori* gastritis. Several studies have found either that *NSAID* intake is present in 25–75% of the *H. pylori*-negative duodenal ulcer patients or that *NSAIDs* are the most frequently identifiable cause in non-infected duodenal ulcers (Gisbert & Calvet, 2009).

### 6.3 Death rates associated with NSAIDs

A very large study carried out by the Spanish National Health System reported a death rate of 15.3 persons per 100,000 *NSAID* users, including aspirin. Approximately 50% of the patients who died in the Spanish study had a prior history of one, or more, of the following risk factors: peptic ulceration, GI bleeding, dyspepsia, cardiac disease, or hypertension. The average age of patients dying from *NSAID* complications was 70±13.5 years and 89.7% of those who died were above age 60 (Lanas et al., 2005). In the United States the reported death rate associated with *NSAIDs* is three times higher than in Spain (Singh & Triadafilopoulos, 1999), probably because this figure was extrapolated from a small sample of rheumatoid arthritis patients and it is well-known that rheumatoid arthritis alone has been associated with increased mortality, independent of *NSAID* use.

## 7. Risk factors for NSAID-related GI complications

Risk factors for GI complications associated with *NSAIDs* have been identified through a series of case–control and cohort studies that compared outcomes for patients taking these agents with those of control groups. A series of nested case–control studies based on incidence rates for hospitalization for GI bleeding in patients above age 65 showed an increased risk not only for this population group (odds ratio 4.7), but also for those on higher doses of *NSAIDs* (odds ratio 8.0), those who had a relatively short-term history of *NSAID* use (less than 1 month; odds ratio 7.2), and those concurrently taking corticosteroids (odds ratio 4.4) or anticoagulants (odds ratio 12.7) (Griffin et al., 1991; Griffin et al., 1988; Piper et al., 1991; Shorr et al., 1993) . In a large study series based on autopsy findings on patients with a history of *NSAID* use, gastric and duodenal ulcers were found to be more common among those who had consumed *NSAIDs* for less than 3 months (Allison et al., 1992). Although the risk of ulcer complications decreases after the first few months of *NSAID* use, it does not disappear with long-term therapy. One approach to risk stratification has been proposed (Table 2) (Lanza et al., 2009). Gastrointestinal risk is arbitrarily stratified into low (i.e., no risk factors), moderate (presence of one or two risk factors), and high-risk groups (multiple risk factors, a history of ulcer complications, or concomitant use of corticosteroids or anticoagulants).

## 8. Treatment and prevention of NSAID-related GI complications

If a patient develops an ulcer while on *NSAIDs*, the relevant *NSAID(s)* should be stopped if at all possible and traditional ulcer therapy with a PPI or an H2 antagonist started. PPIs are generally preferred as they are associated with more rapid healing. As in all patients with peptic ulcers, the individual's *H. pylori* status should also be assessed; if positive, appropriate therapy should be instituted. For patients who must remain on *NSAID* therapy or on low-dose aspirin, randomized trials have shown that ulcer healing occurs more rapidly with a PPI rather than with an H2 antagonist (Agrawal et al., 2000; Yeomans et al., 1998), misoprostol (Hawkey et al., 1998), or sucralfate (Bianchi Porro et al., 1998).

## 8.1 Prevention

Most experts in the field agree that patients with a recent complicated peptic ulcer are at very high risk and it is best in such cases to avoid *NSAID* treatment entirely; however, if anti-inflammatory treatment must be undertaken, a COX-2 inhibitor plus misoprostol or a PPI therapy should be employed. Patients with a history of peptic ulcer disease, with or without complications, at any time in the past, and concurrent use of aspirin (including low

---

*High risk*

    1.   History of a previously complicated ulcer, especially if recent

    2.   Multiple (>2) risk factors

*Moderate risk (1-2)*

    1.   Age > 65

    2.   High-dose NSAID therapy

    3.   A previous history of an uncomplicated ulcer

    4.   Concurrent use of aspirin (including low dose), corticosteroids, or anticoagulants

*Low risk*

    1.   No risk factors

*H. pylori* is an independent and additive risk factor and needs to be addressed separately

---

Table 2. Patients at increased risk for NSAID GI toxicity (Guidelines for the Prevention of NSAID-related Ulcer Complications) (Lanza et al., 2009)

dose), antiplatelet drugs (e.g., clopidrogel), anticoagulants (e.g., warfarin), or corticosteroids, or two or more risk factors also fall in the high-risk categories; here, treatment should consist of a COX-2 inhibitor and either misoprostol or PPI therapy (Lanza et al., 2009). As shown in Table 2, patients considered to be at moderate risk must be treated with a COX-2 inhibitor alone or with an *NSAID* plus misoprostol or a PPI. Patients without risk factors are at low risk for *NSAID*-related peptic ulcer complications and no protective measures are required (Lanza et al., 2009) (Table 3).

As mentioned above, multiple studies have evaluated the relationship between *H. pylori* and the risk of gastric ulcers in *NSAID* users. Based upon the available evidence, patients with a history of uncomplicated or complicated peptic ulcers (gastric, duodenal) should be tested for *H. pylori* prior to beginning a course of *NSAIDs* or low-dose aspirin therapy. If present,

| Gastrointestinal risk level | | |
|---|---|---|
| Low | Moderate | High |
| NSAID alone (the least ulcerogenic NSAID at the lowest effective dose) | NSAID + PPI/misoprostol | Alternative therapy if possible or COX-2 inhibitor+PPI/misoprostol |

Table 3. Treatment recommendations (Guidelines for the Prevention of NSAID-related Ulcer Complications) (Lanza et al., 2009)

*H. pylori* should be treated with the appropriate therapy, even if it is believed that the prior ulcer was due to *NSAIDs*. In asymptomatic patients who have no history of ulcers and who are not currently taking a *NSAID*, physicians can consider *H. pylori* testing prior to beginning long-term therapy with a *NSAID*. One review of this topic found that eradication of *H. pylori* was beneficial in patients who were naïve to *NSAIDs*, while little benefit was observed in patients already taking and tolerating *NSAIDs* (Kiltz et al., 2008). This "test-and-treat" approach may be more useful in populations with a relatively high prevalence of *H. pylori* infection.

### 8.2 Misoprostol

Misoprostol is a synthetic prostaglandin $E_1$ analog that replaces the protective prostaglandins ingested during prostaglandin-inhibiting therapies. It was the first agent approved for the prevention of *NSAID*-related ulceration. Early studies in normal volunteers showed a marked reduction in the primary prevention of gastroduodenal lesion in patients receiving *NSAIDs* in combination with misoprostol, compared with those who received *NSAIDs* and a placebo (Lanza et al., 1989). A more recent meta-analysis revealed that co-therapy with misoprostol reduced the incidence of duodenal ulcers by 53% and gastric ulcers by 74%, when compared with placebo therapy (Rostom et al., 2002). Another study that compared a standard dose of misoprostol (200 mcg q.i.d.) with the PPI lansoprazole (in doses of 15 and 30 mg daily) in long-term *NSAID* users showed that 93% of patients taking misoprostol were protected from developing a gastric ulcer compared with 80% and 82% in the two lansoprazole groups, respectively, over 12 weeks, and without any statistical significance among treated groups. Patients who were ulcer free after 12 weeks of therapy were kept on the same regimen for another 12 weeks, and at the end of that time 43% of those on placebo, 83% on misoprostol, 83% on lansoprazole 30 mg, and 89% on lansoprazole 15 mg were still ulcer free (Graham et al., 2002) .

Although misoprostol has proven to be effective in the prevention of GI complications induced by *NSAIDs*, it should be noted that its usefulness is limited in clinical settings by the occurrence of GI side effects, primarily cramping and diarrhea, and by compliance problems related to multiple dosage.

### 8.3 Proton pump inhibitors (PPIs)

PPIs have been utilized extensively as a co-therapy for the prevention of *NSAID*-induced peptic ulcers. Two large randomized controlled trials (Hawkey et al., 1998; Yeomans et al., 1998) have been performed in osteoarthritis and rheumatoid arthritis patients comparing omeprazole with placebo therapy, misoprostol, and ranitidine in the secondary prevention and healing of gastric and duodenal ulcers. In the first study, omeprazole (20 mg or 40 mg daily) co-therapy resulted in a significant reduction in the total number of NSAID-related ulcers when compared to ranitidine (150 mg orally twice a day). In the second study, omeprazol (20 mg daily) was more effective than misoprostol (800 mg daily) in preventing duodenal ulcers and in reducing gastric ulcers.

The results of two similar multicenter randomized controlled trials have recently been published jointly (Scheiman et al., 2006). They compared esomeprazole 20 or 40 mg/daily with placebo therapy in preventing ulcers in patients taking NSAIDs or COX-2 inhibitors over a 6-month period. In the first study, which involved 844 patients, ulcer rates were 20.4%, 5.3%, and 4.7% for placebo, esomeprazole 20 mg, and esomeprazole 40 mg, respectively. In the second study, which involved 585 patients, the respective ulcer rates were 12.3%, 5.2%, and 4.4 %. Patients in both studies were H. pylori-negative and were considered at-risk on the basis of age (above 60), or due to a history of documented gastric or duodenal ulcerations within 5 years of entry into the study. Both studies concluded that in at-risk patients, esomeprazole was effective at preventing ulcers in long-term users of NSAIDs, including COX-2 inhibitors.

Thus, although full-dose misoprostol (200 mcg q.i.d.) is very effective in preventing NSAID-related ulcers and their complications, as stated above, GI side effects limit its clinical use. Lower doses of misoprostol are not associated with cramps or diarrhea, but appear to be no more effective than standard PPI therapy. For all of these reasons, PPIs have assumed a dominant role in NSAID-related upper GI injury prophylaxis and therapy. A randomized trial of NSAID users who had H. pylori infection and prior ulcer bleeding (Chan et al., 2001) demonstrated that co-therapy with omeprazole was effective at preventing recurrent ulcer bleeding. Data from observational studies and secondary analyses of a large-scale randomized trial also indicate that PPIs reduce the risk of NSAID-associated ulcer bleeding. Maintenance therapy is indicated in patients who remain on or who resume NSAID treatment.

There is no data suggesting that any of the available PPIs is more effective than another in treating NSAID-related GI damage.

### 8.4 H2 receptor antagonists

In most reports, standard doses of H2 receptor antagonists have shown no effectiveness in preventing NSAID-induced gastric ulcers. Systematic reviews have shown that double-dose (e.g., famotidine 40 mg two times daily) but not single-dose H2 receptor antagonists are effective at reducing the risk of NSAID-induced endoscopic gastric ulcers (Leontiadis et al., 2007; Rostom et al., 2002). In patients taking low-dose aspirin, famotidine 20 mg twice daily can reduce the development of oesophagitis, gastric and duodenal ulcers by 80% in an average-risk population, when compared with placebo therapy (Taha et al., 2009). In contrast, a separate study from Hong Kong showed that high-dose famotidine (40 mg twice daily) was inferior to pantoprazole (20mg daily) in the prevention of gastroduodenal ulcers in patients at high risk of aspirin-related ulcers. Recurrent symptomatic or bleeding ulcers (20% versus 0%) and gastrointestinal bleeding (7.7% versus 0%) were more common in patients on famotidine than in those on pantoprazole (Ng et al., 2010). However, economic modeling suggests that co-therapy with H2 receptor antagonists may be a cost-effective strategy for the prevention of ulcer bleeding in NSAID users (Brown et al., 2006). Like PPIs, there have not been any randomized, clinical outcome trials that evaluate the efficacy of H2 receptor antagonists in chronic NSAID users.

## 9. Conclusions

In high-risk patients, gastrointestinal complications associated with the use of NSAIDs are often caused by the concomitant use of aspirin or multiple NSAIDs, a failure to properly identify a patient's risk factors, and the underutilization of gastroprotective agents. The latter includes the use of PPIs in patients at high risk of gastrointestinal bleeding and the eradication of *H. pylori* in patients with a prior history of ulcers. PPIs have been shown to significantly reduce both gastric and duodenal ulcers and their attendant complications in patients taking not only NSAIDs, but also COX-2 inhibitors. Misoprostol, when given at full doses (800 mg/day) is very effective in preventing ulcers, and ulcer complications, in patients taking NSAIDs. However, its usefulness is limited in clinical practice due to its GI side effects. COX-2 inhibitors are associated with a significantly lower incidence of gastric and duodenal ulcers when compared to traditional NSAIDs. However, these beneficial effects are abrogated when the patient is concomitantly taking low-dose aspirin.

## 10. References

Abramson, S. B. & Weissmann, G., (1989). The mechanisms of action of nonsteroidal antiinflammatory drugs. *Arthritis Rheum*, Vol. 32, No. 1, (Jan), pp. 1-9, ISBN 0004-3591

Agrawal, N. M., Campbell, D. R., Safdi, M. A., Lukasik, N. L., Huang, B. & Haber, M. M., (2000). Superiority of lansoprazole vs ranitidine in healing nonsteroidal anti-inflammatory drug-associated gastric ulcers: results of a double-blind, randomized, multicenter study. NSAID-Associated Gastric Ulcer Study Group. *Arch Intern Med*, Vol. 160, No. 10, (May 22), pp. 1455-61, ISBN 0003-9926

Allison, M. C., Howatson, A. G., Torrance, C. J., Lee, F. D. & Russell, R. I., (1992). Gastrointestinal damage associated with the use of nonsteroidal antiinflammatory drugs. *N Engl J Med*, Vol. 327, No. 11, (Sep 10), pp. 749-54, ISBN 0028-4793

Amin, A. R., Vyas, P., Attur, M., Leszczynska-Piziak, J., Patel, I. R., Weissmann, G. & Abramson, S. B., (1995). The mode of action of aspirin-like drugs: effect on inducible nitric oxide synthase. *Proc Natl Acad Sci U S A*, Vol. 92, No. 17, (Aug 15), pp. 7926-30, ISBN 0027-8424

Bazzoli, F., De Luca, L. & Graham, D. Y., (2001). Helicobacter pylori infection and the use of NSAIDs. *Best Pract Res Clin Gastroenterol*, Vol. 15, No. 5, (Oct), pp. 775-85, ISBN 1521-6918

Berger, J. S., Brown, D. L. & Becker, R. C., (2008). Low-dose aspirin in patients with stable cardiovascular disease: a meta-analysis. *Am J Med*, Vol. 121, No. 1, (Jan), pp. 43-9, ISBN 1555-7162

Bianchi Porro, G., Lazzaroni, M., Manzionna, G. & Petrillo, M., (1998). Omeprazole and sucralfate in the treatment of NSAID-induced gastric and duodenal ulcer. *Aliment Pharmacol Ther*, Vol. 12, No. 4, (Apr), pp. 355-60, ISBN 0269-2813

Bombardier, C., Laine, L., Reicin, A., Shapiro, D., Burgos-Vargas, R., Davis, B., Day, R., Ferraz, M. B., Hawkey, C. J., Hochberg, M. C., Kvien, T. K. & Schnitzer, T. J., (2000). Comparison of upper gastrointestinal toxicity of rofecoxib and naproxen in patients with rheumatoid arthritis. VIGOR Study Group. *N Engl J Med*, Vol. 343, No. 21, (Nov 23), pp. 1520-8, ISBN 0028-4793

Brooks, P. M. & Day, R. O., (1991). Nonsteroidal antiinflammatory drugs--differences and similarities. *N Engl J Med*, Vol. 324, No. 24, (Jun 13), pp. 1716-25, ISBN 0028-4793

Brown, T. J., Hooper, L., Elliott, R. A., Payne, K., Webb, R., Roberts, C., Rostom, A. &
    Symmons, D., (2006). A comparison of the cost-effectiveness of five strategies for the
    prevention of non-steroidal anti-inflammatory drug-induced gastrointestinal toxicity:
    a systematic review with economic modelling. *Health Technol Assess*, Vol. 10, No. 38,
    (Oct), pp. 1-183, ISBN 1366-5278
Catella-Lawson, F., Reilly, M. P., Kapoor, S. C., Cucchiara, A. J., DeMarco, S., Tournier, B.,
    Vyas, S. N. & FitzGerald, G. A., (2001). Cyclooxygenase inhibitors and the antiplatelet
    effects of aspirin. *N Engl J Med*, Vol. 345, No. 25, (Dec 20), pp. 1809-17, ISBN 0028-4793
Cryer, B. & Feldman, M., (1992). Effects of nonsteroidal anti-inflammatory drugs on
    endogenous gastrointestinal prostaglandins and therapeutic strategies for prevention
    and treatment of nonsteroidal anti-inflammatory drug-induced damage. *Arch Intern
    Med*, Vol. 152, No. 6, (Jun), pp. 1145-55, ISBN 0003-9926
Chan, F. K., Chung, S. C., Suen, B. Y., Lee, Y. T., Leung, W. K., Leung, V. K., Wu, J. C., Lau, J.
    Y., Hui, Y., Lai, M. S., Chan, H. L. & Sung, J. J., (2001). Preventing recurrent upper
    gastrointestinal bleeding in patients with Helicobacter pylori infection who are taking
    low-dose aspirin or naproxen. *N Engl J Med*, Vol. 344, No. 13, (Mar 29), pp. 967-73,
    ISBN 0028-4793
Chan, H. L., Wu, J. C., Chan, F. K., Choi, C. L., Ching, J. Y., Lee, Y. T., Leung, W. K., Lau, J. Y.,
    Chung, S. C. & Sung, J. J., (2001). Is non-Helicobacter pylori, non-NSAID peptic ulcer
    a common cause of upper GI bleeding? A prospective study of 977 patients.
    *Gastrointest Endosc*, Vol. 53, No. 4, (Apr), pp. 438-42, ISBN 0016-5107
Chow, D. K. & Sung, J. J., (2007). Is the prevalence of idiopathic ulcers really on the increase?
    *Nat Clin Pract Gastroenterol Hepatol*, Vol. 4, No. 4, (Apr), pp. 176-7, ISBN 1743-4386
de Abajo, F. J. & Garcia Rodriguez, L. A., (2001). Risk of upper gastrointestinal bleeding and
    perforation associated with low-dose aspirin as plain and enteric-coated
    formulations. *BMC Clin Pharmacol*, Vol. 1, No. pp. 1, ISBN 1472-6904
Diaz-Gonzalez, F., Gonzalez-Alvaro, I., Campanero, M. R., Mollinedo, F., del Pozo, M. A.,
    Munoz, C., Pivel, J. P. & Sanchez-Madrid, F., (1995). Prevention of in vitro neutrophil-
    endothelial attachment through shedding of L-selectin by nonsteroidal
    antiinflammatory drugs. *J Clin Invest*, Vol. 95, No. 4, (Apr), pp. 1756-65, ISBN 0021-
    9738
Douthwaite, A. H. & Lintott , G. A. M., (1938). Gastroscopic observation of the effect of aspirin
    and certain other substances on the stomach. *Lancet*, Vol. 2, No. pp. 1222-5,
Garcia Rodriguez, L. A. & Hernandez-Diaz, S., (2001). Relative risk of upper gastrointestinal
    complications among users of acetaminophen and nonsteroidal anti-inflammatory
    drugs. *Epidemiology*, Vol. 12, No. 5, (Sep), pp. 570-6, ISBN 1044-3983
Gisbert, J. P. & Calvet, X., (2009). Review article: Helicobacter pylori-negative duodenal ulcer
    disease. *Aliment Pharmacol Ther*, Vol. 30, No. 8, (Oct 15), pp. 791-815, ISBN 1365-2036
Graham, D. Y., Agrawal, N. M., Campbell, D. R., Haber, M. M., Collis, C., Lukasik, N. L. &
    Huang, B., (2002). Ulcer prevention in long-term users of nonsteroidal anti-
    inflammatory drugs: results of a double-blind, randomized, multicenter, active- and
    placebo-controlled study of misoprostol vs lansoprazole. *Arch Intern Med*, Vol. 162,
    No. 2, (Jan 28), pp. 169-75, ISBN 0003-9926
Graham, D. Y., Lew, G. M., Klein, P. D., Evans, D. G., Evans, D. J., Jr., Saeed, Z. A. & Malaty, H.
    M., (1992). Effect of treatment of Helicobacter pylori infection on the long-term

recurrence of gastric or duodenal ulcer. A randomized, controlled study. *Ann Intern Med*, Vol. 116, No. 9, (May 1), pp. 705-8, ISBN 0003-4819

Griffin, M. R., Piper, J. M., Daugherty, J. R., Snowden, M. & Ray, W. A., (1991). Nonsteroidal anti-inflammatory drug use and increased risk for peptic ulcer disease in elderly persons. *Ann Intern Med*, Vol. 114, No. 4, (Feb 15), pp. 257-63, ISBN 0003-4819

Griffin, M. R., Ray, W. A. & Schaffner, W., (1988). Nonsteroidal anti-inflammatory drug use and death from peptic ulcer in elderly persons. *Ann Intern Med*, Vol. 109, No. 5, (Sep 1), pp. 359-63, ISBN 0003-4819

Hawkey, C. J., (1995). Future treatments for arthritis: new NSAIDs, NO NSAIDs, or no NSAIDs? *Gastroenterology*, Vol. 109, No. 2, (Aug), pp. 614-6, ISBN 0016-5085

Hawkey, C. J., Karrasch, J. A., Szczepanski, L., Walker, D. G., Barkun, A., Swannell, A. J. & Yeomans, N. D., (1998). Omeprazole compared with misoprostol for ulcers associated with nonsteroidal antiinflammatory drugs. Omeprazole versus Misoprostol for NSAID-induced Ulcer Management (OMNIUM) Study Group. *N Engl J Med*, Vol. 338, No. 11, (Mar 12), pp. 727-34, ISBN 0028-4793

Hernandez-Diaz, S. & Rodriguez, L. A., (2000). Association between nonsteroidal anti-inflammatory drugs and upper gastrointestinal tract bleeding/perforation: an overview of epidemiologic studies published in the 1990s. *Arch Intern Med*, Vol. 160, No. 14, (Jul 24), pp. 2093-9, ISBN 0003-9926

Huang, J. Q., Sridhar, S. & Hunt, R. H., (2002). Role of Helicobacter pylori infection and non-steroidal anti-inflammatory drugs in peptic-ulcer disease: a meta-analysis. *Lancet*, Vol. 359, No. 9300, (Jan 5), pp. 14-22, ISBN 0140-6736

Hung, L. C., Ching, J. Y., Sung, J. J., To, K. F., Hui, A. J., Wong, V. W., Leong, R. W., Chan, H. L., Wu, J. C., Leung, W. K., Lee, Y. T., Chung, S. C. & Chan, F. K., (2005). Long-term outcome of Helicobacter pylori-negative idiopathic bleeding ulcers: a prospective cohort study. *Gastroenterology*, Vol. 128, No. 7, (Jun), pp. 1845-50, ISBN 0016-5085

Jones, R., (2001). Nonsteroidal anti-inflammatory drug prescribing: past, present, and future. *Am J Med*, Vol. 110, No. 1A, (Jan 8), pp. 4S-7S, ISBN 0002-9343

Kiltz, U., Zochling, J., Schmidt, W. E. & Braun, J., (2008). Use of NSAIDs and infection with Helicobacter pylori--what does the rheumatologist need to know? *Rheumatology (Oxford)*, Vol. 47, No. 9, (Sep), pp. 1342-7, ISBN 1462-0332

Kopp, E. & Ghosh, S., (1994). Inhibition of NF-kappa B by sodium salicylate and aspirin. *Science*, Vol. 265, No. 5174, (Aug 12), pp. 956-9, ISBN 0036-8075

Krause, M. M., Brand, M. D., Krauss, S., Meisel, C., Vergin, H., Burmester, G. R. & Buttgereit, F., (2003). Nonsteroidal antiinflammatory drugs and a selective cyclooxygenase 2 inhibitor uncouple mitochondria in intact cells. *Arthritis Rheum*, Vol. 48, No. 5, (May), pp. 1438-44, ISBN 0004-3591

Laine, L., (1996). Nonsteroidal anti-inflammatory drug gastropathy. *Gastrointest Endosc Clin N Am*, Vol. 6, No. 3, (Jul), pp. 489-504, ISBN 1052-5157

Laine, L., (2001). Approaches to nonsteroidal anti-inflammatory drug use in the high-risk patient. *Gastroenterology*, Vol. 120, No. 3, (Feb), pp. 594-606, ISBN 0016-5085

Laine, L., (2002). The gastrointestinal effects of nonselective NSAIDs and COX-2-selective inhibitors. *Semin Arthritis Rheum*, Vol. 32, No. 3 Suppl 1, (Dec), pp. 25-32, ISBN 0049-0172

Laine, L., Curtis, S. P., Cryer, B., Kaur, A. & Cannon, C. P., (2007). Assessment of upper gastrointestinal safety of etoricoxib and diclofenac in patients with osteoarthritis and rheumatoid arthritis in the Multinational Etoricoxib and Diclofenac Arthritis Long-term (MEDAL) programme: a randomised comparison. *Lancet*, Vol. 369, No. 9560, (Feb 10), pp. 465-73, ISBN 0140-6736

Lanas, A., Perez-Aisa, M. A., Feu, F., Ponce, J., Saperas, E., Santolaria, S., Rodrigo, L., Balanzo, J., Bajador, E., Almela, P., Navarro, J. M., Carballo, F., Castro, M. & Quintero, E., (2005). A nationwide study of mortality associated with hospital admission due to severe gastrointestinal events and those associated with nonsteroidal antiinflammatory drug use. *Am J Gastroenterol*, Vol. 100, No. 8, (Aug), pp. 1685-93, ISBN 0002-9270

Lanza, F. L., Chan, F. K. & Quigley, E. M., (2009). Guidelines for prevention of NSAID-related ulcer complications. *Am J Gastroenterol*, Vol. 104, No. 3, (Mar), pp. 728-38, ISBN 1572-0241

Lanza, F. L., Fakouhi, D., Rubin, A., Davis, R. E., Rack, M. F., Nissen, C. & Geis, S., (1989). A double-blind placebo-controlled comparison of the efficacy and safety of 50, 100, and 200 micrograms of misoprostol QID in the prevention of ibuprofen-induced gastric and duodenal mucosal lesions and symptoms. *Am J Gastroenterol*, Vol. 84, No. 6, (Jun), pp. 633-6, ISBN 0002-9270

Larkai, E. N., Smith, J. L., Lidsky, M. D. & Graham, D. Y., (1987). Gastroduodenal mucosa and dyspeptic symptoms in arthritic patients during chronic nonsteroidal anti-inflammatory drug use. *Am J Gastroenterol*, Vol. 82, No. 11, (Nov), pp. 1153-8, ISBN 0002-9270

Leontiadis, G. I., Sreedharan, A., Dorward, S., Barton, P., Delaney, B., Howden, C. W., Orhewere, M., Gisbert, J., Sharma, V. K., Rostom, A., Moayyedi, P. & Forman, D., (2007). Systematic reviews of the clinical effectiveness and cost-effectiveness of proton pump inhibitors in acute upper gastrointestinal bleeding. *Health Technol Assess*, Vol. 11, No. 51, (Dec), pp. 1-164, ISBN 1366-5278

Mahmud, T., Rafi, S. S., Scott, D. L., Wrigglesworth, J. M. & Bjarnason, I., (1996). Nonsteroidal antiinflammatory drugs and uncoupling of mitochondrial oxidative phosphorylation. *Arthritis Rheum*, Vol. 39, No. 12, (Dec), pp. 1998-2003, ISBN 0004-3591

Malfertheiner, P., Megraud, F., O'Morain, C., Hungin, A. P., Jones, R., Axon, A., Graham, D. Y. & Tytgat, G., (2002). Current concepts in the management of Helicobacter pylori infection--the Maastricht 2-2000 Consensus Report. *Aliment Pharmacol Ther*, Vol. 16, No. 2, (Feb), pp. 167-80, ISBN 0269-2813

McQueen, E. G., Facoory, B. & Faed, J. M., (1986). Non-steroidal anti-inflammatory drugs and platelet function. *N Z Med J*, Vol. 99, No. 802, (May 28), pp. 358-60, ISBN 0028-8446

Mingatto, F. E., Santos, A. C., Uyemura, S. A., Jordani, M. C. & Curti, C., (1996). In vitro interaction of nonsteroidal anti-inflammatory drugs on oxidative phosphorylation of rat kidney mitochondria: respiration and ATP synthesis. *Arch Biochem Biophys*, Vol. 334, No. 2, (Oct 15), pp. 303-8, ISBN 0003-9861

Moncada, S., Ferreira, S. H. & Vane, J. R., (1973). Prostaglandins, aspirin-like drugs and the oedema of inflammation. *Nature*, Vol. 246, No. 5430, (Nov 23), pp. 217-9, ISBN 0028-0836

Ng, F. H., Wong, S. Y., Lam, K. F., Chu, W. M., Chan, P., Ling, Y. H., Kng, C., Yuen, W. C., Lau, Y. K., Kwan, A. & Wong, B. C., (2010). Famotidine is inferior to pantoprazole in preventing recurrence of aspirin-related peptic ulcers or erosions. *Gastroenterology*, Vol. 138, No. 1, (Jan), pp. 82-8, ISBN 1528-0012

O'Brien, J. R., (1968). Effect of anti-inflammatory agents on platelets. *Lancet*, Vol. 1, No. 7548, (Apr 27), pp. 894-5, ISBN 0140-6736

Ortiz, M. I., Granados-Soto, V. & Castaneda-Hernandez, G., (2003). The NO-cGMP-K+ channel pathway participates in the antinociceptive effect of diclofenac, but not of indomethacin. *Pharmacol Biochem Behav*, Vol. 76, No. 1, (Aug), pp. 187-95, ISBN 0091-3057

Patrono, C., Garcia Rodriguez, L. A., Landolfi, R. & Baigent, C., (2005). Low-dose aspirin for the prevention of atherothrombosis. *N Engl J Med*, Vol. 353, No. 22, (Dec 1), pp. 2373-83, ISBN 1533-4406

Piper, J. M., Ray, W. A., Daugherty, J. R. & Griffin, M. R., (1991). Corticosteroid use and peptic ulcer disease: role of nonsteroidal anti-inflammatory drugs. *Ann Intern Med*, Vol. 114, No. 9, (May 1), pp. 735-40, ISBN 0003-4819

Rainsford, K. D., (1980). Aspirin, Prostaglandins and mucopolysaccharide/glycoprotein secretion. *Agents Actions*, Vol. 10, No. 6, (Dec), pp. 520-1, ISBN 0065-4299

Ramakrishnan, K. & Salinas, R. C., (2007). Peptic ulcer disease. *Am Fam Physician*, Vol. 76, No. 7, (Oct 1), pp. 1005-12, ISBN 0002-838X

Robert, A., Nezamis, J. E., Lancaster, C. & Hanchar, A. J., (1979). Cytoprotection by prostaglandins in rats. Prevention of gastric necrosis produced by alcohol, HCl, NaOH, hypertonic NaCl, and thermal injury. *Gastroenterology*, Vol. 77, No. 3, (Sep), pp. 433-43, ISBN 0016-5085

Rostom, A., Dube, C., Wells, G., Tugwell, P., Welch, V., Jolicoeur, E. & McGowan, J., (2002). Prevention of NSAID-induced gastroduodenal ulcers. *Cochrane Database Syst Rev*, No. 4, pp. CD002296, ISBN 1469-493X

Rostom, A., Muir, K., Dube, C., Jolicoeur, E., Boucher, M., Joyce, J., Tugwell, P. & Wells, G. W., (2007). Gastrointestinal safety of cyclooxygenase-2 inhibitors: a Cochrane Collaboration systematic review. *Clin Gastroenterol Hepatol*, Vol. 5, No. 7, (Jul), pp. 818-28, ISBN 1542-7714

Scheiman, J. M., Yeomans, N. D., Talley, N. J., Vakil, N., Chan, F. K., Tulassay, Z., Rainoldi, J. L., Szczepanski, L., Ung, K. A., Kleczkowski, D., Ahlbom, H., Naesdal, J. & Hawkey, C., (2006). Prevention of ulcers by esomeprazole in at-risk patients using non-selective NSAIDs and COX-2 inhibitors. *Am J Gastroenterol*, Vol. 101, No. 4, (Apr), pp. 701-10, ISBN 0002-9270

Schnitzer, T. J., Burmester, G. R., Mysler, E., Hochberg, M. C., Doherty, M., Ehrsam, E., Gitton, X., Krammer, G., Mellein, B., Matchaba, P., Gimona, A. & Hawkey, C. J., (2004). Comparison of lumiracoxib with naproxen and ibuprofen in the Therapeutic Arthritis Research and Gastrointestinal Event Trial (TARGET), reduction in ulcer complications: randomised controlled trial. *Lancet*, Vol. 364, No. 9435, (Aug 21-27), pp. 665-74, ISBN 1474-547X

Shorr, R. I., Ray, W. A., Daugherty, J. R. & Griffin, M. R., (1993). Concurrent use of nonsteroidal anti-inflammatory drugs and oral anticoagulants places elderly persons at high risk for hemorrhagic peptic ulcer disease. *Arch Intern Med*, Vol. 153, No. 14, (Jul 26), pp. 1665-70, ISBN 0003-9926

Silverstein, F. E., Faich, G., Goldstein, J. L., Simon, L. S., Pincus, T., Whelton, A., Makuch, R., Eisen, G., Agrawal, N. M., Stenson, W. F., Burr, A. M., Zhao, W. W., Kent, J. D., Lefkowith, J. B., Verburg, K. M. & Geis, G. S., (2000). Gastrointestinal toxicity with celecoxib vs nonsteroidal anti-inflammatory drugs for osteoarthritis and rheumatoid

arthritis: the CLASS study: A randomized controlled trial. Celecoxib Long-term
    Arthritis Safety Study. *Jama*, Vol. 284, No. 10, (Sep 13), pp. 1247-55, ISBN 0098-7484
Simon, L. S. & Mills, J. A., (1980). Nonsteroidal antiinflammatory drugs (second of two parts).
    *N Engl J Med*, Vol. 302, No. 22, (May 29), pp. 1237-43, ISBN 0028-4793
Singh, G. & Triadafilopoulos, G., (1999). Epidemiology of NSAID induced gastrointestinal
    complications. *J Rheumatol Suppl*, Vol. 56, No. (Apr), pp. 18-24, ISBN 0380-0903
Soll, A. H., Weinstein, W. M., Kurata, J. & McCarthy, D., (1991). Nonsteroidal anti-
    inflammatory drugs and peptic ulcer disease. *Ann Intern Med*, Vol. 114, No. 4, (Feb
    15), pp. 307-19, ISBN 0003-4819
Sung, J. J., Kuipers, E. J. & El-Serag, H. B., (2009). Systematic review: the global incidence and
    prevalence of peptic ulcer disease. *Aliment Pharmacol Ther*, Vol. 29, No. 9, (May 1), pp.
    938-46, ISBN 1365-2036
Taha, A. S., McCloskey, C., Prasad, R. & Bezlyak, V., (2009). Famotidine for the prevention of
    peptic ulcers and oesophagitis in patients taking low-dose aspirin (FAMOUS): a
    phase III, randomised, double-blind, placebo-controlled trial. *Lancet*, Vol. 374, No.
    9684, (Jul 11), pp. 119-25, ISBN 1474-547X
Talley, N. J., Evans, J. M., Fleming, K. C., Harmsen, W. S., Zinsmeister, A. R. & Melton, L. J.,
    3rd, (1995). Nonsteroidal antiinflammatory drugs and dyspepsia in the elderly. *Dig
    Dis Sci*, Vol. 40, No. 6, (Jun), pp. 1345-50, ISBN 0163-2116
van Oijen, M. G., Dieleman, J. P., Laheij, R. J., Sturkenboom, M. C., Jansen, J. B. & Verheugt, F.
    W., (2008). Peptic ulcerations are related to systemic rather than local effects of low-
    dose aspirin. *Clin Gastroenterol Hepatol*, Vol. 6, No. 3, (Mar), pp. 309-13, ISBN 1542-
    7714
Vergara, M., Catalan, M., Gisbert, J. P. & Calvet, X., (2005). Meta-analysis: role of Helicobacter
    pylori eradication in the prevention of peptic ulcer in NSAID users. *Aliment Pharmacol
    Ther*, Vol. 21, No. 12, (Jun 15), pp. 1411-8, ISBN 0269-2813
Wallace, J. L., (1997). Nonsteroidal anti-inflammatory drugs and gastroenteropathy: the second
    hundred years. *Gastroenterology*, Vol. 112, No. 3, (Mar), pp. 1000-16, ISBN 0016-5085
Warner, T. D., Giuliano, F., Vojnovic, I., Bukasa, A., Mitchell, J. A. & Vane, J. R., (1999).
    Nonsteroid drug selectivities for cyclo-oxygenase-1 rather than cyclo-oxygenase-2 are
    associated with human gastrointestinal toxicity: a full in vitro analysis. *Proc Natl Acad
    Sci U S A*, Vol. 96, No. 13, (Jun 22), pp. 7563-8, ISBN 0027-8424
Wolfe, M. M., (1996). NSAIDs and the gastrointestinal mucosa. *Hosp Pract (Minneap)*, Vol. 31,
    No. 12, (Dec 15), pp. 37-44, 47-8, ISBN 2154-8331
Yeomans, N. D., Tulassay, Z., Juhasz, L., Racz, I., Howard, J. M., van Rensburg, C. J., Swannell,
    A. J. & Hawkey, C. J., (1998). A comparison of omeprazole with ranitidine for ulcers
    associated with nonsteroidal antiinflammatory drugs. Acid Suppression Trial:
    Ranitidine versus Omeprazole for NSAID-associated Ulcer Treatment
    (ASTRONAUT) Study Group. *N Engl J Med*, Vol. 338, No. 11, (Mar 12), pp. 719-26,
    ISBN 0028-4793
Yuan, Y., Padol, I. T. & Hunt, R. H., (2006). Peptic ulcer disease today. *Nat Clin Pract
    Gastroenterol Hepatol*, Vol. 3, No. 2, (Feb), pp. 80-9, ISBN 1743-4378
Zhou, Y., Dial, E. J., Doyen, R. & Lichtenberger, L. M., Effect of indomethacin on bile acid-
    phospholipid interactions: implication for small intestinal injury induced by
    nonsteroidal anti-inflammatory drugs. *Am J Physiol Gastrointest Liver Physiol*, Vol. 298,
    No. 5, (May), pp. 722-31, ISBN 1522-1547

# 4

# Effects of *Helicobacter pylori* and Non-Steroidal Anti-Inflammatory Drugs on Peptic Ulcer

Wang G.Z.[1,2] and Wang J.F.[1]
*[1]College of Life Science, Zhejiang University*
*[2]Institute of Medicine, Qiqihaer Medical College*
*P. R. China*

## 1. Introduction

Peptic ulcer (PU) was a local gastrointestinal lesion due to gastric fluid, gastric acid and pepsin insult. The lesion may involve in mucosal layer, submucosal or even muscle and plasma layer in duodenum and stomach. It was characterized as not only easy to relapse but also hard to prevent (Wang *et al.*, 1998). Its etiology and mechanism was very sophisticated due to the imbalance between offensive factors (gastric acid, pepsin, *H. pylori* and NSAIDs) and defensive factors (gastric mucus, bicarbonates and blood flow of gastric mucosa) ( Hoogerwerf & Pasricha, 2006). There were at least 3 defensive barriers in the gastric wall to resist gastric acid and pepsin: the mucus-bicarbonates barrier that includes mucus and the bicarbonates grade in the mucus, the mucosa barrier that is the tight conjunction structure among gastric epithelial cells, and the blood flow in mucosa that provides oxygen and nutrition to mucosa and support the turnover of gastric epithelium and mucus. *H. pylori* and NSAIDs were gastric mucosa's offensive factors (Tytgat, 2000). Although they cause peptic ulcer by destroying the gastric barrier function, the mechanism was not clear. There were arguments for their simultaneous effects on peptic ulcer (Fendrick *et al.*, 2001). Therefore, it is important to clarify the relationship between *H. pylori* and NSAIDs, especially when both cause simultaneously the damage to gastric mucosa.

## 2. *H. pylori* and peptic ulcer

*H. pylori* results in peptic ulcer through damaging gastric mucus and mucosa barriers, and enhancing gastric acid secretion.

### 2.1 Damages of gastric mucus and mucosa barriers

When *H. pylori* infects the stomach, it can produce cytotoxin-associated gene A protein (CagA), vacuolating cytotoxin A (VacA), urease, mucus enzyme, lipase and phospholipase to injure the gastric mucus and mucosa barriers, and finally results in the peptic ulcer with the combination of gastric acid and pepsin.

Vacuolating cytotoxin and cytotoxin-associated protein: VacA is expressed in *H. pylori* and results in vacuolar degeneration in gastric epithelium through interfering ion transport protein, eg. vacuolar ATPase (Leunk *et al.*, 1988). CagA is up-regulated in VacA+ strain and related to VacA activity. 60~70% of *H. pylori* strains express CagA and thereby induce host cells to produce cytokines, enhance inflammatory reaction and damage the gastric mucosa (Ghira *et al.*, 1995). CagA is immunogenic and induces gastric epithelial cell to produce interleukine-8 (IL-8) that causes strong immunoreactions and results in gastric mucosa injury (Ernst *et al.*, 1994).

Urease: *H. pylori* can produce urease. This enzyme locates on the *H. pylori's* surface and introcytoplasma (Phadnis *et al.*, 1996; Bode *et al.*, 1989) and hydrolyses urea into ammonia. Ammonia can decrease the content of mucin in mucus and destroy the integrity of the ion in mucus, and finally decline the function of mucus barrier that results in the diffusion of hydrogen ion back to the stomach wall and the erosion of mucosa layer (Hazell *et al.*, 1986). Ammonia can also deprive alpha-ketoglutaric acid that is a middle metabolic substance in Kreb's cycle, and thus, this cycle is blocked and the metabolism of cells is interfered, and finally the ATP production decreases and the $Na^+$-$K^+$ pump on the cellular membrane is out of order. It may result in cellular edema, degeneration and necrosis, and the barriers of mucus and mucosa are finally destroyed and the ulcer is formed (Marshall, 1994). The hydroxy created from ammonia and water has cytotoxic effect on gastric mucosa. A high concentration of ammonia can cause cellular vacuolar degeneration (Xu *et al.*, 1990). Urease can also cause directly the tissue damage of host (Windsor *et al.*, 2000). *H. pylori* can stimulate neutrophils and cause oxidative burst, and thereby result in the production of $H_2O_2$ and oxygenate oxy-chloride ion. This ion can further combine ammonia and form more toxic monochloramine that participates in the process of mucosa injury (Sarosiek *et al.*, 1989). The urea may serve as leukocyte chemotactic factor to attract inflammatory cells, cause local inflammation in the stomach, and damage indirectly the gastric epithelium.

Mucus enzyme and pepsin: *H. pylori* can produce mucolytic enzyme that causes the gastric mucous degradation. The degraded mucus losses its viscosity and elasticity and thus, allows the diffusion of hydrogen ion back to the stomach wall and the erosion of mucosa layer. The decreased viscosity of mucus benefits the movement of *H. pylori* and makes *H. pylori* easier to plant on the stomach wall. The decomposed mucus can also provide nutrition necessary to *H. pylori* (Beales *et al.*, 1996). *H. pylori* can also generate an extracellular protease that was able to split the polymer of glycoprotein in gastric mucus and wipe out the gastric mucous barrier so as to allow the gastric epithelium to contact directly with attack factors such as gastric acid, pepsin, cholic acid and drugs. Finally, the gastric epithelial erosion appears (Kawano *et al.*, 1990).

Lipase and phospholipase: the normal cell membrane is composed of double phospholipid layers. *H. pylori* can produce phospholipase A that hydrolyzes palmityl lecithin into free palmitic acid and lysolecithin and thereby destroy the integrity of the cellular membrane (Goggin *et al.*, 1991). The lipid and phospholipid in the gastric mucus play an important role in the maintenance of mucous viscosity and hydrophobic characters and in the prevention of hydrogen ion from diffusion back to the stomach wall (Goggin *et al.*, 1991). The lipase and phospholipase A can hydrolyze lipid and phospholipid in the mucus and thus obliterate the function of mucous barrier. Phospholipase A can also enhance the release of arachidonic acid and generate inflammatory media such as prostaglandin and thromboxane that induce inflammatory reaction. The metabolism of phospholipid, such as lysolecithin, also has cytotoxic effect (Lewis *et al.*, 1990).

Alcoholic dehydrogenase: Alcoholic dehydrogenase generated by *H. pylori* can oxygenate alcohol into acetaldehyde that is a strong oxidizer and causes the injury of mucosa.

Lipopolysaccharide (LPS): LPS produced by *H. pylori* can stimulate gastric epithelial cell to secrets IL-8 that can induce local inflammatory reaction in infected stomach. LPS also stimulates the pepsinogen secretion in gastric epithelium. Pepsin hydrolyses the protein in gastric epithelium, originates epithelial injury and causes ulceration (Young *et al.*, 1992). LPS from *H. pylori* has similar antigenic determinants to human being, such as Lewis type 2, e.g. Lewis X and Lewis Y. These similar antigenic determinants also distribute in the surface of parietal cell and gastric gland. The patient with *H. pylori* infection may generate antibody for Lewis antigenic determinants. Therefore, the mucosa barrier will be injured by autoimmune reaction (Appelmelk *et al.*, 1996).

Free radical: When *H. pylori* infects the stomach, it can adhere to gastric epithelium via its surface structure such as N-acetylneuraminic lactose fibril haemogglutinin, extra cellular S adhesin and Lewis B blood-group antigen adhesin, etc (Lundstrom *et al.*, 2001; Domingo *et al.*, 1999; Dundon *et al.*, 2001; McGee *et al.*, 1999) . Neutrophil chemotactic factors such as VacA, CagA and neutrophil activating protein (NAP) are released (Atherton *et al.*, 1997; Naito *et al.*, 2002; Satin *et al.*, 2000; Yoshikawa *et al.*, 2000). Furthermore, *H. pylori* stimulates gastric epithelium to secret interleukin-8 (Shiotani *et al.*, 2002; Bhattacharyya *et al.*, 2002) that is a strong neutrophil chemotactic factor. These white blood chemotactic factors result in the occurrence of inflammation. Neutrophils, monocytes, lymphocytes and macrophage may infiltrate into mucosa and release a big amount of free radicals. Lipids and proteins in epithelium are peroxidized, and the cellular structure and function were damaged, and finally the epithelial barrier was destroyed.

Hemolysin: *H. pylori* can secret hemolysin that has cytotoxic effects, induces inflammatory reaction, and results in the injury of epithelial barrier (Wetherall *et al.*, 1989).

In addition, *H.pylori* inhibits the expression of constitutive nitric oxide (cNOS) and enhances the expression of inducible NOS (iNOS) that may lead to the overproduction of NO and the excessive generation of toxic radical peroxynitrate the is involved in the gastric cell inflammatory response and cellular damage (Brzozowski *et al.*, 2006).

### 2.2 Increases of gastric acid

*H. pylori* causes the release of urease and the formation of ammonia. Ammonia increases the pH on the surface of epithelial. Consequently, the gastrin secretion increases. Gastrinemia stimulates parietal cell to secret gastric acid. Persistent gastrinemia causes the proliferation of parietal cell and the further production of gastric acid. Gastric acid is a strong attack factor and causes ulceration formation (Levi *et al.*, 1989). Other study demonstrated that *H. pylori* inhibit the secretion of somatostatin (SS) in sinus ventriculi D cells. SS inhibits the secretion of gastrin in sinus ventriculi G cells. The reduction of somatostatin weakens the control of gastrin secretion and thus prolongs the postprandial gastric acid secretion and causes ulceration (Kaneko *et al.*, 1992) . *H. pylori* has a growth inhibitory factor that inhibits the turnover of mucous epithelial cells.

### 3. NSAIDs and ulceration

NSAIDs, such as aspirin and indometacin, are effective drugs for anti-inflammation, anti-rheumatics, antipyretics and analgesics. Furthermore, NSAIDs, due to their effect on anti platelet aggregation, are regular prophylaxis drugs for cardiac and brain vascular diseases (Tarnawski *et al.*, 2003). NSAIDs can also decrease the rate of colonial and rectal cancer (Husain *et al.*, 2002) and Alzheimer disease (Tarnawski *et al.*, 2003b). Therefore, NSAIDs are widely used. NSAIDs, however, have a serious side-effect causing gastric mucosa damage.

### 3.1 NSAIDs direct mucosa damage

Most of NSAIDs are weak organic acids as non-ion status under acidic environment in the stomach. NSAIDs can freely pass cellular membrane to intracellular where the environment is neutral. Intracellular NSAIDs can be dissociated into water soluble ion status. The intracellular concentration of NSAIDs is much higher than the extracellular one. Therefore, NSAIDs have a direct cytotoxic effect on gastric mucosa cells (Scheiman, 1996). Furthermore, NSAIDs inhibit mitochondrial oxidative phosphorylation so as to interfere energy metabolism, inhibit the expression of heat shock proteins (HSP) related to cellular membrane integrity (Wallace, 1997), originate the injury of epithelium and the cellular exfoliation, induce the release of various inflammatory factors, such as leukotriene B4 and histamine, and finally damage capillary vascular, increase vascular permeability and reduce blood flow into the mucosa (Wallace *et al.*, 1990; Wallace *et al.*, 1995). Another effect is that NSAIDs trigger gastric epithelium to release tumor necrosis factor alpha (TNF-α). TNF-α increases adhesive molecules and activates neutrophils (Wallace *et al.*, 1995), which result in the gastric mucosa neutrophil infiltration, the submucosa capillary vascular constriction, the mucosa ischemia and hypoxia, the abnormal metabolism in epithelial cells, and finally the functional damage of mucus and mucosa barrier.

### 3.2 NSAIDs inhibit the syntheses of prostaglandin

Arachidonic acid may be produced from phospholipids in the membrane under catalysis of phospholipase $A_2$. Arachidonic acid generates leukotrienes through lipoxidase and generates $PGI_2$ and $PGE_2$ through cyclo-oxygenase. Leukotrienes are involved in allergic reaction, leukocyte chemotaxis and inflammation. $PGI_2$ has the effects on vasodilatation and platelet aggregation. $PGE_2$ is capable of inducing inflammation, fever, pain, vasodilatation and gastric mucosa protection (Scheiman, 1996).

NSAIDs may inhibit COX activity, interfere the metabolism of arachidonic acid, and decrease PG syntheses (Figure 1). Therefore, NSAIDs have the effects of anti-inflammation, antipyretics and analgesics. COX has two isoforms, one is constitutive or COX-1 and another is inducible or COX-2. COX-1 constantly expresses in gastrointestinal tract and platelets, controls the syntheses of $PGI_2$, $PGE_2$ and $TXA_2$, regulates angiotasis, protests the mucosa of digestive tract from assault factors, and maintains the mucosa's integrity. There is little or almost no COX-2 in the mucosa of stomach and intestine and the platelets in healthy people. LPS, interleukin-1 (IL-1) and many other inflammatory factors, however, can induce its production. COX-2 can increase dramatically in local inflammatory lesion. It may result in the increase of $PGI_2$ and $PGE_2$ that also participate in inflammatory reaction. The classic NSAIDs had no selective inhibition effect on COX-1 and COX-2. The inhibition of COX-2 results in anti-inflammation, while inhibition of COX-1 causes side effects, i.e. to decrease $PGI_2$ and $PGE_2$ that have mucosa protective effects, decline the blood flow in gastric mucosa, decrease the provision of oxygen and nutrition, slow the turnover of mucosa cells, lessen the syntheses and secretion of mucus, damage the mucus and mucosa barriers, prolong the mucosa reparation, and finally cause mucosa erosion, ulceration and hemorrhage (Pawlik *et al.*, 2002). Besides above effects, aspirin prolongs the recovery of ulceration. Its mechanism underlies on the inhibition of PG syntheses (Wang *et al.*, 1989), the reduction of cellular proliferation (Penney *et al.*, 1994) and the decrease of blood flow at the ulcer margin (Hirose *et al.*, 1991).

## 4. The simultaneous effects of *H. pyori* and NSAIDs on gastric mucosa

From above discussion, we know that *H. pylori* and NSAIDs are two important factors assaulting gastric mucosa and have the pivotal role in the peptic ulcer. Each has a different way to injure the gastric mucosa. It has been confirmed that *H. pylori* and NSAIDs are two independent offending factors (Grymer *et al.*, 1984). However, the exact relationship remains to be clarified (Laine, 2002). *H. pylori* and NSAIDs may be irrelevant, additive or synergistic, or possibly antagonistic (Ji *et al.*, 2003).

### 4.1 *H. pylori* and NSAIDs are irrelevant
Some studies demonstrated that NSAIDs should not impact *H. pylori*'s plantation (Maxton *et al.*, 1990). The infection of *H. pylori* dose not increase the ulcerative risk in long term NSAIDs user (Kim *et al.*, 1994). The epidemic investigation showed that NSAIDs did not affect the patient's susceptibility to *H. pylori* (Graham *et al.*, 1991; Barkin, 1998; Wilcox, 1997). NSAIDs dose not enhance the gastrointestinal toxicity to *H. pylori* carrier (Rybar *et al.*, 2001). Clinical data demonstrated that *H. pylori* infection did not impinge on the degree and type of gastric mucosa injury by NSAIDs (Barkin, 1998; LANZA *et al.*, 1991).

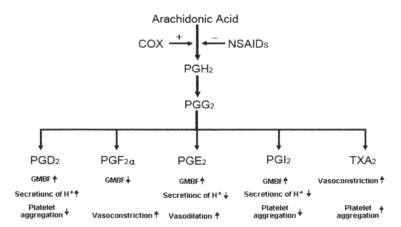

Fig. 1. NSAIDs inhibit COX activity

### 4.2 There is additive or synergistic relationship between *H. pylori* and NSAIDs
*H. pylori* and NSAIDs are strong offensive factors (Chan *et al.*, 1998). Both of them can destroy gastric barrier function. Eradication of *H. pylori* before using NSAIDs reduces the ulcerative rate (Bazzoli *et al.*, 2001). The ulceration is easier to relapse in NSAIDs takers with *H. pylori* than those without *H. pylori* infection (Chan *et al.*, 1998b). Furthermore, both *H. pylori* and NSAIDs increase permeability in the gastric epithelial cellular junction, and thus allow the gastric acid, pepsin and other endogenous offending factors to injure the gastric mucosa (Barr *et al.*, 2000). *H. pylori* and NSAIDs act synergistically through pathways of inflammation in the development of ulcers and in ulcer bleeding (Figure 2).

### 4.3 Antagonistic action between *H. pylori* and NSAIDs

NSAIDs have bacteriostatic and bactericidal activity against *H. pylori* (Shirin *et al.*, 2006). NSAIDs inhibit COX-1 and COX-2. This inhibition declines PG synthesis, while *H. pylori* infection stimulates gastric mucosa to express COX-2 (Takahashi *et al.*, 2000) so as to enhance PG syntheses. *H. pylori* accelerates healing of gastric ulcer induced by NSAIDs in rats due to that *H. pylori* stimulates the overexpression of COX-2 and the increase of PG synthesis, and consequently increases the production of vascular endothelial growth factor (VEGF) and the vascular proliferation. Meanwhile, PG also increases transforming growth factor alpha that causes the increase of cellular proliferation and the decrease of gastric acid (Konturek *et al.*, 2002), and finally enhances the recovery of injured gastric mucosa. The clinical trial also demonstrated that the *H. pylori* infection rate was lower in NSAIDs user than those people without NSAIDs administration (Bianchi *et al.*, 1996). It also verifies that there is antagonistic action between *H. pylori* and NSAIDs.

In conclusion, *H. pylori* and NSAIDs are individual strong factors causing peptic ulcer, and their final mechanism is to wipe out barrier function. However, the investigations are conflicts when *H. pylori* and NSAIDs coexist. The reasons leading to this conflict may be the patient's age, the different type of NSAIDs, the administration length of NSAIDs and the different strain of *H. pylori* and so on.

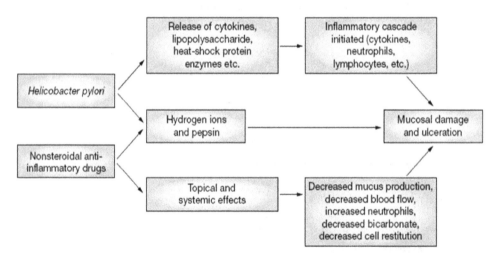

Fig. 2. *Helicobacter pylori* and nonsteroidal anti-inflammatory drugs have synergistic effects on gastric mucosal damage. Both *H. pylori* infection and NSAID use have been found to independently and significantly increase the risk of gastric and duodenal mucosal damage and ulceration. *H. pylori* and NSAIDs act synergistically through pathways of inflammation in the development of ulcers and in ulcer bleeding (Yuan *et al.*, 2006).

## 5. References

Appelmelk, B.J., SimoonsSmit, I., Negrini, R., Moran, A.P., Aspinall, G.O., Forte, J.G., DeVries, T., Quan, H., Verboom, T., Maaskant, J.J., Ghiara, P., Kuipers, E.J., Bloemena, E., Tadema, T.M., Townsend, R.R., Tyagarajan, K., Crothers, J.M.,

Monteiro, M.A., Savio, A., DeGraaff, J. (1996). Potential role of molecular mimicry between Helicobacter pylori lipopolysaccharide and host Lewis blood group antigens in autoimmunity. *Infect Immun*, Vol.64, No.6, pp. 2031-2040, ISSN 0019-9567

Atherton, J.C., Peek, R.M., Tham, K.T., Cover, T.L., Blaser, M.J. (1997). Clinical and pathological importance of heterogeneity in vacA, the vacuolating cytotoxin gene of Helicobacter pylori. *Gastroenterology*, Vol.112, No.1, pp. 92-99, ISSN 0016-5085

Barkin, J. (1998). The relation between Helicobacter pylori and nonsteroidal anti-inflammatory drugs. *Am J Med* Vol.105, No.5, pp. 22S-27S, ISSN 0002-9343

Barr, M., Buckley, M., O'Morain, C. (2000). Review article: non-steroidal anti-inflammatory drugs and Helicobacter pylori. *Aliment Pharm Therap*, Vol.14, pp. 43-47, ISSN 0269-2813

Bazzoli, F., De Luca, L., Graham, D.Y. (2001). Helicobacter pylori infection and the use of NSAIDs. *Best Pract Res Cl Ga*, Vol.15, No. 5, pp. 775-785, ISSN 1521-6918

Bianchi, P.G., Parente, F., Imbesi, V., Montrone, F., Caruso, I. (1996). Role of Helicobacter pylori in ulcer healing and recurrence of gastric and duodenal ulcers in longterm NSAID users. Response to omeprazole dual therapy. *Gut*, Vol.39, No.1, pp. 22-26, ISSN 1468-3288

Bode, G., Malfertheiner, P., Nilius, M., Lehnhardt, G., Ditschuneit, H. (1989). Ultrastructural-localization of urease in outer-membrane and periplasm of campylobacter-pylori. *J Clin Pathol*, Vol.42, No.7, pp.778-779, ISSN 0021-9746

Brzozowski, T., Konturek, P.C., Sliwowski, Z., Kwiecien, S., Drozdowicz, D., Pawlik, M., Mach, K., Konturek, S.J., Pawlik, W.W. (2006). Interaction of nonsteroidal anti-inflammatory drugs (NSAID) with Helicobacter pylori in the stomach of humans and experimental animals. *J Physiol Pharmacol*, Vol.57, Suppl.3, pp. 67-79, ISSN 1899-1505

Chan, F.K., Sung, J.J., Suen, R., Lee, Y.T., Wu, J.C., Leung, W.K., Chan, H.L., Lai, A.C., Lau, J.Y., Ng, E.K., Chung, S.C. (1998a). Does eradication of Helicobacter pylori impairpeptic ulcers? A prospective randomized study. *Aliment Pharmacol Ther*, Vol.12, No.12, pp. 1201-1205, ISSN 1365-2036

Domingo, D., Alarcon, T., Sanz, J.C., Villar, H., Hernandez, J.M., Sanchez, J., Lopez-Brea, M. (1999). The Helicobacter pylori adhesion gene: relation with the origin of the isolates and associated disease. *Enferm Infecc Microbiol Clin*, Vol.17, No.7, pp. 342-346, ISSN 0213-005X

Dundon, W.G., de Bernard, M., Montecucco, C. (2001). Virulence factors of Helicobacter pylori. *Int J Med Microbiol*, Vol.290, No.8, pp. 647-658, ISSN 1438-4221

Ernst, P.B., Jin, Y., Reyes, V.E., Crowe, S.E. (1994). The role of the local immune response in the pathogenesis of peptic ulcer formation. *Scand J Gastroenterol Suppl*, Vol.205, pp. 22-28, ISSN 0085-5928

Fendrick, A.M., Scheiman, J.M. (2001). Helicobacter pylori and NSAID gastropathy: an ambiguous association. *Curr Rheumatol Rep*, Vol.3, No.2, pp. 107-111, ISSN 1523-3774

Ghira, P., Marchetti, M., Blaser, M.J., Tummuru, M., Cover, T.L., Segal, E.D., Tompkins, L.S., Rappuoli, R. (1995). Role of the helicobacter-pylori virulence factors vacuolating cytotoxin, caga, and urease in a mouse model of disease. *Infect Immun*, Vol.63, No.10, pp. 4154-4160, ISSN 0019-9567

Goggin, P.M., Northfield, T.C., Spychal, R.T. (1991). Factors affecting gastric mucosal hydrophobicity in man. *Scand J Gastroenterol Suppl*, Vol.181, pp. 65-73, ISSN 0085-5928

Graham, D.Y., Lidsky, M.D., Cox, A.M., Evans, D.J., Evans, D.G., Alpert, L., Klein, P.D., Sessoms, S.L., Michaletz, P.A., Saeed, Z.A. (1991). Long-term nonsteroidal antiinflammatory drug use and Helicobacter pylori infection. *Gastroenterology*, Vol.100, No.6, pp. 1653-1657, ISSN 0016-5085

Grymer, J., Watson, G.L., Coy, C.H., Prindle, L.V. (1984). Healing of experimentally induced wounds of mammary papilla (teat) of the cow - comparison of closure with tissue adhesive versus nonsutured wounds. *Am J Vet Res*, Vol.45, No.10, pp. 1979-1983, ISSN 0002-9645

Hazell, S.l., Lee, A. (1986). Campylobacter pyloridis, urease, hydrogen-ion back diffusion, and gastric-ulcers. *Lancet*, Vol.2, No.8497, pp. 15-17, ISSN 0140-6736

Hirose, H., Takeuchi, K., Okabe, S. (1991). Effect of indomethacin on gastric-mucosal blood-flow around acetic-acid induced gastric-ulcers in rats. *Gastroenterology*, Vol.100, No.51, pp. 1259-1265, ISSN 0016-5085

Husain, S.S., Szabo, I.L., Tarnawski, A.S. (2002). NSAID inhibition of GI cancer growth: Clinical implications and molecular mechanisms of action. *Am J Gastroentero*, Vol.97, No.3, pp. 542-553, ISSN 0002-9270

Ji, K., Hu, F., Li, A., Li, J. (2003). Interaction of Helicobacter polyri and indomethacin in gastric mucosa injury of Balb/c mice. *Zhonghua Yi Xue Za Zh*, Vol.83, No.9, pp. 726-730, ISSN 0376-2491

Kaneko, H., Nakada, K., Mitsuma, T., Uchida, K., Furusawa, A., Maeda, Y., Morise, K. (1992). Helicobacter-pylori infection induces a decrease in immunoreactive-somatostatin concentrations of human stomach. *Digest Dis Sci*, Vol.37, No.3, pp. 409-416, ISSN 0163-2116

Kawano, S., Tsujii, M., Nagano, K., Ogihara, T., Tanimura, H., Hayashi, N., Ito, T., Sato, N., Kamada, T., Tamura, K., Tanaka, M. (1990). Different effect of helicobacter-pylori on the human gastric antral and body mucosal intracellular mucin. *Scand J Gastroentero*, Vol.25, No.10, pp. 997-1003, ISSN 0036-5521

Kim, J.G., Graham, D.Y. (1994). Helicobacter pylori infection and development of gastric or duodenal ulcer in arthritic patients receiving chronic NSAID therapy. The Misoprostol Study Group. *Am J Gastroenterol*, Vol.89, No.2, pp. 203-207, ISSN 0002-9270

Konturek, P.C., Brzozowski, T., Kwiecien, S., Drozdowicz, D., Harsch, I.A., Meixner, H., Stachura, J., Hahn, E.G., Konturek, S.J. (2002). Effect of Helicobacter pylori on delay in ulcer healing induced by aspirin in rats. *Eur J Pharmacol*, Vol.451, No.2, pp. 191-202, ISSN 0014-2999

Laine, L. (2002). Review article: the effect of Helicobacter pylori infection on nonsteroidala nti-inflammatory drug-induced upper gastrointestinal tract injury. *Aliment Pharm Therap*, Vol.16, pp. 34-39, ISSN 0269-2813

Lanza, F.l, Evans, D.G., Graham, D.Y. (1991). Effect of helicobacter-pylori infection on the severity of gastroduodenal mucosal injury after the acute administration of naproxen or aspirin to normal volunteers. *Am J Gastroenterol*, Vol.86, No.6, pp. 735-737, ISSN 0002-9270

Leunk, R.D., Johnson, P.T., David, B.C., Kraft, W.G., Morgan, D.R. (1988). Cyto-toxic activity in broth-culture filtrates of campylobacter-pylori. *J Med Microbiol*, Vol.26, No.2, pp. 93-99, ISSN 0022-2615

Levi, S., Beardshall, K., Swift, I., Foulkes, W., Playford, R., Ghosh, P., Calam, J. (1989). Antral helicobacter-pylori, hypergastrinemia, and duodenal-ulcers - effect of eradicating the organism. *Brit Med J*, Vol.299, No.6714, pp. 1504-1505, ISSN 0959-8138

Lewis, R.A., Austen, K.F., Soberman, R.J. (1990). Leukotrienes and other products of the 5-lipoxygenase pathway - biochemistry and relation to pathobiology in human-diseases. *New Engl J Med*, Vol.323, No.10, pp. 645-655, ISSN 0028-4793

Lundstrom, A.M., Blom, K., Sundaeus, V., Bolin, I. (2001). HpaA shows variable surface localization but the gene expression is similar in different Helicobacter pylori strains. *Microb Pathogenesis*, Vol.31, No.5, pp. 243-253, ISSN 0882-4010

Marshall, B.J. (1994). Helicobacter-pylori. *Am J Gastroenterol*, Vol.89, No.8, pp. S116-S128, ISSN 0002-9270

Maxton, D.G, Srivastava, E.D., Whorwell, P.J., Jones, D.M. (1990). Do nonsteroidal antiinflammatory drugs or smoking predispose to helicobacter-pylori infection. *Postgrad Med J*, Vol. 66, No.779, pp. 717-719, ISSN 0032-5473

McGee, D.J., Mobley, H. (1999). Mechanisms of Helicobacter pylori infection: Bacterial factors. *Gastroduodenal Disease and Helicobacter Pylori*, Vol.241, pp. 155-180, ISSN 0070-217X

Naito, Y., Yoshikawa, T. (2002). Molecular and cellular mechanisms involved in Helicobacter pylori-induced inflammation and oxidative stress. *Free Radical Bio Med*, Vol.33, No.3, pp. 323-336, ISSN 0891-5849

Pawlik, T., Konturek, P.C., Konturek, J.W., Konturek, S.J., Brzozowski, T., Czesnikiewicz, M., Plonka, M., Bielanski, W., Areny, H. (2002). Impact of Helicobacter pylori and nonsteroidal anti-inflammatory drugs on gastric ulcerogenesis in experimental animals and in humans. *Eur J Pharmacol*, Vol.449, No.1-2, pp. 1-15, ISSN 0014-2999

Penney, A.G., Andrews, F.J., Obrien, P.E. (1994). Effects of misoprostol on delayed ulcer healing induced by aspirin. *Digest Dis Sci*, Vol.39, No.5, pp. 934-939, ISSN 0163-2116

Phadnis, S.H., Parlow, M.H., Levy, M., Ilver, D., Caulkins, C.M., Connors, J.B., Dunn, B.E. (1996). Surface localization of Helicobacter pylori urease and a heat shock protein homolog requires bacterial autolysis. *Infect Immun*, Vol.64, No.3, pp. 905-912. ISSN 0019-9567

Rybar, I., Masaryk, P., Mateicka, F., Kopecky, S., Rovensky, J. (2001). Nonsteroidal antiinflammatory drug-induced mucosal lesions of the upper gastrointestinal tract and their relationship to Helicobacter pylori. *Int J Clin Pharm Res*, Vol.21, No. 3-4, pp. 119-125, ISSN 0251-1649

Sarosiek, J., Bilski, J., Murty, V., Slomiany, A., Slomiany, B.L. (1989). Colloidal bismuth subcitrate (de-nol) inhibits degradation of gastric mucus by campylobacter-pylori protease. *Am J Gastroenterol*, Vol.84, No.5, pp. 506-510, ISSN 0002-9270

Satin, B., Del Giudice, G., Della Bianca, V., Dusi, S., Laudanna, C., Tonello, F., Kelleher, D., Rappuoli, R., Montecucco, C., Rossi, F. (2000). The neutrophil-activating protein (HP-NAP) of Helicobacter pylori is a protective antigen and a major virulence factor. *J Exp Med*, Vol.191, No.9, pp. 1467-1476, ISSN 0022-1007

Scheiman, J.M. (1996). NSAIDs, gastrointestinal injury, and cytoprotection. *Gastroenterol Clin N*, Vol.25, No.2, pp. 279, ISSN 0889-8553

Shiotani, A., Yamaoka, Y., El-Zimaity, H., Saeed, M.A., Qureshi, W.A., Graham, D.Y. (2002). NSAID gastric ulceration - Predictive value of gastric pH, mucosal density of polymorphonuclear leukocytes, or levels of IL-8 or nitrite. *Digest Dis Sci*, Vol.47, No.1, pp. 38-43, ISSN 0163-2116

Shirin, H., Moss, S.F., Kancherla, S., Kancherla, K., Holt, P.R., Weinstein, I.B., Sordillo, E.M. (2006). Non-steroidal anti-inflammatory drugs have bacteriostatic and bactericidal activity against Helicobacter pylori. *J Gastroen Hepatol*, Vol.21, No.9, pp. 1388-1393, ISSN 0815-9319

Takahashi, S., Fujita, T., Yamamoto, A. (2000). Nonsteroidal anti-inflammatory drug-induced acute gastric injury in Helicobacter pylori gastritis in Mongolian gerbils. *Eur J Pharmacol*, Vol.406, No.3, pp. 461-468, ISSN 0014-2999

Tarnawski, A.S., Jones, M.K. (2003a). Inhibition of angiogenesis by NSAIDs: molecular mechanisms and clinical implications. *J Mol Med-Jmm*, Vol.81, No.10, pp. 627-636, ISSN 0946-2716

Tarnawski, A.S., Jones, M.K. (2003b). Inhibition of angiogenesis by NSAIDs: molecular mechanisms and clinical implications. *J Mol Med-Jmm*, Vol.81, No.10, pp. 627-636, ISSN 0946-2716

Tytgat, G. (2000). Ulcers and gastritis. *Endoscopy*, Vol.32, No.2, pp. 108-117, ISSN 0013-726X

Wallace, J.L. (1997). Nonsteroidal anti-inflammatory drugs and gastroenteropathy: the second hundred years. *Gastroenterology*, Vol.112, No.3, pp. 1000-1016, ISSN 0016-5085

Wallace, J.L., Keenan, C.M., Granger, D.N. (1990). Gastric ulceration induced by nonsteroidal anti-inflammatory drugs is a neutrophil-dependent process. *Am J Physiol*, Vol.259, No.3 Pt 1, pp. G462-G467, ISSN 0193-1857

Wallace, J.L., Tigley, A.W. (1995). New insights into prostaglandins and mucosal defense. *Aliment Pharm Therap*, Vol. 9, No.3, pp. 227-235, ISSN 0953-0673

Wang, G.Z., Ru, X., Ding, L.H., Li, H.Q. (1998). Short-term effect of Salvia miltiorrhiza in treating rat acetic acid chronic gastric ulcer and long-term effect in preventing recurrence. *World Journal of Gastroenterology*, Vol.4, NO.2, pp.169-170, ISSN 1007-9327

Wang, J.Y., Yamasaki, S., Takeuchi, K., Okabe, S. (1989). Delayed healing of acetic acid-induced gastric-ulcers in rats by indomethacin. *Gastroenterology*, Vol.96, No.21, pp. 393-402, ISSN 0016-5085

Wetherall, B.L., Johnson, A.M. (1989). Hemolytic-activity of campylobacter-pylori. *Eur J Clin Microbiol*, Vol.8, No.8, pp. 706-710, ISSN 0934-9723

Wilcox, C.M. (1997). Relationship between nonsteroidal anti-inflammatory drug use, Helicobacter pylori, and gastroduodenal mucosal injury. *Gastroenterology*, Vol.113S, No.6, pp. S85-S89, ISSN 0016-5085

Windsor, H.M., O'Rourke, J. (2000). Bacteriology and taxonomy of Helicobacter pylori. *Gastroenterol Clin N*, Vol.29, No.3, pp. 633, ISSN 0889-8553

Yoshikawa, T., Naito, Y. (2000). The role of neutrophils and inflammation in gastric mucosal injury. *Free Radical Res*, Vol.33, No.6, pp. 785-794, ISSN 1071-5762

Young, G.O., Stemmet, N, Lastovica, A., Vandermerwe, E.L., Louw, J.A., Modlin, I.M, Marks, I.N. (1992). Helicobacter-pylori lipopolysaccharide stimulates gastric-mucosal pepsinogen secretion. *Aliment Pharm Therap*, Vol.6, No.2, pp. 169-177, ISSN 0269-2813

Yuan, Y.H., Padol, I.T., Hunt, R.H. (2006). Peptic ulcer disease today. *Nature Clinical Practice Gastroenterology & Hepatology*, Vol.3, No.2, pp. 80-89, ISSN 1743-4378

# 5

# The Etiological Factors of Duodenal and Gastric Ulcers

Ahmet Uyanıkoğlu[1], Ahmet Danalıoğlu[1], Filiz Akyüz[1], Binnur Pınarbaşı[1],
Mine Güllüoğlu[2], Yersu Kapran[2], Kadir Demir[1], Sadakat Özdil[1], Fatih
Beşışık[1], Güngör Boztaş[1], Zeynel Mungan[1] and Sabahattin Kaymakoğlu[1]
*[1]İstanbul University, Faculty of Medicine, Department of Gastroenterohepatology,*
*[2]İstanbul University, Faculty of Medicine, Department of Pathology*
*Turkey*

## 1. Introduction

### 1.1 Background

Peptic ulcer disease (PUD) had a tremendous effect on morbidity and mortality until the last decades of the 20th century. Development of new effective and potent acid suppressants and the discovery of Helicobacter pylori (H. pylori) are two important steps that caused a reduction in the prevalence of peptic ulcer. With the discovery of H. pylori, causes, pathogenesis and treatment of PUD have been defined again in the last 25 years. However, this condition continues to be an important clinical issue because of common use of nonsteroidal anti-inflammatory drugs (NSAID) and acetylsalicylic acid at low doses. The rare but increasingly problematic issue is H pylori-negative and NSAID-negative ulcers (1). Despite progress in diagnosis and treatment, peptic ulcer disease (PUD) remains a common reason for hospitalization and operation (2).

Peptic ulcer disease (PUD) affects 10% of the world population. Helicobacter pylori infection and the use of a nonsteroidal anti-inflammatory drug (NSAID) are the principal factors associated with PUD (3). The declining global prevalence of peptic ulcer disease (PUD) might be because of the decreasing prevalence of Helicobacter pylori (Hp) infection (4). The decreasing prevalence of H. pylori could lead to a relative increase in the number of patients with this NSAID associated and idiopathic peptic ulcer disease (IPUD (5). Another view is that incidence of peptic ulcers decreased and an increasing proportion was related to NSAID and the Mortality was high (6). It is also known that the incidence of idiopathic peptic ulcer disease has increased (7,8).

H pylori infection causes both gastric and duodenal ulcers (35-27). Current data shows that H pylori infection plays a major role in peptic ulcer disease and non-ulcer dyspepsia (9,10). Apart from these diseases, H pylori are thought to play a role in the etiology of atrophic gastritis, gastric adenocarcinoma and lymphoma. In our country, H. pylori prevalence remains an important health problem (11).

The aim of this study is to determine the etiology of patients with duodenal and gastric ulcers.

## 2. Materials-methods

Between April 2002 and April 2009, 140 patients who referred to our endoscopy laboratory with dyspeptic complaints for gastroscopy and diagnosed with peptic ulcer (duodenal and/or gastric) were enrolled to this prospective study. Before the procedure, medical history, cigarette smoking and alcohol consumption and nonsteroidal anti-inflammatory drugs (NSAIDs) and acetylsalicylic acid use within the last month were queried. Patients with a history of gastric operation, with malign ulcer or another malign disease and who were not willing to participate the study were excluded.

Two biopsy specimens were collected from antrum and corpus for histology and one for rapid urease testing and stool samples were analyzed for Helicobacter pylori (H pylori) antigen using Laboquick H pylori antigen test kit. A patient was classified as being H. pylori positive if any of the three test methods were positive. NSAID and/or acetylsalicylic acid use within the last month was associated with ulcer, if any. Inflammatory activity, intestinal metaplasia, atrophy and H. pylori were evaluated in histopathological examination. Serum calcium and gastrin levels were also analyzed.

SPSS 13.0 statistical program was used for statistical assessments. Mean ± standard deviation (SD) or median were used for quantitative variables. For independent group comparisons, intergroup variations were analyzed with non parametrical Mann –Whitney U test. Inter group variations were evaluated using Wilcoxon test (for dependent group comparison). Correlation analyses were performed using Pearson and Spearman correlation tests. Results with "p value" less than 0.05 were accepted as statistically significant.

## 3. Results

82 of the patients (58%) were male and 58% were female (42%). Mean age was 47.70 ± 15.03 (range 16-92). 62 of the patients (44%) were smoking and 18 (13%) were drinking alcohol. 132 of the patients (94%) were from urban whereas 8 (6%) were from rural areas. 14 patients (10%) had a family history of PUD, whereas 4 (0.3%) had a family history of stomach cancer. Ulcer was located in duodenum in 96 patients (69%), in stomach in 40 patients (28%), and both in duodenum and stomach in 4 patients (3%).

Rate of patients tested positive for H pylori antigen in stool, positive in urease testing and tested positive for H. pylory presence in antral and corpus samples were 48%, 52%, 67% and 60% respectively (see Table 1). 107 patients (76%) were positive for H. pylori in one of the test methods.

| Method | Incidence |
|--------|-----------|
| Stool sample for H pylori positive | 48% |
| Rapid urease testing positive | 52% |
| H pylori positive antral histology | 67% |
| H pylori positive corpus histology | 60% |
| H pylori positive with any method | 76% |

Table 1. Incidence of H. pylori in peptic ulcer using various methods.

Among 64 patients (46%) with a story of nonsteroidal antienflammatory drug (NSAID) use within the last 1 month, 48 (75%) were Hp positive and 16 were (25%) negative (see Table 2).

Mean age of patients on NSAID therapy higher 51.26 ± 15.60 (range 21-92) compared to the non-users 45.32 ±14.25 (range 16-80) (p<0.05).

| H pylori positive PUD | 107 | | 76% | |
|---|---|---|---|---|
| NSAID use | 64 | | | (46%) |
|    NSAID+H pylori positive | 48 | | | (75%) |
|    NSAİİ+ H pylori negatifliği | 16 | | 12% | (25%) |
| Idiopathic PUD | 17 | | 12% | |

Table 2. Peptic ulcer (PUD) etiology

Incidence of inflammatory activity, atrophy and intestinal metaplasia were 65%, 17.5% and 11% in antral biopsies and 66%, 6.5% and 1.5% in corpus samples, respectively (see Table 2).

| | Antrum | Corpus |
|---|---|---|
| Inlammatory activity | 65% | 66% |
| Atrophy | 17.5% | 6.5% |
| Intestinal metaplasia | 11% | 1.5% |
| H. pylori incidence | 67% | 60% |

Table 3. Histology findings of the biopsy samples

Histopathologically inflammatory activity was correlated with H. pylori (p<0.05). Mean levels of calcium and gastrin were 9.29 ± 0.40 (7.90-10.20) and 73.96 ± 89.88 (12.86-562.50) respectively. In patients with elevated gastrin levels, no hypersecretory condition was detected. Elevated levels of gastrin were correlated with inflammatory activity and presence of H. pylori (p<0.05).

19 of patients (13.6%) were negative for H pylori, NSAID use and hypersecretory illness and classified as idiopathic. Mean age of these pateints were 51.52 ± 13.88 (range 16-78). Ulcer was located in the duodenum of 13 patients (68%) and in stomach of 6 patients (32%). 11 of the patients (58%) were male and 8% were female (42%). 9 of the patients (47%) were smoking and 3 (16%) were drinking alcohol. 1 patient had a family history of PUD and 1 had a family history of stomach cancer. Mean age of these patients was higher compared to patients with a known etiology (p<0.05), however there were no statistical differences in terms of ulcer location, gender, smoking, alcohol consumption, and family history (p>0.5). Mean gastrin level of 60.07 ± 64.13 (12.86-183.61) was lower compared to the patients with a known etiology (p<0.05) whereas calcium levels of 9.33 ± 0.6 (7.9-10.2) were similar (p>0.5).

## 4. Discussion

54 (19%) of 277 consecutive patients had evidence of peptic ulcer disease (34 gastric ulcer, 14 duodenal ulcer and 6 both gastric and duodenal ulcer) in a similar study where demographic and endoscopic characteristics of patients with Helicobacter pylori positive and negative chronic peptic ulcer disease were evaluated (12). The most common finding in this study was gastric ulcer whereas in our study, among 140 patients with PUD 96 (69%) had duodenal ulcer, 40 had (28%) gastric ulcer and 4 had (3%) both duodenal and gastric

ulcer in our study. These variations may be associated with the regional characteristics, lower number of patients evaluated in the other study and etiological differences.

Helicobacter pylori infection and the use of a nonsteroidal anti-inflammatory drug (NSAID) are the principal factors associated with PUD (3). Similarly, etiologic factor in 88% of patients in our study was H pylori and/or NSAID use.

While incidence of PUD associated with H pylori infection is decreasing especially in western countries (5,7,8), in our country most common cause is H pylori (76%). It may be associated with the fact that H. pylori prevalence remains an important health problem in our country and prevalence in the community is very high. In a study performed in our country with 9239 patients who underwent gastrointestinal endoscopy, H. pylori incidence was 41.44% using the CLO test (11).

In a study where demographic and endoscopic characteristics of peptic ulcer were evaluated, urease, culture, histology and serum anti-H pylori IgG antibody were evaluated in patients and demographic data as well as NSAID use within the last 3 months were assessed. 56% of patients were H pylori positive and 22% were using NSAIDs (70% were H pylori positive) (12). In our study H. pylori was evaluated using urease testing, H pylori antigen in stool and histology and rate of patients who are H pylori positive and using NSAIDs within the last month were higher (76% and 46% respectively). Similarly, some patients using NSAID (75%) were also H pylori positive.

H. pylori induces chronic inflammation of the gastric mucosa, but only a proportion of infected individuals develop peptic ulcer disease or gastric carcinoma Reasons underlying these observations include differences in bacterial pathogenicity as well as in host susceptibility (13). Meta-analyses showed that Helicobacter pylori eradication therapy was effective for healing and prevention of recurrence of peptic ulcers in H. pylori-positive patients and that treatment of H. pylori infection was more effective than antisecretory non-eradicating therapy (with or without long-term maintenance therapy) in preventing recurrent bleeding (14). H pylori eradication has been associated with decreased risk of gastric cancer in patients with peptic ulcer diseases (15). In our study, H pylori were also correlated with inflammatory activity. When it is considered that the H pylori associated PUD is a common disease in our country, we should give more importance to eradication therapy both for effective treatment of PUD and for cancer prophylaxis.

NSAIDs have known detrimental side effects on the gastrointestinal system. The risk is increased with older age and history of PUD. Helicobacter pylori infection and cardioprotective acetylsalicylic acid have additive risks in the presence of NSAID use (16). The development of PUD was observed earlier in the combined H pylori and NSAID group than in patients with only NSAID use and this suggests a synergic effect between the two risks factors in the development of PUD (3). In our study, 75% of patients with history of NSAID therapy were H pylori positive. This finding suggest that H pylori and NSAID usage, when together, increases the risk of PUD.

Apart from H pylori and NSAID, risk factors such as smoking, alcohol intake, age, and male gender were reported as contributing to the gastric and duodenal ulcer development (17-20). In our study, patients who are supporting these findings were at middle or older age and 58% of them were male. Almost half of the patients (44%) were smokers and 13% were drinking alcohol.

Rate of patients classified as idiopathic (H pylori negative, NSAID negative) were reported between 4 and 20% (5, 8, 17). Among 140 patients 19 were (13%) H pylori and NSAID negative. Idiopathic ulcer was reported among younger patients in a study (12) where as 19 patients classified as idiopathic in our study were older compared to patients with a known etiology.

Apart from H pylori, poor socio-economic status has been reported as an important risk factor for PUD infection while genetic factors do not influence the risk of PUD (21). Although the socio-economic status of the patients enrolled in our study has not been investigated in detail, 132 of the patients (94%) were from the urban regions while 8 (6%) were from the rural area and 14 (10%) had a history of ulcer.

As a consequence, most common cause of duodenal and gastric ulcer is H. pylori and is responsible for three-fourths of the cases. About half of the patients had a history of NSAID use and NSAID and H. pylori are both responsible for the ulcer in three-forths of these patients. In one tenth of the patients, NSAİD use was the cause of ulcer alone and about one-tenth of the ulcers were classified as idiopathic.

## 5. References

[1] Malfertheiner P, Chan FK, McColl KE. Peptic ulcer disease. Lancet. 2009 Oct 24;374(9699):1449-61. Epub 2009 Aug 13.

[2] Wang YR, Richter JE, Dempsey DT. Trends and outcomes of hospitalizations for peptic ulcer disease in the United States, 1993 to 2006. Ann Surg. 2010 Jan;251(1):51-8.

[3] Zapata-Colindres JC, Zepeda-Gómez S, Montaño-Loza A, Vázquez-Ballesteros E, de Jesús Villalobos J, Valdovinos-Andraca F. The association of Helicobacter pylori infection and nonsteroidal anti-inflammatory drugs in peptic ulcer disease. Can J Gastroenterol. 2006 Apr;20(4):277-80.

[4] Wong SN, Sollano JD, Chan MM, Carpio RE, Tady CS, Ismael AE, Judan-Ruiz EA, Ang VN, Go JT, Lim VY, Perez JY, Alvarez SZ. Changing trends in peptic ulcer prevalence in a tertiary care setting in the Philippines: a seven-year study. J Gastroenterol Hepatol. 2005 Apr;20(4):628-32.

[5] Arents NL, Thijs JC, van Zwet AA, Kleibeuker JH. Does the declining prevalence of Helicobacter pylori unmask patients with idiopathic peptic ulcer disease? Trends over an 8 year period. Eur J Gastroenterol Hepatol. 2004 Aug;16(8):779-83.

[6] Lassen A, Hallas J, Schaffalitzky de Muckadell OB. Complicated and uncomplicated peptic ulcers in a Danish county 1993-2002: a population-based cohort study. Am J Gastroenterol. 2006 May;101(5):945-53.

[7] Jang HJ, Choi MH, Shin WG, Kim KH, Chung YW, Kim KO, Park CH, Baek IH, Baik KH, Kae SH, Kim HY. Has Peptic Ulcer Disease Changed During the Past Ten Years in Korea? A Prospective Multi-center Study. Dig Dis Sci. 2007 Oct

[8] Arroyo MT, Forne M, de Argila CM, Feu F, Arenas J, de la Vega J, Garrigues V, Mora F, Castro M, Bujanda L, Cosme A, Castiella A, Gisbert JP, Hervas A, Lanas A. The prevalence of peptic ulcer not related to Helicobacter pylori or non-steroidal anti-inflammatory drug use is negligible in southern Europe. Helicobacter. 2004 Jun;9(3):249-54.

[9] Kachintorn U, Luengrojanakul P, Atisook K, Theerabutra C, Tanwandee T, Boonyapisit S, Chinapak O. Helicobacter pylori and peptic ulcer diseases: prevalence and association with antral gastritis in 210 patients. J Med Assoc Thai. 1992 Jul;75(7):386-92.

[10] Itoh T, Seno H, Kita T, Chiba T, Wakatsuki Y. The response to Helicobacter pylori differs between patients with gastric ulcer and duodenal ulcer. Scand J Gastroenterol. 2005 Jun;40(6):641-7.

[11] Sari YS, Sander E, Erkan E, Tunali V.J Gastroenterol Hepatol. Endoscopic diagnoses and CLO test results in 9239 cases, prevalence of Helicobacter pylori in Istanbul, Turkey. 2007 Nov;22(11):1706-11.

[12] Xia HH, Phung N, Kalantar JS, Talley NJ. D.Med J Aust. 2000 Nov 20;173(10):508-9.

[13] Costa AC, Figueiredo C, Touati E. Pathogenesis of Helicobacter pylori infection. Helicobacter. 2009 Sep;14 Suppl 1:15-20.

[14] Satoh K, Sugano K. Helicobacter pylori eradication therapy for peptic ulcer disease. Nippon Rinsho. 2009 Dec;67(12):2322-6.

[15] Wu CY, Kuo KN, Wu MS, Chen YJ, Wang CB, Lin JT. Early Helicobacter pylori eradication decreases risk of gastric cancer in patients with peptic ulcer disease. Gastroenterology. 2009 Nov;137(5):1641-8.e1-2. Epub 2009 Aug 5.

[16] Gupta M, Eisen GM. NSAIDs and the gastrointestinal tract. Curr Gastroenterol Rep. 2009 Oct;11(5):345-53.

[17] Konturek SJ, BielaÅ„ski W, PÅ‚onka M, Pawlik T, Pepera J, Konturek PC, Czarnecki J, Penar A, Jedrychowski W. Helicobacter pylori, non-steroidal anti-inflammatory drugs and smoking in risk pattern of gastroduodenal ulcers. Scand J Gastroenterol. 2003 Sep;38(9):923-30.

[18] Anda RF, Williamson DF, Escobedo LG, Remington PL. Smoking and the risk of peptic ulcer disease among women in the United States. Arch Intern Med. 1990 Jul;150(7):1437-41.

[19] Wu HC, Tuo BG, Wu WM, Gao Y, Xu QQ, Zhao K. Prevalence of peptic ulcer in dyspeptic patients and the influence of age, sex, and Helicobacter pylori infection. Dig Dis Sci. 2008 Oct;53(10):2650-6. Epub 2008 Feb 13.

[20] Salih BA, Abasiyanik MF, Bayyurt N, Sander E. H pylori infection and other risk factors associated with peptic ulcers in Turkish patients: a retrospective study. World J Gastroenterol. 2007 Jun 21;13(23):3245-8.

[21] Rosenstock SJ, JÃ¸rgensen T, Bonnevie O, Andersen LP. Does Helicobacter pylori infection explain all socio-economic differences in peptic ulcer incidence? Genetic and psychosocial markers for incident peptic ulcer disease in a large cohort of Danish adults. Scand J Gastroenterol. 2004 Sep;39(9):823-9.

# 6

# *Helicobacter pylori* –
# Not Only a Gastric Pathogene?

Petr Lukes[1], Jaromir Astl[1], Emil Pavlik[2], Bela Potuznikova[2],
Jan Plzak[1,3], Martin Chovanec[1,3] and Jan Betka[1]
*[1]Charles University in Prague, 1st Faculty of Medicine, Department of
Otorhinolaryngology and Head and Neck Surgery,
Faculty Hospital Motol, Prague
[2]Charles University in Prague, 1st Faculty of Medicine, Institute of
Immunology and Microbiology, Prague
[3]Charles University in Prague, 1st Faculty of Medicine,
Institute of Anatomy, Prague
Czech Republic*

## 1. Introduction

*Helicobacter pylori* is a spiral, microaerophillic, Gram-negative bacterium. Infection by *H. pylori* has been established as the major cause of chronic gastritis and plays important role in the pathogenesis of other gastroduodenal diseases such as peptic ulceration, gastric lymphoma, and gastric cancer (Israel and Peek 2001). *H. pylori* is considered to be the most common chronic bacterial infection in humans (Cave 1996). The prevalence has been estimated to range from 40 to 80% and it varies widely by geographic area, age, race, ethnicity, and socioeconomic status (Bures et al. 2006). In most cases the infection is silent, clinical manifestation appears in only 10-15% of infected individuals. This is due to different strength of virulence of *H. pylori* strains and different host immune system response (Stromberg et al. 2003).

The stomach was supposed to be the only reservoir of infection in humans. Nevertheless *H. pylori* infection was detected in other sites recently. It was found in dental plaque and saliva (Kim et al. 2000) and also in oropharyngeal lymphatic tissue (Pavlik et al. 2007). This finding is of great importance because of known carcinogenic potential of *H. pylori*. It was declared type I carcinogen by IARC (1994). The question of direct contribution of *H. pylori* to oral and oropharyngeal diseases was not resolved yet.

## 2. *H. pylori* pathogenesis

Immunological changes caused by *H. pylori* in the stomach mucosa were explained recently (Tummala et al. 2004). There are no more detailed data about effect of *H. pylori* in the oral or oropharyngeal mucosa. *H. pylori* has several mechanisms to elude host defences (Portal-Celhay and Perez-Perez 2006). It is able to survive the acidic gastric environment by producing the enzyme urease, which metabolizes urea to carbon dioxide and ammonia to buffer the gastric acid. H. *pylori* moves across gastric mucus and can adhere to epithelial cells using a variety of adhesin-like proteins (Sachs et al. 2003). Once adhered to epithelial cells, H. *pylori* induces a strong immune system response (Crabtree 1996). This response does not lead to elimination of the bacterium, but causes development of chronic inflammation. H. *pylori* is not eradicated unless an infected individual is treated with a combination of antibiotics (Portal-Celhay and Perez-Perez 2006). Chemical products of H. *pylori* attract cells of the immune system into lamina propria (Blanchard et al. 2004). It was shown that H. *pylori* can induce the maturation and activation of monocyte-derived dendritic cells. This activity is mediated by TLRs (Toll-like receptors) expressed on antigen presenting cells and leads to promotion of NK and Th1 effector responses (Portal-Celhay and Perez-Perez 2006). IFN – gamma producing Th1 polarized T cells and activated NK cells have been suggested to play an important role for development of severe pathologies (Hafsi et al. 2004).

H. *pylori* infection in gastric mucosa is associated with the production of both proinflammatory and immunomodulatory cytokines. Changes in secretion of IL-8, IL-1beta, IL-6, TNF-alpha, TGF-beta were described (Stromberg et al. 2003). These cytokines are produced by both the immune system and epithelial cells. The response of host cells is dependent on production of H. *pylori* virulence factors (Blanchard et al. 2004). The most important virulence factors, which are associated with gastric diseases, are CagA (cytotoxin associated gene A) and VacA (vacuolizating cytotoxin A).

## 3. *H. pylori* virulence factors

Genome sequence analysis led to identification of genes encoding these virulence factors grouped in the so-called pathogenicity island (cagPAI). It is a genomic region containing about 30 genes including genes for type IV secretion system (Mobley 1996). H. *pylori* strains producing CagA are associated with increased risk of severe gastric pathologies compared with CagA negative strains (Portal-Celhay and Perez-Perez 2006). Injection of bacterial proteins into the gastric cells by a type IV bacterial secretion system (a multi-molecular complex that mediates the translocation of bacterial factors into the host cell) has been described (Segal et al. 1999; Oliveira et al. 2006). In this way, CagA protein can get inside the host cells and stimulate cell signalling through interaction with several host proteins. This interaction leads to increased cytokine and regulatory molecule production (Guillemin et al. 2002) and could be related to initiation of tumour transformation (Segal 1997; Tummala et al. 2004; Hatakeyama 2006).

VacA is another important H. *pylori* virulence factor. This bacterial toxin with multiple activities is inserted into the host cell membrane, inducing cytoplasmic vacuolation (Cover and Blaser 1992). This toxin is coded by *vacA* gene, which is present in all H. *pylori* strains. Only about 50% of strains produce VacA protein. This is due to variability of *vacA* sequence. (Portal-Celhay and Perez-Perez 2006). There are several types of signal region (s1a, s1b, s1c, s2) and two types of midregion (m1 or m2). H. *pylori* strains with different forms of *vacA* differ in association with diseases. Strains with s1 signal sequence allele produce intact VacA toxin, s2 strains have low cytotoxic activity. Strains with s1/m1 allele combination have highest cytotoxic activity and they are associated with gastric ulceration and gastric carcinoma (Miehlke et al. 2000). s1/m2 strains are characterized by medium or low VacA production and s2/m2 strains do not produce VacA at all (Van Doorn et al. 1999). s2/m1 strains was found only sporadically (Letley et al. 1999; Martinez-Gomis et al. 2006).

Other virulence factors are e.g. adhesins, which help *H. pylori* to adhere to mucosal epithelial cells (Gisbert and Pajares 2004). Important is BabA protein which binds Lewis[b] antigen, which is present in individuals with 0 blood group. Presence of *BabA* gene is connected to increased prevalence of gastric ulcers and gastric carcinoma in Lewis[b] positive individuals (Blanchard et al. 2004). *BabA* often coexists with *vacA* s1 and *cagA* alleles (Kusters et al. 2006).

## 4. *H. pylori* induced carcinogenesis

*H. pylori* is a declared type I carcinogen (IARC, 1994). However, the exact way of carcinogenesis is not yet fully understood. There are three supposed ways of *H. pylori* carcinogenic action:

1. *H. pylori* could act as direct mutagen. Interaction of intracellular signalling molecules and *H. pylori* CagA may predispose cells to accumulate multiple genetic and epigenetic changes that promote multistep carcinogenesis (Hatakeyama 2006).
2. *H. pylori* produced VacA can cause immunosuppression by blocking proliferation of T cells (Boncristiano et al. 2003),
3. *H. pylori* can induce cell proliferation by increasing levels of several cytokines and regulatory molecules, which are involved in tumour formation and cell transformation (Konturek et al. 1997; Sakaguchi et al. 1999; Keates et al. 2001; Gobert et al. 2002; Schiemann et al. 2002; Wang et al. 2002). Current information about regulation mechanism of epithelial tissue by cytokines and regulatory molecules focus an interest mainly on Epithelial Growth Factor (EGF), Transforming Growth Factor (TGF) and NO synthases (NOS) (Gallo et al. 1998; Rubin Grandis et al. 1998; Sakaguchi et al. 1999; Gobert et al. 2002; Schiemann et al. 2002).

## 5. Methods of *H. pylori* detection in the oral cavity and pharynx

Diagnostics of *H. pylori* is significantly developed in gastroenterology. Attempts of *H. pylori* detection in other sites encountered diverse success rates (Dowsett and Kowolik 2003). Routinely used tests can be divided into non-invasive and invasive group. When detecting extragastric presence of *H. pylori*, invasive tests must be used based on the detection of bacteria in biopsy specimen. These invasive tests are often used to detect extragastric *H. pylori* presence:

Histology – Several staining methods are in use. These include e.g. haematoxylin and eosin, modified Giemsa, Warthin Starry, Gimenez, and Genta (Rotimi et al., 2000). These staining methods achieve high sensitivity and specificity rates (up to 96%) (Hep 2003) in case of gastric mucosa specimens, where no other bacterial strains are supposed to be present, but provide low specificity in the case of oral specimens, where other bacterial strains are often found (Dowsett and Kowolik, 2003). Differentiation of *H. pylori* from other bacteria can be very difficult.

Rapid Urease Test (RUT) or Campylobacter-like Organism (CLO) test is based on detection of urease production by *H. pylori*. When viable *H. pylori* bacteria are present, urea is being cleaved and the change of pH is visualized by colour indicator (Qureshi et al. 1992). This is very useful method when dealing with gastric mucosa specimens, in case of other specimens results may show high false-positive rate because of some other urease-producing species presence, e.g. *Streptococcus spp., Haemophilus spp.* a *Actinomyces spp.* (Dowsett and Kowolik 2003).

Culture is currently accepted gold standard for the diagnosis of gastric *H. pylori* (Makristathis et al., 2004). This method achieve 80-90% sensitivity and 90-100% specificity rates (Hep 2003). Culture of *H. pylori* from the oral cavity or oropharynx showed to by highly difficult to perform and has met with limited success (Dowsett and Kowolik, 2003). Use of special transport medium, microaerophilic environment, supplemented media for culture and three to seven days incubation is mandatory. Overgrowth by other bacterial species often appears. Direct inhibition of *H. pylori* by oral species in vitro has also been reported (Ishihara et al., 1997). Transformation of *H. pylori* into unculturable, coccoid form in the unfavourable environment was described (Shahamat et al., 2004).

Immunohistochemistry – to detect extragastric *H. pylori* is being used only experimentally. Tissue sections are incubated with rabbit polyclonal anti-*H. pylori* antibodies followed with the use of streptavidin-biotin-peroxidase kit and haematoxylin and eosin counterstaining (Akbayir et al. 2005).

Molecular methods – are currently generating most possibilities of detection and also typing of *H. pylori* strains. Various modifications of the polymerase chain reaction (PCR) are in use. These methods are used only for experimental purposes in the detection of extragastric *H. pylori*. In experiments on the detection of oral and pharyngeal *H. pylori* many variations of PCR diagnosis has been used with a detection rate ranging between 0-90% (Dowsett and Kowolik 2003). The lack of uniformity of laboratory procedures can play a role in the reported inconsistencies. The described modification exerted different primers and probes for the detection of different DNA segments of *H. pylori* DNA. Various primers were used (for example, urease gene, 16S ribosomal RNA genes and others). Specificity and sensitivity of different primers, however, can vary significantly (Song et al., 1999). PCR genotyping makes it possible to distinguish different *H. pylori* strains and their carriage of genes encoding virulence factors (Pavlik et al. 2007). The discrepancy of published PCR results shows the importance of finding suitable PCR assay. Tissue specimens collection and especially immediate immersion into proper transport medium is essential for successful test results (Pavlik et al. 2007). It has to be considered that PCR allows the detection of a low number of bacteria or nonviable bacteria, which cannot influence progress of diseases.

## 6. *H. pylori* in oropharyngeal lymphatic tissue

Several studies have explored the presence of *H. pylori* in tonsillar and adenoid tissue. The results of these studies were inconsistent with different detection rates. The discrepancies are due to different detection methods used. Some of the methods are believed to be unsuitable for detection of extragastric *H. pylori* (e.g. RUT or CLO test). PCR assay is now considered the most appropriate method for detection of pharyngeal *H. pylori*. However, differences in the primers and probes used in published studies do not allow drawing specific conclusions. Table 1. shows an overview of published papers focused on the detection of *H. pylori* in tonsillar and adenoid tissue. According to above mentioned data PCR assay is considered most valuable detection method for extragastric *H. pylori* detection. In their study Di Bonaventura et al. (2001) used PCR for investigation of tonsillar swabs and biopsy specimens with no evidence of *H. pylori* presence. Cirak et al. (2003), Bulut et al. (2006) found *H. pylori* in tonsillar and adenoid tissue by PCR (*16S rRNA* gene and *glmM* gene respectively). They found *H. pylori* strains positive for *cagA* gene. Bitar et al. (2005) investigated adenoid tissue specimens by RUT, histology and nested PCR (*ureA* gene). They found positivity by RUT and histology, but no positivity by nested PCR. In their next study these authors investigated middle ear fluids and adenoid tissue specimens using culture, RUT and PCR (*ureC* and adhesion subunit genes). All middle ear fluids were negative. In adenoids they found positivity by RUT, but none by PCR (Bitar et al. 2006). Yilmaz et al. (2004) found *H. pylori* in middle ear effusions and in one adenoid tissue specimen using PCR (*23S rRNA* gene). Yilmaz et al. (2006) found *H. pylori* in 64% of adenoid and tonsillar specimens by PCR (*16S rRNA* gene). Kusano et al. (2007) showed *H. pylori* positivity in 126 (72.9%) tonsillar specimens using PCR (*16S rRNA* gene). They also demonstrated the presence of coccoid forms of *H. pylori* in tonsillar crypts using immunoelectron microscopy. Eyigor et al. (2009) found 5,5% of adenoid and tonsillar specimens positive for *H. pylori* by RUT, but none of them positive by PCR (*glmM* gene). Vilarinho et al. (2010) found 3 adenoid and tonsillar specimens positive by RUT, 2 positive by immunohistochemistry, but none positive by fluorescence in situ hybridization or PCR (*vacA* gene). Abdel-Monem (2011) found 16 (53.3%) adenoid and tonsillar specimens positive by RUT and 5 (16.6%) specimens positive by PCR (*ureC* gene). Other studies mentioned in Table 1. used different diagnostic methods with different detection rates.

The relationship between *H. pylori* infection and gastric tumour pathogenesis has been well described. It was supposed that *H. pylori* could act the same way in progression of oropharyngeal tumourigenesis. Some authors tried to identify a correlation between *H. pylori* and cancers of head and neck (Table 2.). Tests which determined serum levels of anti-*H. pylori* antibodies in patients with head and neck spinocellular carcinoma (HNSCC) brought inconsistent results (Grandis et al. 1997; Aygenc et al. 2001; Rubin et al. 2003; Nurgalieva et al. 2005). Okuda et al. (2000) proved the presence of *H. pylori* in oral swab specimens and oral cancer specimens using RT PCR (reverse transcriptase polymerase chain reaction) and culture. On the other hand Kanda (2005) found no HNSCC specimen positive using PCR, culture and immunohistochemical analysis. Kizilay et al. (2006) did not find *H. pylori* in laryngeal SCC and non-neoplastic specimens using haematoxylin and eosin stain or modified Giemsa stain. Akbayir et al. (2005) found *H. pylori* in specimens collected from laryngeal cancers and benign laryngeal disorders by histopathological methods, but not by immunohistochemical methods. Only one study performed PCR genotyping of *H. pylori* strains in specimens collected from the oropharynx. Tonsillar tissue specimens were collected from patients with chronic tonsillitis, obstructive sleep apnea syndrome (OSAS) and tonsillar cancer. The detected *H. pylori* strains differ from strains found in the stomachs of Czech patients with gastric diseases (Pavlik et al. 2007).

## 7. Comparison of oral and oropharyngeal genotypes

It is supposed that *H. pylori* is spread from person to person by oral-oral or faecal-oral route (Brown 2000), this hypothesis has not yet been convincingly demonstrated. Assuming the oral cavity and oropharynx as a gateway of infection, we can assume that in the oral cavity and oropharynx of the same individual we can find *H. pylori* strains of the same genotype. Initial works focused on comparison of oral and gastric *H. pylori* strains used endonuklease restriction analysis, single strand conformation polymorphism analysis (SSCP) or PCR (Shames et al. 1989; Khandaker et al. 1993; Zhang and Lu 1997; Kim et al. 2003). Identical strains have been found in gastric mucosa and oral cavity. The first comparison of gastric and oral *H. pylori* strains using PCR genotyping performed Wang et al. (2002) and, consequently, Burgers et al. (2008). Different genotypes in the stomach and oral cavity were found in both studies. PCR assays used by these authors could be considered more accurate

| Author | Year | Subjects | Specimens | Diagnostic Method | Number of Subjects positive for *H.pylori* |
|---|---|---|---|---|---|
| Di Bonaventura | 2000 | 36 | tonsillar swabs | culture, imunohistochemistry | 0 (0%) |
| Di Bonaventura | 2001 | 75 | tonsillar swabs and biopsy | PCR | 0 (0%) |
| Unver et al. | 2001 | 19 | adenoid tissue | CLO test | 11 (58%) |
| Skinner et al. | 2001 | 50 | tonsillar tissue | CLO test, imunocytochemistry | 0 (0%) CLO test and imunocytochem. |
| Uygur-Bayramicli | 2002 | 27 | tonsillar tissue | histology, imunohistochemistry | 0 (0%) histology and imunohistochemistry |
| Cirak | 2003 | 23 | tonsillar and adenoid tissue | PCR (16S ribosomal RNA, CagA) | 7 ( 30%) positive for *H. pylori* 5 of them (71%) positive for Cag A gene |
| Yilmaz et al. | 2004 | 50 | tonsillar and adenoid tissue | CLO test | 0 (0%) |
| Yilmaz et al. | 2005 | 38 | adenoid tissue, middle ear effusions | PCR (23S ribosomal RNA) | 12 (67%) in middle ear effusion. 1 (5%) in adenoid tissue |
| Pitkaranta | 2005 | 20 | adenoid tissue and middle ear fluid | culture | 0 (0%) |
| Khademi et al. | 2005 | 56 | tonsillar and adenoid tissue | CLO test | 27 (48%) |
| Bitar | 2005 | 25 | adenoid tissue | RUT, histology and nested PCR (UreA) | 21 (84%) positive by RUT, 4 (16%) positive by histology 0 (0%) positive by nested PCR |
| Bulut | 2006 | 71 | tonsillar and adenoid tissue | PCR (CagA - glmM gene) | 29 (24,6%) postitive for *H. pylori* 17 of them (58,6%) CagA positive |
| Bitar | 2006 | 28 | adenoid tissue and middle ear fluid | culture, RUT, PCR (urease-C, adhesion subunit genes) | 0 (0%) middle ear fluids 10 (77%) adenoid tissue by RUT 0 (0%) by PCR |
| Yilmaz et al. | 2006 | 22 | middle ear fluid, promontorium mucosa, adenoid and tonsillar tissue | culture, PCR (16S RNA) | middle ear fluids: 2 positive by culture, 7 by PCR mucosa: 1 by culture, 7 by PCR adenoids 11 (50%) by culture, 14 (64%) by PCR tonsillar tissue:12 (55%) by culture, 14 (64% by PCR) |
| Kusano et al. | 2007 | 173 | palatal tonsils | immunohistochemistry, immunoelectron microscopy, in-situ hybridization, PCR (16S RNA gene) | 126 (72,9%) positive |
| Vayisoglu et al. | 2008 | 91 | tonsillar and adenoid tissue | RUT, immunohistochemistry | 2 (2,2%) adenoid tissue, 0 (0%) tonsillar tissue using RUT, 0(0%) immunohostochemistry |
| Eyigor et al. | 2009 | 55 | 35 adenoids, 20 tonsils | RUT, PCR (glmM gene) | RUT 5,5% positive, 0% PCR positive |
| Ozcan | 2009 | 25 | adenoid tissue, middle ear fluid | CLO, immunohistochemistry | 0 (0%) CLO positive, 0 (0%) immunohistochemistry positive |
| Jabbari Moghaddam | 2009 | 285 | tonsillar tissue | RUT, histopathology | 113 (39.6%) positive by histopatology 40 (14%) positive by RUT |
| Vilarinho et al. | 2010 | 62 | adenoid and tonsillar tissue | RUT, immunohistochemistry, fluorescence in situ hybridization (FISH), PCR-DNA hybridization assay (vacA gene) | 3 positive by RUT, 2 positive by immunohistochemistry, 0 positive by FISH, 0 positive by PCR |
| Abdel-Monem | 2011 | 20 | adenoid and tonsillar tissue | RUT, PCR (ureC gene) | 16 (53.3%) positive by RUT, 5 (16.6%) positive by PCR |

Table 1. Studies focused on detection of pharyngeal presence of *H. pylori*

| Author | Year | Subjects | Specimens | Diagnostic Method | Number of Subjects Positive for *H. pylori* |
|---|---|---|---|---|---|
| Grandis et al. | 1997 | 42 | 21 SCC 21 controls without SCC | serology - IgG antibodies | 57% with SCC 62% controls |
| Okuda et al. | 2000 | 116 | 116 gastric and oral samples including 58 oral cancers | RT-PCR, culture | 46,6% gastric samples 12,1% oral swab samples 100% oral cancer swabs |
| Aygenc et al. | 2001 | 58 | 26 laryngeal SCC 32 controls without SCC | serology - IgG antibodies | 73% with SCC 41% controls |
| Rubin et al. | 2003 | 61 | 6 severe laryngeal dysplasia, 5 tonsillar SCC, 50 other SCC | serology | 38 seropositive ( including all tonsillar SCC) |
| Akbayir et al | 2005 | 100 | 50 laryngeal SCC 50 benign laryngeal disorders | histopathological and imunohistochemical methods | 0 (0%) imunihist. 28 SCC, 1 benign by histol. |
| Kanda et al. | 2005 | 31 | 31 SCC | PCR, culture, immunohistochemical analysis, serology - from urine | 21 seropositive 0 PCR, culture , immunohist. |
| Nurgalieva et al. | 2005 | 230 | 119 laryngeal or pharyngeal SCC 111 controls without SCC | serology - IgG antibodies | 32,8% with SCC 27,0% controls |
| Kizilay et al. | 2006 | 99 | 69 laryngeal SCC 30 nonneoplastic controls | histology - HE, modified Giemsa stain | 0% |
| Pavlik et al. | 2006 | 7 | 3 chronic tonsillitis 3 tonsillar SCC 1 OSAS | serology IgA, IgG, IgM PCR genotyping | 2 of 3 chronic tonsillitis serolgicaly 2 of 3 chronic tonsillitis, 3 of 3 SCC and 1 of 1 OSAS by PCR |

Table 2. Studies focused on possible role of *H. pylori* in head and neck carcinogenesis

(Schabereiter-Gurtner et al. 2004). Findings of Lukes et al. (2009) are in concordance with these results. In four of six individuals different genotypes of *H. pylori* strains were found in the stomach and oropharynx. The results also show that from 20 individuals with proven oropharyngeal *H. pylori* infection, only 8 had concurrent gastric infection. This confirms the findings of Burgers et al. (2008), who report that only 38% of persons with demonstrated presence of *H. pylori* in the oral cavity also had the infection in the stomach. These authors also reported the finding of 10 cases with positive *H. pylori* in saliva, with no detectable specific anti-*H. pylori* antibodies in serum. This is consistent with the results obtained by Lukes et. al. (2009). *H. pylori* was found in the oropharynx in 12 patients with no demonstrable antibody response.

## 8. Conclusions

Oral cavity (saliva and dental plaque) is now considered a possible extragastric reservoir of *H. pylori*. The published works dealing with oropharyngeal and nasopharyngeal detection of *H. pylori* infection have yielded contradictory results. Pharyngeal detection of *H. pylori* was reported in the range of 0-90%. Regarding that the various authors used different methods of detection, it is not possible to reach valuable conclusions. Frequently used tests like CLO test and RUT appears to be inappropriate methods for diagnosis of pharyngeal *H. pylori*. The presence of other urease-producing bacterial strains in the pharynx can lead to false positive results. Culture has proved to be very difficult and not very resistant to external influences, which may even prevent a successful detection. Molecular diagnostics (PCR) can be regarded as a method with sufficient sensitivity and specificity. Results achieved by these methods demonstrated the presence of *H. pylori* in the lymphoid tissue of oropharynx and nasopharynx. PCR method allows not only detect the presence of *H. pylori* infection, but also genotyping of strains within the tissue. The fact remains that the PCR methods allow determine the presence of bacterial DNA but can not determine whether the DNA comes from live or dead bacteria. Results of culture despite the very low numbers of positive results indicate the possible presence of viable bacteria capable of reproduction. High susceptibility of *H. pylori* in adverse effects during transport of specimens or during handling in the laboratory can explain low numbers of positive results of culture. Also, a frequent colonisation of oropharyngeal tissue by other bacterial species can have a significant influence on the failure of the culture of *H. pylori*.

The assumption that the oropharyngeal *H. pylori* infection may contribute to oropharyngeal carcinogenesis as a direct mutagen was not confirmed yet. An analogous situation, however, occurs in the stomach, where prevalence of *H. pylori* infection among the population is reported between 40-80%, serious stomach problems such as gastroduodenal ulcer disease or gastric cancer has only 10 -15% of infected.

Virulence of *H. pylori* strains varies according to the production of toxins. This production is due to the presence of virulence factor genes. Most important are the *cagA* gene and *vacA* gene. The main carcinogenic effect of *H. pylori* is declared to be associated with the presence of *cagA* gene and s1/m1 combination of alleles of *vacA* gene. Recent studies indicate that *H. pylori* may exist in the oropharynx independently to the gastric infection. Comparison of genotypes of *H. pylori* in the oral cavity, oropharynx, and stomach showed that an individual can host more than one strain of *H. pylori* in various locations. Differences were found in the presence of *cagA* gene and in the structure of *vacA* gene.

The findings of *H. pylori* in the oral cavity and oropharynx without demonstrable specific anti-*H. pylori* antibodies in serum are remarkable. This could be explained by an early detection of *H. pylori* presence after primary infection, when the antibody response has not started yet. Next, the possibility that *H. pylori* could colonize the oral cavity and the oropharynx without inducing the host immune response must be considered. Another possible explanation is the presence of *H. pylori* coccoid forms. These are viable form of bacteria that can not be cultivated by conventional microbiological techniques and are characterized by a reduced virulence.

The question of transmission of *H. pylori* has not been satisfactorily resolved yet. If we consider the oral-oral or faecal-oral route as a way of transmission, we can assume finding of the same *H. pylori* strains in the oropharynx and stomach in the same individual. The findings of different genotypes in both locations still lack an accurate explanation. Inoculation of mixtures of *H. pylori* strains and consequently their different settlements in the different areas according to sensitivity of the strains could be one of the possible explanations. It can be assumed that the area of the oropharynx is less favourable for *H. pylori*, and can only be colonized by more resistant strains. One of the negative factors for growth and reproduction of *H. pylori* is the presence of other bacterial strains that were able to stop the growth of *H. pylori* during in-vitro experiments. A variety of bacterial colonization in the oral cavity and oropharynx can be assumed.

Epidemiological data on the prevalence of *H. pylori* infection published in the literature are often based on serological detection of specific anti-*H. pylori* antibodies. The prevalence of infection is reported 40-80%. The presence of anti-*H. pylori* antibodies was given in relation only to gastric infection. The newly obtained data prove the possibility of the presence of *H. pylori* infection in other locations independently to the gastric infection. This should be considered in future epidemiological studies. Not only antibodies should be evaluated but also identification of the exact location of the infection must be done.

In the future it would be appropriate to focus attention on local effects of *H. pylori* in oropharyngeal lymphoid tissue. Changes in the expression of some cytokines caused by *H. pylori*, which were described in the gastric mucosa, can be expected in the oropharyngeal tissue. Another study focused on oropharyngeal *H. pylori* genotyping should be done. In case that high virulent *H. pylori* strains can survive in oropharyngeal tissue, translocation of toxins into the oropharyngeal mucosa cells with subsequent cytokine response can be expected. Nevertheless this assumption has not been confirmed nor refuted yet.

## 9. Acknowledgements

This work was supported by grant NT11523 of the Internal Grant Agency of the Ministry of Health of the Czech Republic

## 10. References

Abdel-Monem MH, Magdy EA, Nour YA, Harfoush RA, Ibreak A (2011) Detection of Helicobacter pylori in adenotonsillar tissue of children with chronic adenotonsillitis using rapid urease test, PCR and blood serology: A prospective study. Int J Pediatr Otorhinolaryngol

Akbayir N, Basak T, Seven H, Sungun A, Erdem L (2005) Investigation of Helicobacter pylori colonization in laryngeal neoplasia. Eur Arch Otorhinolaryngol 262:170-172.

Aygenc E, Selcuk A, Celikkanat S, Ozbek C, Ozdem C (2001) The role of Helicobacter pylori infection in the cause of squamous cell carcinoma of the larynx. Otolaryngol Head Neck Surg 125:520-521.

Bitar M, Mahfouz R, Soweid A, Racoubian E, Ghasham M, Zaatari G, Fuleihan N (2006) Does Helicobacter pylori colonize the nasopharynx of children and contribute to their middle ear disease? Acta Otolaryngol 126:154-159.

Bitar MA, Soweid A, Mahfouz R, Zaatari G, Fuleihan N (2005) Is Helicobacter pylori really present in the adenoids of children? Eur Arch Otorhinolaryngol 262:987-992.

Blanchard TG, Drakes ML, Czinn SJ (2004) Helicobacter infection: pathogenesis. Curr Opin Gastroenterol 20:10-15.

Boncristiano M, Paccani SR, Barone S, Ulivieri C, Patrussi L, Ilver D, Amedei A, D'Elios MM, Telford JL, Baldari CT (2003) The Helicobacter pylori vacuolating toxin inhibits T cell activation by two independent mechanisms. J Exp Med 198:1887-1897.

Brown LM (2000) Helicobacter pylori: epidemiology and routes of transmission. Epidemiol Rev 22:283-297.

Bulut Y, Agacayak A, Karlidag T, Toraman ZA, Yilmaz M (2006) Association of cagA+ Helicobacter pylori with adenotonsillar hypertrophy. Tohoku J Exp Med 209:229-233.

Bures J, Kopacova M, Koupil I, Vorisek V, Rejchrt S, Beranek M, Seifert B, Pozler O, Zivny P, Douda T, Kolesarova M, Pinter M, Palicka V, Holcik J (2006) Epidemiology of Helicobacter pylori infection in the Czech Republic. Helicobacter 11:56-65.

Burgers R, Schneider-Brachert W, Reischl U, Behr A, Hiller KA, Lehn N, Schmalz G, Ruhl S (2008) Helicobacter pylori in human oral cavity and stomach. Eur J Oral Sci 116:297-304.

Cave DR (1996) Transmission and epidemiology of Helicobacter pylori. Am J Med 100:12S-17S; discussion 17S-18S.

Cirak MY, Ozdek A, Yilmaz D, Bayiz U, Samim E, Turet S (2003) Detection of Helicobacter pylori and its CagA gene in tonsil and adenoid tissues by PCR. Arch Otolaryngol Head Neck Surg 129:1225-1229.

Cover TL, Blaser MJ (1992) Purification and characterization of the vacuolating toxin from Helicobacter pylori. J Biol Chem 267:10570-10575.

Crabtree JE (1996) Immune and inflammatory responses to Helicobacter pylori infection. Scand J Gastroenterol Suppl 215:3-10.

Di Bonaventura G (2001) Do tonsils represent an extragastric reservoir for Helicobacter pylori infection. J Infect 42(3):221-222.

Dowsett SA, Kowolik MJ (2003) Oral Helicobacter pylori: can we stomach it? Crit Rev Oral Biol Med 14:226-233.

Eyigor M, Eyigor H, Gultekin B, Aydin N (2009) Detection of Helicobacter pylori in adenotonsiller tissue specimens by rapid urease test and polymerase chain reaction. Eur Arch Otorhinolaryngol 266:1611-1613.

Gallo O, Masini E, Morbidelli L, Franchi A, Fini-Storchi I, Vergari WA, Ziche M (1998) Role of nitric oxide in angiogenesis and tumor progression in head and neck cancer. J Natl Cancer Inst 90:587-596.

Gisbert JP, Pajares JM (2004) Review article: C-urea breath test in the diagnosis of Helicobacter pylori infection -- a critical review. Aliment Pharmacol Ther 20:1001-1017.

Gobert AP, Mersey BD, Cheng Y, Blumberg DR, Newton JC, Wilson KT (2002) Cutting edge: urease release by Helicobacter pylori stimulates macrophage inducible nitric oxide synthase. J Immunol 168:6002-6006.

Grandis JR, Perez-Perez GI, Yu VL, Johnson JT, Blaser MJ (1997) Lack of serologic evidence for Helicobacter pylori infection in head and neck cancer. Head Neck 19:216-218.

Guillemin K, Salama NR, Tompkins LS, Falkow S (2002) Cag pathogenicity island-specific responses of gastric epithelial cells to Helicobacter pylori infection. Proc Natl Acad Sci U S A 99:15136-15141.

Hafsi N, Voland P, Schwendy S, Rad R, Reindl W, Gerhard M, Prinz C (2004) Human dendritic cells respond to Helicobacter pylori, promoting NK cell and Th1-effector responses in vitro. J Immunol 173:1249-1257.

Hatakeyama M (2006) The role of Helicobacter pylori CagA in gastric carcinogenesis. Int J Hematol 84:301-308.

Hep A (2003) Současné možnosti diagnostiky Helicobacter pylori. MEDICÍNA PO PROMOCI 4:6-8.

IARC (1994) Schistosomes, liver flukes and Helicobacter pylori. IARC Working Group on the Evaluation of Carcinogenic Risks to Humans. Lyon, 7-14 June 1994. IARC Monogr Eval Carcinog Risks Hum 61:1-241.

Israel DA, Peek RM (2001) pathogenesis of Helicobacter pylori-induced gastric inflammation. Aliment Pharmacol Ther 15:1271-1290.

Kanda T (2005) Investigation of Helicobacter pylori tumor tissue specimens from patients of head and neck tumor. Practica Oto-Rhino-Laryngologica 98:571-575.

Keates S, Sougioultzis S, Keates AC, Zhao D, Peek RM, Jr., Shaw LM, Kelly CP (2001) cag+ Helicobacter pylori induce transactivation of the epidermal growth factor receptor in AGS gastric epithelial cells. J Biol Chem 276:48127-48134.

Khandaker K, Palmer KR, Eastwood MA, Scott AC, Desai M, Owen RJ (1993) DNA fingerprints of Helicobacter pylori from mouth and antrum of patients with chronic ulcer dyspepsia. Lancet 342:751.

Kim JM, Kim JS, Jung HC, Oh YK, Chung HY, Lee CH, Song IS (2003) Helicobacter pylori infection activates NF-kappaB signaling pathway to induce iNOS and protect human gastric epithelial cells from apoptosis. Am J Physiol Gastrointest Liver Physiol 285:G1171-1180.

Kim N, Lim SH, Lee KH, You JY, Kim JM, Lee NR, Jung HC, Song IS, Kim CY (2000) Helicobacter pylori in dental plaque and saliva. Korean J Intern Med 15:187-194.

Kizilay A, Saydam L, Aydin A, Kalcioglu MT, Ozturan O, Aydin NE (2006) Histopathologic examination for Helicobacter pylori as a possible etiopathogenic factor in laryngeal carcinoma. Chemotherapy 52:80-82.

Konturek PC, Ernst H, Konturek SJ, Bobrzynski AJ, Faller G, Klingler C, Hahn EG (1997) Mucosal expression and luminal release of epidermal and transforming growth factors in patients with duodenal ulcer before and after eradication of Helicobacter pylori. Gut 40:463-469.

Kusano K, Tokunaga O, Ando T, Inokuchi A (2007) Helicobacter pylori in the palatine tonsils of patients with IgA nephropathy compared with those of patients with recurrent pharyngotonsillitis. Hum Pathol 38:1788-1797.

Kusters JG, van Vliet AH, Kuipers EJ (2006) Pathogenesis of Helicobacter pylori infection. Clin Microbiol Rev 19:449-490.

Letley DP, Lastovica A, Louw JA, Hawkey CJ, Atherton JC (1999) Allelic diversity of the Helicobacter pylori vacuolating cytotoxin gene in South Africa: rarity of the vacA s1a genotype and natural occurrence of an s2/m1 allele. J Clin Microbiol 37:1203-1205.

Lukes P, Pavlik E, Potuznikova B, Plzak J, Nartova E, Dosedel J, Katra R, Sterzl I, Betka J, Astl J (2009) Comparison of Helicobacter pylori genotypes obtained from the oropharynx and stomach of the same individuals. Unpublished manuscript

Martinez-Gomis J, Diouf A, Lakhssassi N, Sixou M (2006) Absence of Helicobacter pylori in the oral cavity of 10 non-dyspeptic subjects demonstrated by real-time polymerase chain reaction. Oral Microbiol Immunol 21:407-410.

Miehlke S, Kirsch C, Agha-Amiri K, Gunther T, Lehn N, Malfertheiner P, Stolte M, Ehninger G, Bayerdorffer E (2000) The Helicobacter pylori vacA s1, m1 genotype and cagA is associated with gastric carcinoma in Germany. Int J Cancer 87:322-327.

Mobley HL (1996) Defining Helicobacter pylori as a pathogen: strain heterogeneity and virulence. Am J Med 100:2S-9S; discussion 9S-11S.

Nurgalieva ZZ, Graham DY, Dahlstrom KR, Wei Q, Sturgis EM (2005) A pilot study of Helicobacter pylori infection and risk of laryngopharyngeal cancer. Head Neck 27:22-27.

Okuda K, Ishihara K, Miura T, Katakura A, Noma H, Ebihara Y (2000) Helicobacter pylori may have only a transient presence in the oral cavity and on the surface of oral cancer. Microbiol Immunol 44:385-388.

Oliveira MJ, Costa AC, Costa AM, Henriques L, Suriano G, Atherton JC, Machado JC, Carneiro F, Seruca R, Mareel M, Leroy A, Figueiredo C (2006) Helicobacter pylori induces gastric epithelial cell invasion in a c-Met and type IV secretion system-dependent manner. J Biol Chem 281:34888-34896.

Pavlik E, Lukes P, Potuznikova B, Astl J, Hrda P, Soucek A, Matucha P, Dosedel J, Sterzl I (2007) Helicobacter pylori isolated from patients with tonsillar cancer or tonsillitis chronica could be of different genotype compared to isolates from gastrointestinal tract. Folia Microbiol (Praha) 52:91-94.

Portal-Celhay C, Perez-Perez GI (2006) Immune responses to Helicobacter pylori colonization: mechanisms and clinical outcomes. Clin Sci (Lond) 110:305-314.

Qureshi H, Ahmed W, Zuberi SJ, Kazi J (1992) Use of CLO test in the detection of Helicobacter pylori infection and its correlation with histologic gastritis. J Pak Med Assoc 42:292-293.

Rubin Grandis J, Melhem MF, Gooding WE, Day R, Holst VA, Wagener MM, Drenning SD, Tweardy DJ (1998) Levels of TGF-alpha and EGFR protein in head and neck squamous cell carcinoma and patient survival. J Natl Cancer Inst 90:824-832.

Rubin JS, Benjamin E, Prior A, Lavy J (2003) The prevalence of Helicobacter pylori infection in malignant and premalignant conditions of the head and neck. J Laryngol Otol 117:118-121.

Sachs G, Weeks DL, Melchers K, Scott DR (2003) The gastric biology of Helicobacter pylori. Annu Rev Physiol 65:349-369.

Sakaguchi AA, Miura S, Takeuchi T, Hokari R, Mizumori M, Yoshida H, Higuchi H, Mori M, Kimura H, Suzuki H, Ishii H (1999) Increased expression of inducible nitric oxide synthase and peroxynitrite in Helicobacter pylori gastric ulcer. Free Radic Biol Med 27:781-789.

Segal ED (1997) Consequences of attachment of Helicobacter pylori to gastric cells. Biomed Pharmacother 51:5-12.

Segal ED, Cha J, Lo J, Falkow S, Tompkins LS (1999) Altered states: involvement of phosphorylated CagA in the induction of host cellular growth changes by Helicobacter pylori. Proc Natl Acad Sci U S A 96:14559-14564.

Shames B, Krajden S, Fuksa M, Babida C, Penner JL (1989) Evidence for the occurrence of the same strain of Campylobacter pylori in the stomach and dental plaque. J Clin Microbiol 27:2849-2850.

Schabereiter-Gurtner C, Hirschl AM, Dragosics B, Hufnagl P, Puz S, Kovach Z, Rotter M, Makristathis A (2004) Novel real-time PCR assay for detection of Helicobacter pylori infection and simultaneous clarithromycin susceptibility testing of stool and biopsy specimens. J Clin Microbiol 42:4512-4518.

Schiemann U, Konturek J, Assert R, Rembiasz K, Domschke W, Konturek S, Pfeiffer A (2002) mRNA expression of EGF receptor ligands in atrophic gastritis before and after Helicobacter pylori eradication. Med Sci Monit 8:CR53-58.

Stromberg E, Edebo A, Svennerholm AM, Lindholm C (2003) Decreased epithelial cytokine responses in the duodenal mucosa of Helicobacter pylori-infected duodenal ulcer patients. Clin Diagn Lab Immunol 10:116-124.

Tummala S, Keates S, Kelly CP (2004) Update on the immunologic basis of Helicobacter pylori gastritis. Curr Opin Gastroenterol 20:592-597.

Van Doorn LJ, Figueiredo C, Megraud F, Pena S, Midolo P, Queiroz DM, Carneiro F, Vanderborght B, Pegado MD, Sanna R, De Boer W, Schneeberger PM, Correa P, Ng EK, Atherton J, Blaser MJ, Quint WG (1999) Geographic distribution of vacA allelic types of Helicobacter pylori. Gastroenterology 116:823-830.

Vilarinho S, Guimaraes NM, Ferreira RM, Gomes B, Wen X, Vieira MJ, Carneiro F, Godinho T, Figueiredo C (2010) Helicobacter pylori colonization of the adenotonsillar tissue: fact or fiction? Int J Pediatr Otorhinolaryngol 74:807-811.

Wang J, Chi DS, Laffan JJ, Li C, Ferguson DA, Jr., Litchfield P, Thomas E (2002) Comparison of cytotoxin genotypes of Helicobacter pylori in stomach and saliva. Dig Dis Sci 47:1850-1856.

Yilmaz M, Kara CO, Kaleli I, Demir M, Tumkaya F, Buke AS, Topuz B (2004) Are tonsils a reservoir for Helicobacter pylori infection in children? Int J Pediatr Otorhinolaryngol 68:307-310.

Yilmaz T, Ceylan M, Akyon Y, Ozcakyr O, Gursel B (2006) Helicobacter pylori: a possible association with otitis media with effusion. Otolaryngol Head Neck Surg 134:772-777.

Zhang Y, Lu X (1997) [Detection and differentiation of Helicobacter pylori from gastric biopsy and saliva by PCR-SSCP]. Zhonghua Nei Ke Za Zhi 36:446-449.

# Part 2

## Molecular Mechanisms
of Peptic Ulcer Development and Healing

# 7

# Pathophysiology of Gastric Ulcer Development and Healing: Molecular Mechanisms and Novel Therapeutic Options

Matteo Fornai, Luca Antonioli, Rocchina Colucci,
Marco Tuccori and Corrado Blandizzi
*Department of Internal Medicine,*
*University of Pisa, Pisa,*
*Italy*

## 1. Introduction

The stomach plays a pivotal role in the digestion of foods that we eat. With the exception of rare cases, this organ can resist to a large variety of noxious factors, including hydrochloric acid, refluxed bile salts and alcohol, with a wide range of temperatures and osmolality. This high resistance to injuries depends on a number of physiological responses elicited by the mucosal lining against potentially harmful luminal agents, as well as to the ability of rapidly repairing the mucosal damage when it does occur (Laine et al., 2008). Nevertheless, when these protective mechanisms are overwhelmed by injurious factors, a gastric mucosal lesion may develop. Major detrimental effects on gastric mucosa are exerted by non-steroidal anti-inflammatory drugs (NSAIDs). These drugs are able not only to exert gastric injuring effects, but also to delay the healing of ulcer lesions through a variety of local and systemic mechanisms (Musumba et al., 2009).

Since the discovery that prostaglandin biosynthesis could be inhibited by NSAIDs through the blockade of cyclooxygenase enzymes, there has been a great interest in the contribution of prostaglandins to the mechanisms of gastric mucosal defense. Thus, it has been appreciated that these lipidic mediators are able to modulate virtually every factor involved in mucosal protection, and the importance of this contribution is made evident by the increased susceptibility of the stomach to injury following the intake of NSAIDs. Indeed, chronic treatments with these drugs can be associated with the development of ulcers in the stomach, and research over the past two decades has helped to identify some of the key events, triggered by cyclooxygenase blockade, which take part to ulcer formation and/or impairment of ulcer healing. Since many years, it has been recognized that NSAIDs can interfere with gastric mucosal physiology also through injuring mechanisms unrelated to the inhibition of prostaglandin biosynthesis, such as oxidative stress and changes in epithelial cell proliferation/apoptosis balance.

Following the discovery of two isoforms of cyclooxygenase (COX-1 and COX-2), and based on the assumption that COX-2 was an inducible enzyme responsible for inflammation, but devoid of gastroprotective functions (Vane et al., 1998), selective COX-2 inhibitors (coxibs, including celecoxib, rofecoxib, valdecoxib, parecoxib, etoricoxib and lumiracoxib) were clinically developed as novel anti-inflammatory/analgesic drugs characterized by reduced gastric toxicity (Dubois et al., 2004). These advances have then fostered intensive preclinical and clinical research supporting the view that coxibs may confer advantages over conventional non-selective NSAIDs in terms of gastrointestinal risk reduction. Nevertheless, there are still a number of unresolved issues in this field, and the criteria for an appropriate use of coxibs in patients with various degrees of gastrointestinal risk, including ongoing gastric ulcerations, remain matter of discussion.

Another relevant topic, regarding the integrity of gastric mucosa, is represented by the use of proton pump inhibitors (PPIs). These drugs have been proven not only to prevent NSAID-induced upper gastrointestinal injury, but also to promote the healing process once the damage has occurred, even in the presence of a continued NSAID administration. The beneficial effects of PPIs can be largely ascribed to their ability to maintain a sustained inhibition of gastric acid secretion. However, there is also evidence to suggest that pharmacodynamic properties unrelated to acid inhibition may contribute to the therapeutic actions of these drugs (Blandizzi et al., 2008).

Recent research has highlighted the fact that, beside prostaglandins, gastric mucosal protective functions can be accomplished by other mediators, with particular regard for the gaseous mediators nitric oxide (NO) and hydrogen sulfide ($H_2S$). Moreover, anti-inflammatory drugs endowed with dual cyclooxygenase/5-lypooxygenase inhibitory effects, such as licofelone, could represent novel therapeutic strategies helping to drive the development of safer anti-inflammatory drugs and effective therapies to accelerate and improve the quality of ulcer healing (Blandizzi et al., 2009).

This chapter is focused on the available evidence on the molecular mechanisms underlying the pathophysiology of gastric injury development and healing, as well as on novel therapeutic options for prevention and treatment of gastric ulcers.

## 2. Mechanisms of gastric mucosal defense

The mechanisms of gastric mucosal defense include several local and neurohormonal protective factors, which allow the mucosa to resist against frequent exposures to damaging factors (Laine et al., 2008). In the following sections, a detailed description of the mucosal defense mechanisms is provided.

### 2.1 Local mechanisms of gastric mucosal defense
### 2.1.1 Mucus-bicarbonate-phospholipid barrier
The first line of gastric mucosal defense is represented by the mucus-bicarbonate-phospholipid barrier (Lichtenberger, 1999). The surface of gastric mucosa is covered by a layer formed by mucus gel, bicarbonate anions and surfactant phospholipids. This unstirred layer is capable of retaining the bicarbonate ions secreted by surface epithelial cells and maintaining a microenvironment with a pH near to 7 at the mucus-mucosa interface. The mucus layer is also able to prevent the penetration of pepsin, thus avoiding the proteolytic digestion of epithelium (Allen and Flemstrom, 2005). In addition, the luminal surface of mucus gel is covered by a film of surfactant phospholipids which confers hydrophobic properties to the mucus layer (Lichtenberger, 1999).

The mucus gel is secreted by surface epithelial cells and is formed by a large amount of water (about 95%) and various kinds of mucin glycoproteins (i.e., MUC2, MUC5AC, MUC5B and MUC6), the production of which may vary in different regions of the gastric mucosa (Allen and Flemstrom, 2005; Ho et al., 2004). Gel-forming mucin units polymerize into large mucin multimers, which are essential for gel formation. The mucus gel is secreted along with low-molecular weight trefoil factor (CRF) family (TFF) peptides, which play a relevant role in the formation of the mucus layer (Newton et al., 2000). For example, TFF2 is known to increase the viscosity of gastric mucin and stabilize the gel network (Thim et al., 2002). The secretion of gastric mucus is regulated also by various gastrointestinal hormones, including gastrin and secretin, as well as prostaglandins and acetylcholine (Allen and Flemstrom, 2005).

The secretion of bicarbonate into the mucus gel layer is essential to maintain a pH gradient at the epithelial surface, which represents a first line of defense against gastric acid (Allen and Flemstrom, 2005). Bicarbonate secretion from the apical membrane of surface epithelial cells is mediated by a $Cl^-/HCO_3^-$ anion exchanger, and it is stimulated by various factors, including prostaglandins (via $EP_1$ receptors), luminal acid, corticotrophin-releasing factor, melatonin, uroguanylin and orexin A (Allen and Flemstrom, 2005; Montrose et al., 2006).

The mucus-bicarbonate barrier is the only system which segregates the epithelium from the gastric lumen. Therefore, when this protective barrier breaks down during pathological events or upon detrimental actions by injuring agents, a second line of protective mechanisms comes into play. They include intracellular acid neutralization, rapid epithelial repair, and maintenance of mucosal blood flow.

### 2.1.2 Epithelial cells

The continuous layer of surface epithelial cells represents the next line of mucosal defense. This epithelial tissue is responsible for the production of mucus, bicarbonate and other components of the gastric mucosal barrier. These cells are hydrophobic in nature, being able to repel acid- and water-soluble injuring agents, owing to the presence of phospholipids on their surface (Lichtenberger, 1999). Surface epithelial cells are also closely interconnected by tight junctions, forming a continuous barrier, which prevents back diffusion of acid and pepsin (Allen and Flemstrom, 2005). Another relevant protective factor, available in the epithelial cells, is represented by heat shock proteins, which are activated in response to stress, including temperature increments, oxidative stress and cytotoxic agents (Tanaka et al., 2007). These proteins can prevent protein denaturation and protect cells against injury. Cathelicidin and beta-defensin are cationic peptides which play a relevant role in the innate defensive system at the mucosal surface, preventing bacterial colonization (Yang et al., 2006). In addition, TFFs secreted by epithelial cells regulate the re-epithelization process and exert mucosal protective actions (Taupin and Podolsky, 2003).

### 2.1.3 Mucosal cell renewal

The integrity of gastric epithelium is maintained by a continuous process of cell renewal ensured by mucosal progenitor cells. These cells are subjected to a continuous, well coordinated and controlled proliferation, which ensures the replacement of damaged or aged cells on the epithelial surface. The process of complete epithelial renewal takes about 3-7 days, while the overall glandular cell replacement requires months. However, the restitution of surface epithelium after damage occurs very quickly (i.e., few minutes) and results by migration of preserved cells located in the neck area of gastric glands (Laine et al., 2008).

The process of cell turnover is regulated by growth factors. In particular, a marked expression of epidermal growth factor receptor (EGF-R) has been detected in gastric progenitor cells. Such a receptor can be activated by mitogenic growth factors, such as transforming growth factor-α (TGF-α) and insulin-like growth factor-1 (IGF-1) (Nguyen et al., 2007). In addition, $PGE_2$ and gastrin are able to transactivate the EGF-R and promote the activation of mitogen-activated protein kinase (MAPK) pathway, with consequent stimulation of cell proliferation (Pai et al., 2002). Notably, the presence of EGF has not been detected in the normal mucosa, although it is contained in the gastric juice, as a product of salivary and esophageal glands, and can stimulate mucosal cell proliferation in case of injury (Milani and Calabrò, 2001). In addition, mucosal progenitor cells do express survivin, an antiapoptotic factor, which inhibits apoptotic cell death (Chiou et al., 2005).

### 2.1.4 Mucosal blood flow

Mucosal blood flow is essential to deliver oxygen and nutrients and to remove toxic metabolites from gastric mucosa. Arteries embedded into the muscularis mucosae branch into capillaries, which then enter the lamina propria and travel toward the proximity of glandular epithelial cells. Endothelial cells, lining these microvessels, produce NO and prostacyclin ($PGI_2$), which act as potent vasodilators, thus protecting the gastric mucosa against damage and counteracting the detrimental effects of various vasoconstrictors, including leukotriene $C_4$, thromboxane $A_2$, and endothelin. In addition, NO and $PGI_2$ maintain the viability of endothelial cells and inhibit platelet and leukocyte adhesion to the microvasculature, thus preventing the occurrence of microischaemic phenomena (Laine et al., 2008).

When the gastric mucosa is exposed to irritants or acid back-diffusion, a massive and rapid increase in mucosal blood flow occurs. This process allows removal and dilution of back-diffusing acid or noxious agents. The increase in blood flow is regarded as a pivotal mechanism for preventing gastric mucosal cell injury, and its decrease results in the development of tissue necrosis. The increase in mucosal blood flow is mediated by NO release, and there is experimental evidence demonstrating that NO protects the gastric mucosa against injury induced by ethanol or endothelin 1, while the inhibition of NO synthase enhances mucosal injury (Holzer, 2006). It has been also observed that another endogenous compound, $H_2S$, can exert protective actions against gastric mucosal injury. In particular, this compound has been shown to reduce the expression of tumor necrosis factor α (TNF-α), to decrease leukocyte adhesion to vascular endothelium, and to prevent NSAID-induced gastric mucosal damage (Fiorucci et al., 2006).

### 2.1.5 Sensory innervation

The vasculature of gastric mucosa and submucosa is innervated by extrinsic primary afferent sensory neurons, which are arranged in a plexus at the base of the mucosal layer (Holzer, 2007). The nerve fibers stemming from this plexus run along with capillary vessels and reach the basal membrane of surface epithelial cells. These nerves can detect luminal acidity or back-diffusing acid through acid-sensing channels. The activation of such sensory nerves modulates the contractile tone of submucosal arterioles, thus regulating the mucosal blood flow. In particular, the stimulation of sensory nerves leads to the release of calcitonin gene-related peptide (CGRP) and substance P from nerve terminals surrounding large submucosal vessels (Holzer, 2007). CGRP then contributes to the maintenance of mucosal integrity through the vasodilation of submucosal vessels mediated by NO release. Sensory innervation plays a prominent role in the protection of gastric mucosa from injury, as demonstrated by studies where the ablation of sensory transmission (i.e., with capsaicin) impaired the vasodilatatory response and increased the sensitivity of gastric mucosa to injuring agents (Holzer, 2007).

### 2.1.6 Prostaglandins

The gastric mucosa represents a source of continuous prostaglandin production, such as $PGE_2$ and $PGI_2$, which are regarded as crucial factors for the maintenance of mucosal integrity and protection against injuring factors (Halter et al., 2001; Brzozowski et al., 2005a). It has been demonstrated that prostaglandins have the potential to stimulate almost all the mucosal defense mechanisms. In particular, they reduce acid output, stimulate mucus, bicarbonate and phospholipid production, increase mucosal blood flow, and accelerate epithelial restitution and mucosal healing (Brzozowski et al., 2005a). Prostaglandins are also known to inhibit mast cell activation as well as leukocyte and platelet adhesion to the vascular endothelium (Halter et al., 2001; Brzozowski et al., 2005a). The beneficial actions exerted by $PGE_2$ have been shown to be mediated by activation of specific EP receptor subtypes. In particular, the activation of $EP_1$ receptors mediates the most important protective effects of prostaglandins, through an increase in bicarbonate secretion and mucosal blood flow in the damaged mucosa and a decrease in gastric motility (Takeuchi et al., 2002). Other EP receptor subtypes are also involved in the protective actions of $PGE_2$. For example, $EP_3$ receptors inhibit the gastric acid secretion, while $EP_4$ receptors stimulate the secretion of mucus (Kato et al., 2005).

### 2.2 Neurohormonal mechanisms

Gastric mucosal defense is supported by mechanisms activated, at least in part, by the central nervous system and hormonal factors (Laine et al., 2008). Experimental studies have demonstrated that central vagal activation stimulates mucus secretion and increases intracellular pH in the surface epithelial cells of in the stomach. In addition, while the CRF pathway is involved in endocrine responses to stress (Chatzaki et al., 2006). In addition, peripheral CRF contributes significantly to the regulation of gastric defense mechanisms, in particular, the CRF2 receptor is known to mediate antiapoptotic effects in gastric epithelial cells as well as to inhibit gastric emptying and motility (Chatzaki et al., 2006).

Other hormone mediators, including gastrin-17, cholecystokinin, thyrotropin-releasing hormone, bombesin, EGF, peptide YY and neurokinin A, play significant roles in the regulation of gastric protective mechanisms, which can be blunted by afferent nerve ablation, CGRP receptor blockade, and inhibition of NO synthase (Peskar, 2001; Moszik et al., 2001). Ghrelin, a hormone peptide produced by gastric A-like cells in rodents and P/D1 cells in humans, is involved in the regulation of growth hormone secretion and appetite stimulation (Brzozowski et al., 2005b). Moreover, it is also able to exert significant protective effects at gastric level, including the enhancement of mucosal blood flow via stimulation of NO and CGRP release from sensory afferent nerves (Brzozowski et al., 2005b).

Glucocorticoids have been shown to support the mechanisms of protection at gastric level. These hormones are involved in the response to stress, and represent potent gastroprotective factors against injury (Filaretova et al., 1998). Consistently with this contention, glucocorticoid antagonists enhanced the severity of stress-induced erosions, further supporting a protective role of these hormones during stress (Filaretova et al., 2001). The mechanisms through which glucocorticoids exert their protective effects include the maintenance of glucose homeostasis, the increase in mucosal blood flow and mucus secretion, and the attenuation of both enhanced gastric motility and microvascular permeability (Filaretova et al., 2007).

## 3. Mechanisms of gastric mucosal damage

Gastric mucosal injury may occur as a consequence of various conditions, including alcohol intake, refluxed bile salts, stress, aging and *Helicobacter pylori* infection, although the most important agents known to impair the mechanisms of gastric mucosal defense are represented by NSAIDs. For this reason, in the following sections a detailed description of NSAID-related mechanisms of gastric injury is provided.

### 3.1 Effects of NSAIDs on gastric mucosa

The pathophysiology of gastric injury associated with NSAID administration depends partly on cyclooxygenase inhibition and partly on cyclooxygenase-independent mechanisms, which result mainly from local direct actions (Scarpignato and Hunt, 2010). Cyclooxygenase blockade has been shown to increase the susceptibility of gastric mucosa to NSAID-induced injury by suppression of a number of prostaglandin-mediated protective functions. For instance, prostaglandins reduce the activation of neutrophils and the local release of reactive oxygen species (ROS). The production of prostacyclin by the endothelium of mucosal microcirculation is also highly relevant in ensuring a tonic inhibition of neutrophil adhesion. Therefore, NSAIDs can shift the mucosal balance toward the recruitment and endothelial adhesion of circulating neutrophils through the inhibition of prostaglandin biosynthesis (Whittle, 2002). Once adhered, neutrophils clog the microvasculature causing a local decrease in mucosal blood flow and a marked release of tissue damaging factors, including proteolytic enzymes and leukotrienes, which enhance the vascular tone, exacerbate tissue ischaemia, stimulate the production of ROS, and promote the destruction of intestinal matrix, leading to a severe degree of focal tissue necrosis, particularly in the presence of a low luminal pH (Whittle, 2002; Jimenez et al., 2004).

As anticipated above, cyclooxygenase-dependent inhibition of bicarbonate secretion contributes also to the gastric mucosal injury elicited by NSAIDs. Indeed, the secretion of bicarbonate ions in the mucus gel layer generates a pH gradient on the mucosal surface, thus providing a first line defense against luminal acid (Allen and Flemstrom, 2005). A number of studies have demonstrated the expression of bicarbonate/chloride ion exchangers in the apical membranes of gastric surface epithelial cells, and shown that cyclooxygenase-derived prostaglandins stimulate bicarbonate secretion via activation of $EP_1$ receptors (Takeuchi et al., 1997; Rossmann et al., 1999).

Most NSAIDs are weakly acidic in nature and this property accounts for their local cyclooxygenase-independent injuring actions on the gastric mucosa. In the presence of gastric acidity, the undissociated lipophilic form of acidic NSAIDs can impair the hydrophobic surface barrier of the stomach. This transformation of the gastric mucosal surface from a non-wettable to a wettable state appears to be linked with the ability of acidic NSAIDs to destabilize the extracellular lining of zwitterionic phospholipids, particularly phosphatidylcholine, which are present within and on surface of the mucus gel layer (Lichtenberger et al., 2007). Previous studies have demonstrated that such an effect contributes significantly to NSAID-induced gastric injury in experimental models, and that it can persist for prolonged periods after discontinuation of NSAID administration (Lichtenberger, 2001). There is also consistent evidence that the protonophore actions of aspirin and other acidic NSAIDs take a significant part in the topical damage to gastric mucosa. In particular, upon exposure to the acidic environment of gastric lumen, the undissociated lipid-soluble form of aspirin is able to penetrate cell membranes and accumulate into epithelial cells, where the inner pH is at a physiological level of 7.4. At this pH value, aspirin dissociates and remains segregated within cells. This accumulation enhances the inhibition of prostaglandin biosynthesis, and it brings also into play other properties of aspirin, such as the uncoupling of mitochondrial oxidative phosphorylation. The consequences of such mitochondrial dysfunction are a decrease in ATP production and an increase in AMP and ADP levels, which are then responsible for increments of intracellular calcium concentration. These changes are followed by mitochondrial injury, increased generation of ROS and alterations in the $Na^+/K^+$ balance, which lead to weakening of the mucosal barrier and cellular necrosis (Wallace, 2001; Bjarnson et al., 2007).

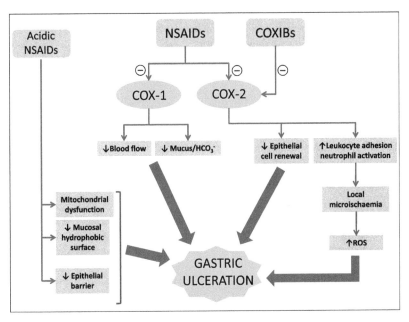

Fig. 1. Pathophysiology of gastric injury induced by non-selective NSAIDs. These anti-inflammatory drugs exert their detrimental effects on the gastric mucosa through two key mechanisms: simultaneous inhibition of COX-1 and COX-2, and direct topic cytotoxic effects. The topic injuring actions depend on the acidic chemical structure of NSAIDs. Coxibs do not harm the gastric mucosa owing to their ability to selectively inhibit COX-2, while not affecting the protective functions of COX-1. ROS: reactive oxygen species.

An additional mechanism, involved in the injurious effects of NSAIDs on gastrointestinal mucosa, is related to the detrimental actions of these drugs on the integrity of epithelial tight junctions, which are known to segregate the apical from basolateral cell surface domains, in order to establish cell polarity and provide a barrier function against the back diffusion of acid and other solutes through the paracellular space (Schneeberger and Lynch, 2004). It has been suggested that cyclooxygenase inhibition may be implicated in NSAID-induced alterations of intercellular epithelial permeability (Joh et al., 2003). However, recent evidence indicates that aspirin can elicit gastric epithelial barrier dysfunction through down-regulation of claudin-7, a member of the claudin protein family, which play important roles in the formation of tight junctions (Oshima et al., 2008).

Coxibs do not alter the integrity of normal gastric mucosa in preclinical models, and their clinical development was based on the assumption that COX-2 is not expressed in the gastric mucosa (Laine et al., 2008). However, this initial hypothesis has not been supported by subsequent observations, demonstrating the constitutive presence of both COX-1 and COX-2 in human and rodent gastric mucosa (Zimmermann et al., 1998). In addition, studies on COX-1-knockout mice have provided no evidence of spontaneous gastric injury and demonstrated the ability of NSAIDs to damage the gastric mucosa via COX-2-dependent mechanisms (Langenbach et al., 1995). Wallace et al. (2000) investigated further the functional roles of COX isoforms in the gastric mucosa, showing that COX-1-dependent prostaglandins are involved in the maintenance of mucus/bicarbonate secretion and blood flow, while COX-2 protects the mucosa from leucocyte endothelial adhesion and supports epithelial renewal. In addition, these Authors observed that selective COX-1 or COX-2 inhibitors did not damage the stomach when tested alone, while NSAIDs or the combined administration of COX-1 plus COX-2 selective inhibitors resulted in gastric erosions (Wallace et al., 2000). A schematic diagram illustrating the mechanisms of gastric mucosal injury exerted by cyclooxygenase inhibitors is provided in Figure 1. Overall, it is currently acknowledged that NSAIDs can impair gastric protection via a concomitant blockade of COX-1 and COX-2, while coxibs lack damaging actions on gastric mucosa by preserving COX-1-dependent prostaglandin production (Wallace, 2006).

## 4. Mechanisms of gastric ulcer healing

Gastric ulcer results from mucosal tissue necrosis triggered primarily by ischemia, with cessation of nutrient delivery and ROS formation. Tissue necrosis and subsequent release of arachidonic acid metabolites from injured cells, including leukotrienes B, attract leukocytes and macrophages, which then phagocitize the necrotic tissue and release pro-inflammatory cytokines, which in turn activate local fibroblasts, endothelial cells and epithelial cells to attempt a tissue restoration (Cotran et al., 1999; Tarnawski, 2005). Morphologically, gastric ulcer consists of two components: the margin, sorrounded by adjacent non-necrotic mucosa, and the base, consisting of granulation tissue, which is a connective tissue rich in macrophages, fibroblasts and proliferating microvessels (Cotran et al., 1999). Ulcer healing is a complex process, in which the tissue repairs itself after injury, attempting a restitution towards integrity. It has been proposed that such a process can be distinguished in sequential, partly overlapping, phases: haemostasis, inflammation, proliferation and remodeling (Stadelmann et al., 1998). According to Schmassmann (1998), the phases and time course of ulcer healing can be described as follows: ulcer development phase (within 3 days from injury), characterized by tissue necrosis, inflammatory infiltration, formation of ulcer margin (de-differentiation) and development of granulation tissue; healing phase (after 3-10 days from injury), which includes an early healing (rapid migration of epithelial cells and contraction of ulcer base) followed by a late healing (angiogenesis in ulcer bed, remodeling of granulation tissue and complete re-epithelialization of ulcer crater); reconstruction phase (day 20-40 after ulceration) consisting of the reconstruction of glands, muscularis mucosae and muscularis propria; maturation phase (40-150 days after ulceration), characterized by maturation and differentiation of specialized cells (Schmassmann, 1998).

In general, following the ulcerative injury, a set of complex biochemical events takes place to provide support for cellular migration from ulcer margin and attachment to the ulcer base, with subsequent cellular proliferation and restoration of the epithelial layer. Ulcer healing is initiated by formation of the 'healing zone', consisting of dilated glands, whose cells undergo de-differentiation, express epidermal growth factor receptor (EGF-R) and starts to actively proliferate. At this stage, inflammatory infiltration occurs closely to the necrotic tissue and ulcer crater. In response to growth factors, the ulcer margin is formed, cells adjacent to the margin de-differentiate, and granulation tissue develops at the ulcer base. During healing, the granulation tissue undergoes continuous remodeling, contraction and changes in cellular composition, whereby the inflammatory cells, appeared in the early phase of healing, are replaced by fibroblasts and microvessels in the late healing phase (Cotran et al., 1999). Wong et al. (2000) analyzed the sequential expression of various genes during ulcer healing and were able to distinguish the following arrays: *genes involved in early response* (EGF-R, c-fos, c-jun, egr-1, sp-1, trefoil factor-2/spasmolytic peptide [TFF-2/SP]), which are all activated shortly after ulcer formation (i.e., within 30 minutes-2 hours); *intermediate response genes* (EGF, basic fibroblast growth factor [bFGF], platelet derived growth factor [PDGF] and vascular endothelial growth factor [VEGF]), which become activated within 6 hours-2 days; *late response genes* (hepatocyte growth factor [HGF], intestinal trefoil factor [ITF], c-met/hepatocyte growth factor receptor [HGF-R]), which are activated within 14 days (Wong et al., 2000). The subsequent proliferation step is initiated within 3 days from ulceration, and it is essential for the healing process, since it supplies the epithelial cells needed for re-epithelialization mucosal surface and gland reconstruction of (Cotran et al., 1999). There is evidence that mucosal ulceration leads to the development of a novel cell lineage designated as *ulcer associated-cell lineage,* which stems from the base of surviving crypts (Cotran et al., 1999). These cells, which express EGF-R and initiate the synthesis of EGF, HGF, trefoil peptides and other growth factors, promote epithelial tube formation, migration and invasion of granulation tissue, and ultimately drive gland reconstruction within the ulcer scar (Tarnawski, 2005). Time-sequence analysis has shown that trefoil peptides are expressed much earlier than EGF following the induction of tissue ulceration. Furthermore, receptor analysis, using radioligand binding assays and immunohistochemistry, has shown a rapid increase in EGF-R expression and a rapid decrease in somatostatin receptor density in the ulcer margin (Reubi et al., 1994).

The major stimuli for cell migration and ulcer re-epithelialization are mediated by growth factors which are produced by platelets, injured tissue and macrophages. Current evidence suggests also that the epithelium of ulcerated mucosa can be regenerated by bone marrow-derived adult stem cells, since biopsy specimens of gastric mucosa, obtained from female patients receiving bone marrow transplants from male donors, were found to contain cells equipped with chromosome Y (Okamoto et al., 2002). The migration of epithelial cells from the ulcer margin, to restore the continuity of epithelial lining, is essential for ulcer healing, and it is subjected to a fine regulation, since it generates a barrier protecting the granulation tissue from any mechanical and chemical damage. Notably, cell migration requires complex cytoskeletal rearrangements. In particular, it has been appreciated that cytoplasmic microfilaments, consisting of G-actin, polymerize into F-actin and the latter, together with myosin II, provides contractile bundles through which cell motility can take place (Chai et al., 2004). A schematic diagram showing the main factors involved in gastric ulcer healing is provided in Figure 2.

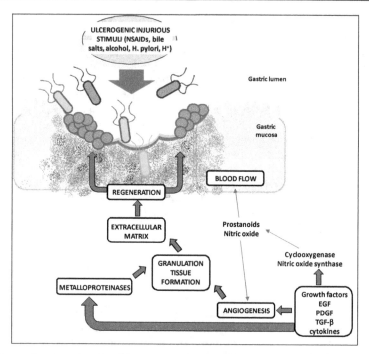

Fig. 2. Main mechanisms involved in gastric ulcer healing. EGF: epidermal growth factor; PDGF: platelet-derived growth factor; TGF-β: transforming growth factor- β.

## 4.1 Early primary response genes: protooncogenes

Ulcer healing depends on a long-term array of responses, which requires de novo mRNA and protein synthesis as well as cell replication. Changes in gene regulation, in response to wounding or ulceration, result in an increase in cell proliferation to replace lost cells. To accomplish this task, the damaged tissue induces early primary response genes, belonging to the family of protooncogenes, which code for sequence-specific DNA-binding nuclear proteins, having the potential of directly influencing the expression of specific genes at the transcriptional level. Although a low basal expression of the nuclear protooncogenes *c-fos*, *c-jun* and *c-myc* is usually observed in most cells, their expression can be rapidly and transiently up-regulated following tissue wounding (Wang and Johnson, 1994). In the rat stress ulcer model, it has been demonstrated that exposure to stress resulted in a rapid increase in *c-fos* and *c-myc* mRNA levels, up to 3-4-fold the basal value. The change in the expression of these protooncogenes was found to precede an increased rate of DNA synthesis (Wang e Johnson, 1994). In another study, based on in situ ibridization, Ito et al. (1990) examined the changes in protooncogenes expression during gastric regeneration after stress injury. In this setting, cells expressing *c-myc* mRNA were identified as mucous neck, parietal, chief and enterochromaffin-like cells, and the distribution of cells in S-phase coincided with that of protooncogene expressing cells (Ito et al., 1990). The exact signal transduction pathways, leading to protooncogene up-regulation following tissue injury, are still unclear, but they  are thought to result from modulation of gene transcription by the polyamines, spermine, spermidine and putrescine. These low-molecular-weight organic cations are ubiquitous in eukariotic cells and able to bind negatively charged macromolecules, such as DNA, RNA and proteins, thus influencing the chromatin structure and sequence-specific DNA-protein interactions, with consequent changes in the regulation of initiation, elongation and termination of gene transcription (Li et al., 2001).

## 4.2 Angiogenesis and angiogenic growth factors

Following gastric ulcerative insults, all mucosal components, including microvessels, undergo destruction within the necrotic area. The healing of such deep mucosal lesions requires the reconstruction of surface epithelium and glandular epithelial structures, the restoration of lamina propria and the reconstruction of mucosal microvascular network, which is essential for delivery of oxygen and nutrients to the healing site (Tarnawski, 2005). The latter goal is achieved through angiogenesis, a finely regulated process, in which microvascular endothelial cells migrate from preserved microvessels at the wound edge, proliferate and attempt to re-establish a microvascular network through de novo vessel formation (Folkman and D'Amore, 1996). Angiogenesis occurs via a series of sequential steps, which include: degradadation of capillary basement membranes by activation of matrix metalloproteinases (MMPs); endothelial cell migration into the perivascular space and proliferation; formation of microvascular tubes followed by anastomoses; establishment of lamina propria and basement membranes and, ultimately, formation of a novel capillary network (Folkman and D'Amore, 1996). The growth of granulation tissue and generation of new microvessels through angiogenesis is stimulated by bFGF, VEGF, PDGF, angiopoietins, other growth factors and cytokines, including IL-1 and TNF-$\alpha$ (Risau, 1997). Gastric mucosal angiogenesis is strongly stimulated by prostacyclin and human recombinant bFGF. Furthermore, the induction of mucosal injury triggers the activation of bFGF and its receptors, and enhances bFGF protein expression in the mucosa-bordering necrosis (Tarnawski, 2005).

VEGF is a pivotal regulator of angiogenesis. It binds at least two specific receptors, VEGF-R1 or flt-1 and VEGF-R2 or flk/KDR, which are expressed mainly on endothelial cells and initiate the phosphorylation of cytosolic proteins involved in signal transduction promoting endothelial cell proliferation, migration and microvascular formation (Ferrara, 2004). VEGF production is stimulated by PDGF, TGF-$\alpha$, cytokines, NO and prostaglandin $E_2$. Hypoxia is one of the best characterized  stimuli for the induction of VEGF expression, acting via a hypoxia-inducible factor (HIF)-1 binding site located on the VEGF gene promoter (Ferrara, 2004). Jones et al. (1999) demonstrated a 4-6 fold increase in VEGF mRNA and protein in the mucosa-bordering necrosis after 24 hours from the induction of ulcer by intragastric ethanol instillation. In this study, the quantitative assessment of angiogenesis demonstrated that almost 10% of microvessels in the mucosa-bordering necrosis displayed endothelial sprouting, reflecting the ongoing angiogenesis. Moreover, treatment with anti-VEGF neutralizing antibody reduced the angiogenic response and delayed ulcer healing (Jones et al., 1999). The activation of MAPK (Erk1 and Erk2) signal transduction pathway is crucial for VEGF-induced stimulation of angiogenesis in ulcer healing, and NSAIDs have been found to interfere with the angiogenic process in part by inihibiting the MAPK/Erk pathway (Jones et al., 1999). In normal gastric microvascular cells it has been demonstrated that prostaglandins can induce VEGF mRNA through transactivation of JNK by Erk2 (Pai et al., 2001). Moreover, this stimulant effect of prostaglandins is likely to be amplified via a positive feedback mechanism, since VEGF, once induced, activates COX-2 expression via an autocrine and paracrine action (Tamura et al., 2002).

## 4.3 Platelets

It is becoming increasingly appreciated that the platelet has the potential of performing a large array of functions, in addition to its role in haemostasis. Tissue repair is initiated with the aggregation of platelets, formation of fibrin clot and release of growth factors from platelets, injured cells and extracellular matrix. Platelets represent one of the largest source of growth factors in the body, and it is through the release of these growth factors that, at least in part, platelets are capable of markedly influencing the processes of tissue healing. Several potent angiogenic stimulators are stored in platelets, including VEGF, platelet derived endothelial growth factor (PDEGF), EGF and PDGF (Perini et al., 2005). These factors account for the ability of platelets to stimulate endothelial cell proliferation and capillary-like formation. Factors that influence the platelet content of pro- versus antiangiogenic factors, or their release from platelets, have the potential to markedly affect angiogenesis and ulcer healing. For example, treatment of rats for 1 week with ticlopidine, an antiplatelet drug acting as adenosine diphosphate receptor antagonist, resulted in a marked increase in platelets and serum levels of endostatin, without affecting platelet VEGF levels. Moreover, this treatment resulted in a marked delay in gastric ulcer healing (Ma et al., 2001). Notably, among a number of receptors, that are important in regulating platelet adhesion, aggregation and secretion, platelet membranes have been found to express proteinase-activated receptors (PARs), which are G protein–coupled receptors, activated by proteinase cleavage at a specific site in their extracellular NH2-terminus. Four PARs have been cloned to date. The activation of $PAR_1$ by thrombin stimulates the release of VEGF, while inhibiting the release of endostatin. By contrast, the activation of $PAR_4$ mediates opposite effects on VEGF release (Ma et al., 2005). The balance in platelet and serum levels of pro- and antiangiogenic factors may influence the healing processes of gastric ulcer and raises the possibility that a selective modulation of PARs could be a viable pharmacological strategy for modulating ulcer healing.

## 4.4 Heat shock proteins

In response to environmental or physical stress, such as heat or ethanol, eukaryotic cells induce the synthesis of intracellular proteins designated as heat shock proteins (HSPs) or stress proteins (Tsukimi and Okabe, 2001). These proteins function as molecular chaperones, which participate in the folding and assembly of nascent proteins, the refolding of partial damaged functional proteins, and the delivery of precursor proteins to mitochondria (Hightower, 1991). HSPs are classified into four major families according to their biological activities and apparent molecular weights: HSP90, HSP70, HSP60, which are constitutively expressed, and small HSPs, including HSP27 and HSP10, which are inducible by various conditions, including oxidative stress (Hightower, 1991). Tsukimi and Okabe (2001) found that the level of HSP70 in normal mucosa was quite low, while it was significantly higher in the ulcer base at the time of ulcer development. HSP70 is expressed in proliferating cells during re-epithelialization (Soncin and Calderwood, 1996), and thus it is likely to be involved in the regeneration of ulcerated mucosa. The induction of HSP70 in the ulcer base might either contribute to the de novo synthesis of proteins or regulate the activity of key enzymes involved in ulcer healing through a molecular chaperone activity. Of note, Ethridge et al. (1998) reported that the overexpression of COX-2 by transfected cDNA inhibited the expression of HSP70 and the activation of heat shock factor-1 (HSF-1) in response to heat shock in rat intestinal epithelial cells. Such inhibition was antagonized by the COX-2 inhibitor NS-398. Accordingly, Ethridge et al. (1998) proposed that prostaglandins derived from COX-2 might be associated with HSP70 induced by heat shock, suggesting an inverse relationship between COX-2 expression and HSP70 induction. HSP47 is a 47 kDa stress protein that specifically binds collagen (Nagata et al., 1988). Collagen biosynthesis represents an essential step for granulation tissue formation. In this regard, HSP47 was found to be expressed in the ulcer base at the time of ulcer development, and its expression decreased with the progress of ulcer healing. Based on these results, it has been suggested that HSP47 might be involved in ulcer healing by playing a role in collagen biosynthesis (Tsukimi and Okabe, 2001).

### 4.5 Annexin-1

Annexin-1 is a 37-kDa member of the annexin family of proteins, which bind and activate 'formyl-peptide' receptors (FPR), known to mediate immune and anti-inflammatory responses. These receptors are expressed on the surface on a variety of cells, including subepithelial myofibroblasts, smooth muscle cells, leukocytes, mast cells and T cells (Chiang et al., 2006). Annexin-1 can also exert its anti-inflammatory actions after proteolitic removal of its NH2 terminus (Martin et al., 2008). The expression of annexin-1, designated also as lipocortin, can be induced by glucocorticoids and it has been shown to contribute to their anti-inflammatory effects (Hannon et al., 2003). In mice, annexin-1 is expressed in the healthy gastric mucosa, and it is markedly up-regulated following ulcer induction by acetic-acid. In this setting, treatment of mice with an annexin-1 mimetic peptide improved gastric ulcer healing. Furthermore, although annexin-1 deficient mice did not exhibit any difference from wild-type mice in terms of susceptibility to indomethacin-induced gastric damage, the healing of such lesions was impaired in annexin-1-deficient mice (Martin et al., 2008). These data are consistent with the hypothesis that annexin-1 contributes to ulcer repair through mechanisms depending on its anti-inflammatory actions. Consistently with this view, Martin et al. (2008) observed an increased expression of the 33-kDa cleavage product of annexin-1 in concomitance with the up-regulation of annexin-1 in the gastric ulcer of mice. The expression of this cleavage product was not observed in healthy stomachs, and therefore it is likely that annexin-1 cleavage, probably due to elevated protease levels, occurred as a consequence of factors induced during the inflammatory or repair process to generate peptide retaining anti-inflammatory properties (Martin et al., 2008).

### 4.6 Extracellular matrix and tissue remodeling

The replacement of granulation tissue with a connective tissue scar, as well as the reconstruction of mucosal architecture, involves tissue remodeling and changes in the composition of extracellular matrix (ECM). ECM consists of fibrous structural proteins, such as collagens and elastins, adhesive glycoproteins, including fibronectin and laminin, and an amorphous gel composed by proteoglycan and hyaluronan. ECM provides the supporting structure for epithelial, endothelial and smooth muscle cells and it is an essential component of connective tissue (Cotran et al., 1999). In the acetic acid-induced gastric ulcer model, Shahin et al. (2001) demonstrated a marked increase in procollagen I 3 days after ulcer induction. Procollagen gene expression remained elevated up to day 15, while returning to the initial levels on day 30. The highest procollagen transcript levels were found in the intact submucosa surrounding the ulcer margins, followed by the muscularis propria and serosa, with the lamina propria displaying the lowest transcript levels (Shahin et al., 1997). Beside collagens, other important components of ECM are spatially and temporally regulated during ulcer healing. MMPs include collagenases, which cleave the fibrillar collagens. These enzymes are produced by several cell types, such as fibroblast, macrophages, neutrophils, endothelial cells and some epithelial cells, and their secretion is induced by growth factors, cytokines or steroids (Cotran et al., 1999). Activated MMPs are rapidly inhibited by specific tissue inhibitors, designated as tissue inhibitors of metalloproteinase (TIMP), to prevent uncontrolled actions by proteinases (Cotran et al., 1999). It has been reported that MMP-2 RNA expression can be detected as early as 24 hours after ulcer induction, a time point that coincides with the clearance of necrotic tissue (Shahin et al., 2001). Its further enhancement at the ulcer margin, after 48 hours, parallels the increment of ulcer diameter observed after the sloughing of necrotic tissue. TIMP-1 expression has been found to be enhanced at 72 hours, suggesting that MMP-2 may promote the ulceration process through local degradation of matrix and tissue proteolysis (Shahin et al., 2001).

## 5. Effects of NSAIDs and coxibs on gastric ulcer healing

The pharmacological modulation of cellular and molecular targets involved in the healing process can alter ulcer repair. Cell renewal in the ulcer margin and angiogenesis in the ulcer base have been found to be significantly impaired during NSAID treatment, with significant delay in ulcer healing (Levi et al., 1990). In the acetic acid-induced ulcer rat model, Sanchez-Fidalgo et al., (2004) found that the ulcerated area was characterized by increased bFGF expression and microvessel density in the granulation tissue at the ulcer base, in concomitance with increments of both apoptotic cell death and expression of proliferation cellular nuclear antigen (PCNA), a marker of cell proliferation. In this setting, both rofecoxib (a selective COX-2 inhibitor) and ibuprofen (a non selective NSAID) delayed ulcer healing, but only rofecoxib was found to reduce all the above mentioned parameters. More recently, indomethacin was tested for its effects on ulcer healing, PCNA and activated caspase-3 expression in acetic acid-induced gastric ulcers. In this study, indomethacin was found to delay ulcer healing, and to up-regulate caspase-3 but not PCNA in ulcerated tissues, suggesting that apoptotic cell death represents a relevant mechanism whereby NSAIDs can impair ulcer repair (Colucci et al., 2009).

Prostaglandins are known to stimulate angiogenesis in vivo and in vitro (Mehrabi et al., 2001; Cheng et al., 1998). Therefore, it is likely that drugs acting as cyclooxygenase blockers, such as NSAIDs, can interfere with angiogenesis in the setting of gastric ulcer healing. Tsujii et al. (1998) showed that aspirin, a non selective NSAID, and NS398, a selective COX-2 inhibitor, blocked angiogenesis in cultured human umbilical vein endothelial cells. Some clinical and experimental data support the view that both non-selective NSAIDs and COX-2 selective inhibitors can delay gastric ulcer healing, partly by inhibiting angiogenesis in the granulation tissue at the ulcer base (Tarnawski and Jones, 2003). In particular, indomethacin significantly reduced (by >37%) the number of microvessels in the ulcer granulation tissue, and the selective COX-2 inhibitors L-745,337, celecoxib and NS398 were found to exert similar effects (Tarnawski and Jones, 2003). The mechanisms by which NSAIDs inhibit angiogenesis appear to include a local change in angiogenic growth factor expression, alterations in key regulators of VEGF, increased endothelial cell apoptosis, inhibition of endothelial cell migration and recruitment of inflammatory cells and platelets (Tarnawski and Jones, 2003). In rat primary aortic endothelial cells, indomethacin and NS398 markedly inhibited the tube formation and Erk2 nuclear translocation. Incubation with prostaglandins partly prevented the NS398-induced effects, but not those exerted by indomethacin, suggesting that both COX-1 and COX-2 are important for the regulation of ulcer angiogenesis, and that the inhibitory action of NSAIDs on angiogenesis depends on both prostaglandin-dependent and prostaglandin-independent mechanisms (Tarnawski and Jones, 2003). Pai et al. (2001) have proposed that NSAIDs can arrest endothelial cell proliferation by suppressing cell cycle proteins, since indomethacin was found to significantly inhibit bFGF-stimulated endothelial cell proliferation by reducing cyclin D1 and increasing p21 protein expression. Furthermore, in a study carried on microvascular endothelial cells, indomethacin and NS398 were found to be able to inhibit VEGF-induced early growth response factor (Egr) 1 gene activation, which is a transcription factor activated by hypoxia in angiogenesis (Szabo et al., 2001). Ma et al. (2002) examined the effects of cyclooxygenase inhibitors on the healing of gastric ulcer in rats, angiogenesis in granulation tissue, and serum levels of VEGF and endostatin. In this study, both celecoxib, a selective COX-2 inhibitor, and flurbiprofen, a non-selective NSAID, significantly impaired angiogenesis, delayed ulcer healing and increased serum endostatin levels (Ma et al., 2002). There is also evidence that NSAIDs can interfere with ulcer healing by both acid-dependent and acid-independent mechanisms (Schmassmann, 1998). In this respect, an experimental study has shown that: the thick granulation tissue below the ulcer crater was transformed into a thinner mature scar within 2 weeks from ulceration; in the presence of NSAIDs, the thickness of granulation tissue progressively increased, indicating an inhibition of its maturation process, and the ulcer healing was delayed; such detrimental effect of NSAIDs on the remodeling of granulation tissue could be reversed by omeprazole, suggesting the involvement of acid-dependent mechanisms (Schmassmann et al., 1995).

As anticipated above, preclinical studies have shown that the impairing actions of NSAIDs on ulcer healing can be shared by COX-2 selective inhibitors, suggesting a role for COX-2 in the process of ulcer repair. However, there is also evidence supporting the view that factors other than COX-2 could be important in the detrimental effects of NSAIDs and selective COX-2 inhibitors on ulcer healing (Blandizzi et al., 2009). First of all, data regarding COX-2 expression in gastric ulcer tissue are conflicting. Furthermore, Schmassmann et al. (2006) observed that treatment with selective COX-1 inhibitors did not delay ulcer healing in COX-1 knockout mice and wild type animals. However, in the same study, the combination of selective COX-1 and COX-2 inhibitors impaired ulcer healing to a higher extent than selective COX-2 inhibitors alone, suggesting that COX-1 could also contribute to ulcer healing process under a condition of COX-2 inhibition. It has been suggested also that the detrimental action of aspirin in combination with celecoxib on ulcer healing could result from the ability of aspirin to alter surface phospholipids, without significant involvement of the cyclooxygenase pathways (Lichtenberg et al., 2007). More recently, we have obtained preliminary evidence that the ulcer healing impairing effects exerted by treatment with indomethacin (COX-1/COX-2 inhibitor) or DFU (selective COX-2 inhibitor) could depend on the ability of these drugs to induce the expression of NSAID activated gene-1 (NAG-1), which is known to promote apoptosis (Colucci et al., 2008).

## 6. Effects of PPIs on gastric mucosal protection and ulcer healing

Several preclinical and clinical lines of evidence have demonstrated that PPIs are highly effective in promoting the healing of gastric damage induced by NSAIDs, even in the presence of a continued NSAID administration, through the activation of both acid-dependent and -independent mechanisms (Blandizzi et al., 2008).

PPIs are substituted benzimidazole derivatives (Figure 3) endowed with potent inhibitory effects on gastric acid secretion.

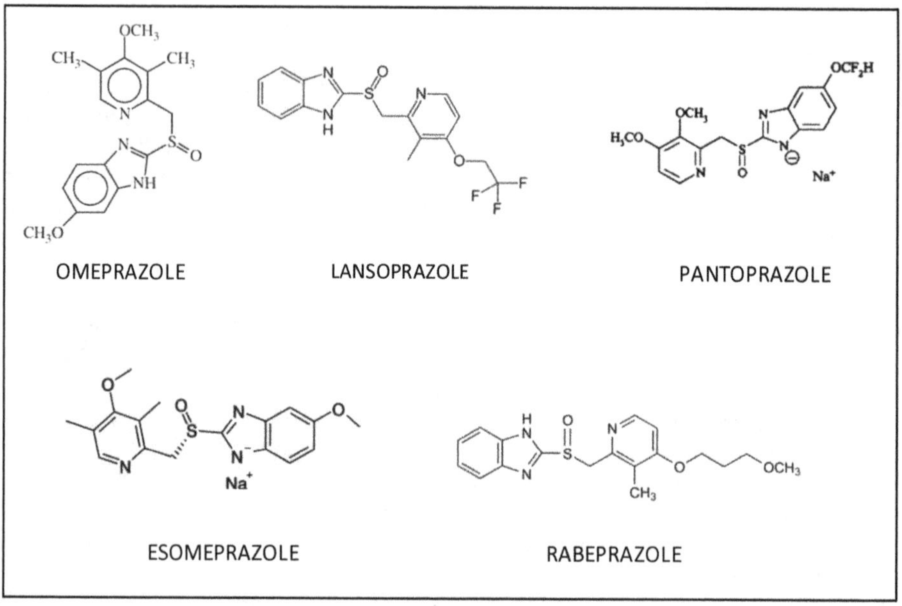

Fig. 3. Chemical structure of proton pump inhibitors (PPIs)

These drugs act primarily through the blockade of the enzyme H+/K+-adenosine triphosphatase (H+/K+-ATPase, the so-called "proton pump"), which is activated during the final step of acid secretion by the parietal cells of the stomach. PPIs are weak basic compounds, with acid dissociation constant (pKa) values ranging from 3.9 to 5.0. For this reason, they accumulate massively in the highly-acidic secretory canalicula of parietal cells, where they are rapidly converted into their active cyclic sulfenamide form. This highly reactive sulfenamide derivative binds sulfidryl groups of H+/K+-ATPase, leading to permanent enzyme inhibition and subsequent potent reduction of acid secretion (Boparai et al., 2008). Some studies have suggested that the beneficial effects of PPIs on ulcer healing could be ascribed to a marked inhibition of acid secretion, which can lead to a consistent increase in plasma gastrin levels, a peptide actively involved in the regulation of mucosal cell proliferation (Koh and Chen, 2000). However, the evidence supporting the involvement of gastrin in the healing action of PPIs is conflicting and there is no general consensus on the significance of this mechanism. Ito et al. (1994) initially showed that omeprazole was effective in increasing the healing rate of acetic acid-induced gastric ulcers in rats, and that this effect was related to a marked increase in serum gastrin levels. In a subsequent study, Schmassmann and Reubi (2000) observed that both omeprazole, inducing hypergastrinaemia, and exogenous gastrin-17 enhanced cell proliferation in the ulcer margin, with an acceleration of the healing process. Since these ameliorative effects were reversed by treatment with a gastrin receptor antagonist, the authors suggested that omeprazole promoted ulcer healing through an increase in cell proliferation secondary to hypergastrinaemia. However, Okabe and Amagase (2005) provided evidence that a somatostatin analogue significantly decreased the omeprazole-induced hypergastrinaemia in rats with gastric ulcers, while not affecting the ability of this PPI to stimulate ulcer healing. In addition, the healing effect of omeprazole was not modified by gastrin receptor antagonists, thus suggesting that gastrin, released in response to omeprazole, played a marginal role in the mechanisms underlying the ulcer healing action of this PPI.

Besides the marked inhibition of gastric acid secretion, increasing evidence indicates that the beneficial effects of PPIs against NSAID-induced gastric injury could depend on acid-independent mechanisms. For instance, it has been shown that these drugs are able to counteract tissue oxidative damage in a direct or indirect manner (Lapenna et al., 1996; Natale et al., 2004). In particular, several in vitro experiments demonstrated a direct antioxidant activity of PPIs, showing that pantoprazole (Fornai et al., 2005) and lansoprazole (Blandizzi et al., 2005) concentration-dependently reduced copper-induced oxidation of human native low density lipoproteins (LDLs), while omeprazole behaved as a scavenger of hypochlorous acid (an oxidant compound generated by phagocytes) (Lapenna et al., 1996). Other studies have shown that pantoprazole is able to scavenge hydroxyl radicals, produced during a Fenton reaction, through the interaction with the hydroxyl radical generating system (Simon et al., 2006). Interestingly, in vitro experiments demonstrated that omeprazole and lansoprazole protected DNA from oxidative damage generated by hydroxyl radicals (Biswas et al., 2003). When considering the indirect antioxidant mechanisms, it has been observed that PPIs can significantly counteract the oxidative stress arising from polymorphonuclear cell activation. In this regard, omeprazole was shown to reduce neutrophil functions (Wandall, 1992), including adhesion processes to endothelial cells (Suzuki et al., 1999), phagocytosis and acidification of phagolysosomes (Agastya et al., 2000), and the production of ROS (Zedtwitz-Liebenstein et al., 2002). In addition, lansoprazole inhibited the release of free oxygen radicals from neutrophils activated by *Helicobacter pylori* (Suzuki et al., 1995). Recently, Martins de Oliveira et al. (2007) showed that omeprazole and pantoprazole inhibited $H^+K^+$-ATPase in neutrophils, resulting in cationic flow disturbances and subsequent suppression of migration and intracellular events, such as calcium influx and p38 MAPK activation. On the same line, Pastoris et al. (2008) demonstrated that, in addition to inhibiting acid secretion, the effects exerted by esomeprazole against indomethacin-induced gastric damage can be partly ascribed to a reduction in gastric oxidative injury.

It is also worthy to mention a novel mechanism contributing to the acid-independent beneficial effects of PPIs, which are able to induce and subsequently increase the catalytic activity of heme oxygenase-1 (HO-1) (Becker et al., 2006). The antioxidant, anti-inflammatory, anti-apoptotic, and vasodilatory properties of HO-1 pathway products, such as bilirubin and carbon monoxide, can counteract the main mechanisms of gastric damage. In particular, HO-1 plays a key role in the physiological tissue defense as well as in the modulation of ulcer healing process (Becker et al., 2006).

Mucosal depletion of sulphydryl radicals has been found to take part to the pathogenesis of gastric lesions evoked by different NSAIDs (Villegas et al., 2002), and reduced glutathione (GSH) concentrations have been detected in mucosal biopsies from patients with NSAID-induced gastric bleeding (Savoye et al., 2001). Consistently with these findings, gastric injury evoked by indomethacin in rats was shown to be associated with a significant decrease in mucosal GSH concentration, and treatment with esomeprazole protected the gastric mucosa against indometacin-induced damage by restoring mucosal GSH levels (Pastoris et al., 2008).

The involvement of cyclooxygenase/prostaglandin pathways in the ulcer healing mechanisms activated by PPIs has been investigated with conflicting evidence. Some reports suggested that gastric mucosal levels of $PGE_2$ were unaffected by treatment with PPIs (Natale et al., 2004; Fornai et al., 2011). By contrast, Tsuji et al. (2002) reported that lansoprazole increased gastric COX-2 expression and $PGE_2$ production after repeated administrations in rats, and suggested that such increments resulted from a lansoprazole-induced increase in gastrin secretion.

Some studies have investigated the modulating effects of PPIs on several molecular markers of cell proliferation and apoptosis, in order to better characterize the mechanisms contributing to their ulcer healing actions. In this respect, Colucci et al. (2009) observed that the ability of esomeprazole to counteract the detrimental action of indomethacin on ulcer repair was ascribable to an enhancement of NF-kB activation and to a decrease in caspase-3-dependent apoptosis. Interestingly, these effects were found to likely depend on acid-independent mechanisms, since they were not reproduced by the histamine $H_2$ receptor antagonist famotidine, administered at an equivalent acid-inhibiting dose. More recently, in another experimental model of gastric ulceration, elicited by chronic indomethacin administration, it was confirmed that esomeprazole can exert antiapoptotic actions on gastric mucosal cells in the setting of ulcer repair (Fornai et al., 2011). In the same study, treatment with esomeprazole was also associated with a significant increase in mucosal expression of PCNA and Ki-67, both regarded as markers of cell proliferation. The beneficial influence of esomeprazole on ulcer repair has been related to mechanisms which are likely to be independent from the inhibition of acid secretion and ascribable to antioxidant properties (Fornai et al., 2011). This view is in line with previous studies reporting that both the antioxidant compound ascorbic acid and omeprazole enhanced the expression of growth factors, including TGF-$\alpha$, in the gastric mucosa of rats treated with aspirin (Jainu and Mohan, 2008). In addition, these preclinical findings are consistent with the clinical evidence provided by Tsuji et al. (1995), who showed that lansoprazole, but not famotidine, induced the expression of bFGF in the gastric ulcer margin, and that PPI was more effective than famotidine in promoting ulcer healing. Other reports have suggested that several growth factors are involved in the ulcer healing effects of PPIs. In this regard, Kinoshita et al. (1998) observed that the gastric levels of HGF were enhanced by omeprazole in rats with indomethacin-induced gastric damage. Moreover, the expression of EGF was found to be increased in the gastric mucosa of mice with indomethacin-induced injury, and further enhanced by omeprazole (Banerjee et al., 2008).

## 6.1 Effects of PPIs on gastric ulcer healing: clinical evidence

Several clinical studies have been performed to investigate the efficacy of PPIs in promoting the healing of mucosal lesions in patients who unavoidably need to continue NSAID therapy. In a multicentre study, a subgroup of 68 gastric ulcer patients, who continued using NSAIDs, showed rapid ulcer healing when receiving omeprazole 20 and 40 mg/day, with a therapeutic advantage of 31% and 43%, respectively, after 8 weeks as compared with ranitidine 300 mg (Walan et al., 1989). Subsequently, in the ASTRONAUT trial, two doses of omeprazole (20 and 40 mg/day) were compared with ranitidine (150 mg twice daily) in patients with both gastric and duodenal ulcers. In this study, treatment with omeprazole was more effective than the $H_2$-receptor antagonist in terms of ulcer healing (Yeomans et al.,

1998). The clinical effectiveness of omeprazole has also been documented in comparative studies with other protective drugs. For example, a therapeutic gain of 18% in gastric ulcer patients and 22% in duodenal ulcer patients taking NSAIDs has been estimated when comparing omeprazole with sucralfate (Bianchi Porro et al., 1998). By contrast, the OMNIUM study did not display significant differences between omeprazole (20 and 40 mg/day) and misoprostol (200 μg four times daily) in terms of ulcer healing (Hawkey et al., 1998). Similar results were observed for lansoprazole (15 or 30 mg/day) in comparison with ranitidine (150 mg twice daily). Both doses of lansoprazole were significantly more effective than ranitidine for promoting the healing of gastric ulcers, in patients taking NSAIDs, after 4 and 8 weeks of treatment. In particular, after 8 weeks, the healing rate was 74% in patients treated with lansoprazole 30 mg, and 50% in patients treated with ranitidine 150 mg twice daily (Agrawal et al., 2000; Campbell et al., 2002). In a double-blind, placebo-controlled, randomized trial, patients, treated with low-dose aspirin and affected by upper digestive symptoms, were assigned to treatment with rabeprazole (20 mg once daily) or placebo for 4 weeks. At the end of this period, 47% of patients treated with rabeprazole and 43% of patients given placebo reported a complete relief of upper gastrointestinal symptoms (Laheij et al., 2003). Subsequently, two studies were performed to compare esomeprazole (20 or 40 mg once daily) with ranitidine (Goldstein et al., 2005; 2007). In the first study, gastric ulcer healing occurred in significantly higher proportions of patients treated with either 20 or 40 mg of esomeprazole, as compared with ranitidine at both 4 and 8 weeks. In particular, at the end of the 8-week treatment, the healing rate was 74% in the ranitidine group, 88% with esomeprazole 20 mg and 92% with esomeprazole 40 mg (Goldstein et al., 2005). The second study, performed by the same Authors, highlighted a significant difference in favor of both esomeprazole doses only after 4 weeks. By contrast, after 8 weeks, the healing rates were similar for esomeprazole (20 and 40 mg/day) in comparison with ranitidine (Goldstein et al., 2007).

## 7. Novel therapeutic options for prevention and treatment of gastric ulcer

Although the control of gastric acid secretion represents a cornerstone for the promotion of ulcer healing, an increasing interest is growing up about the characterization of the mechanisms supporting the process of ulcer repair, and the possibility that both the speed and quality of ulcer healing can be pharmacologically modulated.

At present, novel pharmacological strategies are being investigated to counteract the detrimental actions of traditional NSAIDs on the gastrointestinal tract. The main options currently under active evaluation are: (i) dual inhibitors of cyclooxygenase and 5-lipooxygenase (5-LOX), in order to prevent the mucosal injury resulting from the enhanced biosynthesis of leukotrienes, arising from the shift of arachidonic acid metabolism towards the leukotriene pathway as a consequence of cyclooxygenase inhibition; (ii) traditional NSAIDs associated with phosphatidylcholine, to minimize the destabilizing action of these drugs on the extracellular mucosal lining of zwitterionic phospholipids; (iii) NO donating NSAIDs, designated as cyclooxygenase inhibitors/NO donors (CINODs) and aimed at preventing the injurious actions of NSAIDs through the gastroprotective activity of exogenous NO; (iv) NSAIDs releasing $H_2S$, a gaseous mediator actively involved in the maintenance of digestive mucosal integrity and blood flow (Blandizzi et al., 2009). Some of the above mentioned drugs are under clinical development. In particular, licofelone, a dual cyclooxygenase/5-LOX inhibitor, has been shown to spare the human gastric mucosa (endoscopic endpoint) when administered for 4–12 weeks to healthy volunteers or patients with osteoarthritis in phase II or phase III trials controlled with placebo or naproxen (Bias et al., 2004; Becker et al., 2004). In a 4-day study, performed on healthy volunteers, the gastric injuring action of aspirin, assessed through endoscopic examination, was significantly reduced in subjects administered with soy phosphatidylcholine, although in both treatment groups prostaglandin levels in gastric biopsies were significantly reduced (Anand et al., 1999). Recently, Lanza et al. (2008) evaluated the digestive safety of ibuprofen chemically combined with phosphatidylcholine in osteoarthritic patients, observing a better tolerability of this association in comparison with ibuprofen alone.

CINODs have been developed exploiting the concept that NO, released locally in the gastric mucosa, would enhance the mucosal blood flow and reduce leukocyte adherence in the gastric microcirculation. Based on this assumption, aspirin and other traditional NSAIDs have been coupled to a nitroxybutyl or nitrosothiol group to yield novel anti-inflammatory entities which release discrete amounts of NO (Fiorucci et al., 2007). At present, the pharmacokinetic profile of these novel pharmacological entities remains unclear and deserve further investigations. However, encouraging results about the gastric safety profiles of these novel drugs arise from studies performed on healthy volunteers. In this regard, an endoscopic study demonstrated that healthy subjects treated for 7 days with NCX-4016, an NO-donating aspirin, did not display gastrointestinal toxicity (Fiorucci et al., 2003). On the same line, a trial performed on 31 healthy volunteers showed that upper gastrointestinal endoscopic events following oral administration of AZD 3582, a novel NO donating naproxen, for 12 days were significantly reduced in comparison with traditional naproxen (Hawkey et al., 2003). Moreover, Wilder-Smith et al. (2006) investigated the effects of equimolar doses of AZD3582 and traditional naproxen in healthy volunteers treated for 12 days, observing that treatment with the CINOD was endowed with a better gastroduodenal safety profile in comparison with naproxen. Clearly, further clinical studies are needed to establish whether CINODs confer actual advantages over traditional NSAIDs in terms of upper digestive safety.

Recently, an increasing attention has been paid to the beneficial effects of $H_2S$ on the gastric mucosa. This gaseous compound, previously regarded as a toxic agent, is emerging as an endogenous modulator which seems to share almost all the beneficial actions of NO on several physiological processes. In particular, it has been demonstrated that $H_2S$ is produced by the gastric mucosa, and that it contributes to the ability of this tissue to resist against damage induced by luminal agents (Fiorucci et al., 2007). Interestingly, several lines of evidence have shown that $H_2S$ donors can prevent the decrease in gastric blood flow induced by NSAIDs, and reduce NSAID-induced leukocyte accumulation and adhesion in gastric microvessels, thus providing a rationale for the synthesis of $H_2S$-releasing NSAID derivatives as novel anti-inflammatory drugs (Fiorucci et al., 2007). As previously observed with CINODs, an $H_2S$-releasing derivative of diclofenac was shown to be better tolerated, in terms of gastric damage, than traditional NSAIDs. Moreover, the addition of the $H_2S$-releasing moiety has been found to increase the anti-inflammatory activity of diclofenac (Wallace, 2007; Li et al., 2007). Additional strategies for the prevention of NSAID-induced upper digestive damage include the ongoing clinical development of pharmaceutical products containing fixed combinations of a NSAID with a gastroprotective drug, such as naproxen/omeprazole, naproxen/lansoprazole, naproxen/esomeprazole and ibuprofen/famotidine (Blandizzi et al., 2009).

Several studies have focused their attention toward novel approaches to promote the healing of gastric ulcer. It has been widely recognized that the healing process requires angiogenesis in the granulation tissue at the ulcer base, followed by a sustained proliferation of epithelial cells in ulcer margins and a subsequent re-arrangement of tissue architecture (Wallace, 2005). As discussed in this chapter, this complex process is finely regulated. In particular, it has been demonstrated PARs play important roles in the modulation of ulcer repair. In particular, preclinical studies have suggested PAR1 as a potential therapeutic target for promoting ulcer healing (Ma et al., 2005).

## 8. References

Agastya, G., et al. (2000). Omeprazole inhibits phagocytosis and acidification of phagolysosomes of normal human neutrophils in vitro. *Immunopharmacol Immunotoxicol*, Vol.22, No.2, (May 2000), pp. 357-372

Agrawal, N.M., et al. (2000). Superiority of lansoprazole vs ranitidine in healing nonsteroidal anti-inflammatory drug-associated gastric ulcers: results of a double-blind, randomized, multicenter study. NSAID Associated Gastric Ulcer Study Group. *Arch Intern Med*, Vol.160, No.10, (May 2000), pp. 1455-1461

Allen, A., & Flemström, G. (2005). Gastroduodenal mucus bicarbonate barrier: protection against acid and pepsin. *Am J Physiol Cell Physiol*, Vol.288, No.1, (January 2005), pp.C1–C19

Anand, B.S., et al. (1999). Phospholipid association reduces the gastric mucosal toxicity of aspirin in human subjects. *Am J Gastroenterol*, Vol.94, No.7, (July 1999), pp. 1818-1822

Banerjee, D., et al. (2008). Angiogenic and cell proliferating action of the natural diarylnonanoids, malabaricone B and malabaricone C during healing of indomethacin-induced gastric ulceration. *Pharm Res*, Vol.25, No.7, (July 2008), pp. 1601–1609

Becker, J.C., et al. (2004). Current approaches to prevent NSAID-induced gastropathy-- COX selectivity and beyond. *Br J Clin Pharmacol*, Vol.58, No.6, (December 2004), pp. 587-600

Becker, J.C., et al. (2006). Beyond gastric acid reduction: proton pump inhibitors induce heme oxygenase-1 in gastric and endothelial cells. *Biochem Biophys Res Commun*,Vol.345, No.3, (July 2006), pp. 1014–1021

Bianchi Porro, G., et al. (1998). Omeprazole and sucralfate in the treatment of NSAID-induced gastric and duodenal ulcer. *Aliment Pharmacol Ther*, Vol. 12, No.4, (April 1998), pp. 355-360

Bias, P., et al. (2004). The gastrointestinal tolerability of the LOX/COX inhibitor, licofelone, is similar to placebo and superior to naproxen therapy in healthy volunteers: results from a randomized, controlled trial. *Am J Gastroenterol*, Vol.99, No.4, (April 2004), pp. 611-618

Biswas, K., et al. (2003). A novel antioxidant and antiapoptotic role of omeprazole to block gastric ulcer through scavenging of hydroxyl radical. *J Biol Chem*, Vol.278, No.13, (March 2003), pp. 10993-11001

Bjarnason, I., et al. (2007). Determinants of the short-term gastric damage caused by NSAIDs in man. *Aliment Pharmacol Ther*, Vol.26, No.1, (July 2007), pp. 95–106

Blandizzi, C., et al. (2005). Lansoprazole prevents experimental gastric injury induced by non-steroidal anti-inflammatory drugs through a reduction of mucosal oxidative damage. *World J Gastroenterol*, Vol.11, No.26, (July 2005), pp. 4052-4060

Blandizzi, C., et al. (2008). Clinical efficacy of esomeprazole in the prevention and healing of gastrointestinal toxicity associated with NSAIDs in elderly patients. *Drugs Aging*, Vol.25, No.3, (March 2008), pp. 197-208

Blandizzi, C., et al. (2009). Role of coxibs in the strategies for gastrointestinal protection in patients requiring chronic non-steroidal anti-inflammatory therapy. *Pharmacol Res*, Vol.59, No.2, (February 2009), pp. 90-100

Boparai, V., et al. (2008). Guide to the use of proton pump inhibitors in adult patients. *Drugs*, Vol.68, No.7, (May 2008), pp. 925-947

Brzozowski, T., et al. (2005a). Role of prostaglandins in gastroprotection and gastric adaptation. *J Physiol Pharmacol*, Vol.56, No.Suppl 5, (September 2005), pp. 33–55

Brzozowski, T., et al. (2005b). Role of central and peripheral ghrelin in the mechanism of gastric mucosal defence. *Inflammopharmacology*, Vol.13, No.1-3, (January 2005), pp. 45– 62

Campbell, D.R., et al. (2002). Effect of H. pylori status on gastric ulcer healing in patients continuing nonsteroidal anti-inflammatory therapy and receiving treatment with lansoprazole or ranitidine. *Am J Gastroenterol*, Vol.97, No.9, (September 2002), pp. 2208-2214

Chai J., et al. (2004). Serum response factor promotes re-epitelialization and muscular structure restoration during gastric ulcer healing. *Gastronterology*, Vol.126, No.7, (June 2004), pp. 1809-1818

Chatzaki, E., et al. (2006). Corticotropin-releasing factor (CRF) receptor type 2 in the human stomach: protective biological role by inhibition of apoptosis. *J Cell Physiol*, Vol.209, No.3 (December 2006), pp. 905–911

Cheng, T., et al. (1998). Prostaglandin $E_2$ induces vascular endothelial growth factor and basic fibroblast growth factor mRNA expression in cultured rat Muller cells. *Invest Ophthalmol Vis Sci*, Vol.39, No.3, (March 1998), pp. 581-591

Chiang, N., et al. (2006). The lipoxin receptor ALX: potent ligand-specific and stereoselective actions in vivo. *Pharmacol Rev*, Vol.58, No.3, (September 2006), pp. 463-487

Chiou, S.K., et al. (2005). Survivin: a novel target for indomethacin-induced gastric injury. *Gastroenterology*, Vol. 128, No.1, (January 2005), pp. 63–73

Colucci R., et al. (2008). NSAID activated gene-1 (NAG-1) plays a role in the impairing effects of cyclooxygenase inhibitors on gastric ulcer repair. *Gastroenterology*, Vol.134, No. suppl.1, (April 2008), pp. A738

Colucci, R., et al. (2009). Characterization of mechanisms underlying the effects of esomeprazole on the impairment of gastric ulcer healing with addition of NSAID treatment. *Dig Liver Dis*, Vol.41, No.6, (June 2009), pp. 395-405

Cotran, R.S., et al. (1999). Gastric ulceration, In: *pathologic basis of disease*, Cotran, V Kumar, SL Robbins, pp. 298-299, Saunders, Philadelphia

Dubois, R.W., et al. (2004). Guidelines for the appropriate use of non-steroidal anti-inflammatory drugs, cyclooxygenase-2-specific inhibitors and proton pump inhibitors in patients requiring chronic anti-inflammatory therapy. *Aliment Pharmacol Ther*, Vol.19, No.2, (January 2004), pp. 197–208

Ethridge, R.T., et al. (1998). Inhibition of heat-shock protein 70 induction in intestinal cells overexpressing cyclooxygenase-2. *Gastroenterology*, Vol.115, No.6, (December 1998), pp. 1454-1463

Ferrara, N. (2004). Vascular endothelial growth factor: basic science and clinical progress. *Endocr Rev*, Vol.25, No.4, (August 2004), pp. 581-611

Filaretova, L.P., et al. (1998). Corticosterone increase inhibits stress-induced gastric erosions in rats. *Am J Physiol Gastrointest Liver Physiol*, Vol.274, No.6 pt 1, (June 1998), pp. G1024–G1030

Filaretova, L., et al. (2001). Various ulcerogenic stimuli are potentiated by glucocorticoid deficiency in rats. *J Physiol (Paris)*, Vol.95, No.1-6, (January-December 2001), pp. 59– 65

Filaretova, L., et al. (2007). Gastroprotective role of glucocorticoid hormones. *J Pharmacol Sci*, Vol.104, No.3, (July 2007), pp. 195–201

Fiorucci, S., et al. (2003). Gastrointestinal safety of NO-aspirin (NCX-4016) in healthy human volunteers: a proof of concept endoscopic study. *Gastroenterology*, Vol.124, No.3, (March 2003), pp.600–607

Fiorucci, S., et al. (2006). The emerging roles of hydrogen sulfide in the gastrointestinal tract and liver. *Gastroenterology*, Vol.131, No.1, (July 2006), pp. 259–271

Fiorucci, S., et al. (2007). NSAIDs, coxibs, CINOD and $H_2S$-releasing NSAIDs: what lies beyond the horizon. *Dig Liver Dis*, Vol.39, No.12, (December 2007), pp. 1043-1051

Folkman, J., & D'Amore, P.A. (1996). Blood vessel formation: what is its molecular basis? *Cell*, Vol.87, No.7, (December 1996), pp. 1153-1155

Fornai, M., et al. (2005). Mechanisms of protection by pantoprazole against NSAID-induced gastric mucosal damage. *Naunyn Schmiedebergs Arch Pharmacol*, Vol.372, No.1, (July 2005), pp. 79-87

Fornai, M., et al. (2011). Effects of esomeprazole on healing of nonsteroidal anti-inflammatory drug (NSAID)-induced gastric ulcers in the presence of a continued NSAID treatment: Characterization of molecular mechanisms. *Pharmacol Res*, Vol.63, No.1, (January 2011), pp. 59-67

Goldstein, J.L., et al. (2005). Healing of gastric ulcers with esomeprazole versus ranitidine in patients who continued to receive NSAID therapy: a randomized trial. *Am J Gastroenterol*, Vol.100, No.12, (December 2005), pp. 2650-2657

Goldstein, J.L., et al. (2007). Clinical trial: healing of NSAID-associated gastric ulcers in patients continuing NSAID therapy. A randomized study comparing ranitidine with esomeprazole. *Aliment Pharmacol Ther*, Vol.26, No.8, (October 2007), pp. 1101-1111

Halter, F., et al. (2001). Cyclooxygenase-2 implications on maintenance of gastric mucosal integrity and ulcer healing: controversial issues and perspectives. *Gut*, Vol.49, No.3, (September 2001), pp. 443– 453

Hannon, R., et al. (2003). Aberrant inflammation and resistance to glucocorticoids in annexin 1-/- mouse. *Faseb J*, Vol.17, No.2, (February 2003), pp. 253-255

Hawkey, C.J., et al. (1998). Omeprazole compared with misoprostol for ulcers associated with nonsteroidal anti-inflammatory drugs. Omeprazole versus Misoprostol for NSAID-induced Ulcer Management (OMNIUM) Study Group. *N Engl J Med*, Vol.338, No.11, (March 1998), pp. 727-734

Hawkey, C.J., et al. (2003). Gastrointestinal safety of AZD3582, a cyclooxygenase inhibiting nitric oxide donor: proof of concept study in humans. *Gut*, Vol.52, No.11, (November 2003), pp. 1537-1542

Hightower, L.E. (1991). Heat shock, stress proteins, chaperones and proteotoxicity. *Cell*, Vol.66, No.2, (July 1991), pp. 191-197

Ho, S.B., et al. (2004). The adherent gastric mucous layer is composed of alternating layers of MUC5AC and MUC6 mucin proteins. *Dig Dis Sci*, Vol.49, No.10, (October 2004), pp. 1598-1606

Holzer P. (2006). Neural regulation of gastrointestinal blood flow, In: *Physiology of the gastrointestinal tract.*, Johnson LR, pp. 817– 839, Academic Press, New York

Holzer, P. (2007). Role of visceral afferent neurons in mucosal inflammation and defense. *Curr Opin Phamacol*, Vol.7, No.6, (December 2007), pp. 563–569

Ito, T., et al. (1990). Sequential protooncogene expression during regeneration in rat stomach. *Gastroenterology*, Vol.98, No.6, (June 1990), pp. 1525-1531

Ito, M., et al. (1994). Cimetidine and omeprazole accelerate gastric ulcer healing by an increase in gastrin secretion. *Eur J Pharmacol*, Vol.263, No.3, (October 1994), pp. 253-259

Jainu, M., & Mohan, K.V. (2008). Protective role of ascorbic acid isolated from Cissus quadrangularis on NSAID-induced toxicity through immunomodulating response and growth factors expression. *Int Immunopharmacol*, Vol.8, No.13-14, (December 2008), pp. 1721-1727

Jimènez, M.D., et al. (2004). Role of L-arginine in ibuprofen-induced oxidative stress and neutrophil infiltration in gastric mucosa. *Free Radic Res*, Vol.38, No.9, (September 2004), pp. 903–911

Joh, T., et al. (2003). The protective effect of rebamipide on paracellular permeability of rat gastric epithelial cells. *Aliment Pharmacol Ther*, Vol.18, No.Suppl 1, (July 2003), pp. 133–138

Jones, M.K., et al. (1999). Activation of VEGF and Ras genes in gastric mucosa during angiogenic response to ethanol injury. *Am J Physiol Gastrointest Liver Physiol*, Vol.276, No.6 pt 1, (June 1999), pp. G1345-G1355

Kato, S., et al. (2005). Dual action of prostaglandin $E_2$ on gastric acid secretion through different EP receptor subtypes in the rat. *Am J Physiol Gastrointest Liver Physiol*, Vol.89, No.1, (July 2005), pp. G64–G69

Kinoshita, Y., et al. (1998). Increased hepatocyte growth factor content in rat stomach during omeprazole treatment. *Digestion*, Vol.59, No.2, (March-April 1998), pp. 102–109

Koh, T.J., & Chen, D. (2000). Gastrin as a growth factor in the gastrointestinal tract. *Regul Pept*, Vol.93, No.1-3, (September 2000), pp. 37-44

Laheij, R.J., et al. (2003). Proton-pump inhibitor therapy for acetylsalicylic acid associated upper gastrointestinal symptoms: a randomized placebo-controlled trial. *Aliment Pharmacol Ther,* Vol.18, No.1, (July 2003), pp. 109-115

Laine L., et al. (2008). Gastric mucosal defense and cytoprotection: bench to bedside. *Gastroenterology,* Vol.135, No.1, (July 2008), pp.41-60

Langenbach, R., et al. (1995). Prostaglandin synthase 1 gene disruption in mice reduces arachidonic acid-induced inflammation and indomethacin-induced gastric ulceration. *Cell,* Vol.83, No.3, (November 1995), pp. 483–492

Lanza, F.L., et al. (2008). Clinical trial: comparison of ibuprofen-phosphatidylcholine and ibuprofen on the gastrointestinal safety and analgesic efficacy in osteoarthritic patients. *Aliment Pharmacol Ther,* Vol.28, No.4, (August 2008), pp. 431-442

Lapenna, D., et al. (1996). Antioxidant properties of omeprazole. *FEBS Lett,* Vol.382, No.1-2, (March 1996), pp. 189-192

Levi S., et al. (1990). Inhibitory effect of non-steroidal anti-inflammatory drugs on mucosal cell proliferation associated with gastric ulcer healing. *Lancet,* Vol.336, No.8719, (October 1990), pp. 840-843

Li, L., et al. (2001). Polyamine depletion stabilizes p53 resulting in inhibition of normal intestinal epithelia proliferation. *Am J Physiol Cell Physiol,* Vol.281, No.3, (September 2001), pp. C941-C953

Li, L., et al. (2007). Anti-inflammatory and gastrointestinal effects of a novel diclofenac derivative. *Free Radic Biol Med,* Vol.42, No.5, (March 2007), pp. 706-719

Lichtenberger, L.M. (1999). Gastroduodenal mucosal defense. *Curr Opin Gastroenterol,* Vol.15, No.6, (November 1999), pp. 463- 472

Lichtenberger, L.M. (2001). Where is the evidence that cyclooxygenase inhibition is the primary cause of nonsteroidal anti-inflammatory drug (NSAID)-induced gastrointestinal injury? Topical injury revisited. *Biochem Pharmacol,* Vol.61, No.6, (March 2001), pp. 631–637

Lichtenberger, L.M., et al. (2007). Surface phospholipids in gastric injury and protection when a selective cyclooxygenase-2 inhibitor (Coxib) is used in combination with aspirin. *Br J Pharmacol,* Vol. 150, No.7, (April 2007), pp. 913–919

Ma, L., et al. (2001). Platelets modulate gastric ulcer healing: role of endostatin and vascular endothelial growth factor release. *Proc Natl Acad Sci USA,* Vol.98, No.11, (May 2001), 6470-6475

Ma, L., et al. (2002). Divergent effects of new cyclooxygenase inhibitors on gastric ulcer healing: shifting the angiogenic balance. *Proc Natl Acad Sci USA,* Vol.99, No.20, (October 2002), pp. 13243-13247

Ma, L., et al. (2005). Proteinase-activated receptors 1 and 4 counterregulate endostatin and VEGF release from human platelets. *Proc Natl Acad Sci USA,* Vol.102, No.1, (January 2005), pp. 216-220

Martin, G.R., et al. (2008). Annexin-1 modulates repair of gastric mucosal injury. *Am J Physiol Gastrointest Liver Physiol,* Vol.294, No.3, (March 2008), pp. G764-G769

Martins de Oliveira, R., et al. (2007). The inhibitory effects of $H^+/K^+$-ATPase inhibitors on human neutrophils in vitro: restoration by a $K^+$ ionophore. *Inflamm Res,* Vol.56, No.3, (March 2007), pp. 105-111

Mehrabi, M.R., et al. (2001). Angiogenesis stimulation in explanted hearts from patients pretreated with intravenous prostaglandin E. *J Heart Lung Transplant*, Vol.20, No.4, (April 2001), pp. 465-473

Milani, S., & Calabrò, A. (2001). Role of growth factors and their receptors in gastric ulcer healing. *Microsc Res Tech*, Vol.53, No.5, (June 2001), pp. 360-371

Montrose, M.H., et al. (2006). Gastroduodenal mucosal defense, In: *Physiology of the gastrointestinal tract*, Johnson LR, pp. 1259-1291, Academic Press, New York

Mózsik, G., et al. (2001). The key-role of vagal nerve and adrenals in the cytoprotection and general gastric mucosal integrity. *J Physiol (Paris)*, Vol.95, No.1-6, (January-December 2001), pp. 229-237

Musumba, C., et al. (2009). Review article: cellular and molecular mechanisms of NSAID-induced peptic ulcer. *Aliment Pharmacol Ther*, Vol.30, No.6, (September 2009), pp. 517-531

Nagata, K., et al. (1988). Characterization of a novel transformation-sensitive heat-shock protein (HSP47) that binds to collagen. *Biochem Biophys Res Commun*, Vol.153, No.1, (May 1998), 428-434

Natale, G., et al. (2004). Mechanisms of gastroprotection by lansoprazole pretreatment against experimentally induced injury in rats: role of mucosal oxidative damage and sulfhydryl compounds. *Toxicol Appl Pharmacol*, Vol.195, No.1, (February 2004), pp. 62-72

Newton, J., et al. (2000). The human trefoil peptide, TFFl, is present in different molecular forms that are intimately associated with the adherent mucus gel in normal stomach. *Gut*, Vol.46, No.3, (March 2000), pp. 312-320

Nguyen, T., et al. (2007). Novel roles of local IGF-1 activation in rat gastric ulcer healing: promotes actin polymerization, cell proliferation, reepithelialization and induces COX-2 in a PI3K-dependent manner. *Am J Pathol*, Vol.170, No.4, (April 2007), pp. 1219-1228

Okabe, S., & Amagase, K. (2005). An overview of acetic acid ulcer models--the history and state of the art of peptic ulcer research. *Biol Pharm Bull*, Vol.28, No.8, (August 2005), pp. 1321-1341

Okamoto, R., et al. (2002). Damaged epithelial regenerated by bone marrow-derived cells in the human gastrointestinal tract. *Nature Med*, Vol.8, No.9, (September 2002), pp. 1011-1017

Oshima, T., et al. (2008). Aspirin induces gastric epithelial barrier dysfunction by activating p38 MAPK via claudin-7. *Am J Physiol Cell Physiol*, Vol.295, No.3, (September 2008), pp. C800–C806

Pai, R., et al. (2001). $PGE_2$ stimulates VEGF expression in endothelial cells via ERK2/JNK1 signaling pathways. *Biochem Biophys Res Comm*, Vol.286, No.5, (September 2001), pp. 923-928

Pai, R., et al. (2002). Prostaglandin $E_2$ transactivates EGF receptor: a novel mechanism for promoting colon cancer growth and gastrointestinal hypertrophy. *Nat Med*, Vol.8, No.3, (March 2002), pp. 289–293

Pastoris, O., et al. (2008). Effects of esomeprazole on glutathione levels and mitochondrial oxidative phosphorylation in the gastric mucosa of rats treated with indomethacin. *Naunyn Schmiedebergs Arch Pharmacol*, Vol.378, No.4, (October 2008), pp. 421-429

Perini, R., et al. (2005). Roles of platelets and proteinase-activated receptors in gastric ulcer healing. *Dig Dis Sci*, Vol.50, No.suppl 1, (October 2005), pp. S12-S15

Peskar, B.M. (2001). Neural aspects of prostaglandin involvement in gastric mucosal defense. *J Physiol Pharmacol*, Vol.52, No.4 pt 1, (December 2001), pp. 555–568

Reubi, J.C., et al. (1994). Persistent lack of somatostatin receptors in gastric mucosa of healing ulcers in rat. *Gastroenterology*, Vol.107, No.2, (August 1994), pp. 339-346

Risau, W. (1997). Mechanism of angiogenesis. *Nature*, Vol.386, No.6626, (April 1997), pp. 671-673

Rossmann, H., et al. (1999). $Na^+/HCO_3^-$ cotransport and expression of NBC1 and NBC2 in rabbit gastric parietal and mucous cells. *Gastroenterology*, Vol.116, No.6, (June 1999), pp. 1389–1398

Sánchez-Fidalgo, S., et al. (2004). Angiogenesis, cell proliferation and apoptosis in gastric ulcer healing. Effect of a selective cox-2 inhibitor. *Eur J Pharmacol*, Vol.505, No.1-3, (November 2004), pp. 187-194

Savoye, G., et al. (2001). Low levels of gastric mucosal glutathione during upper gastric bleeding associated with the use of nonsteroidal anti-inflammatory drugs. *Eur J Gastroenterol Hepatol*, Vol.13, No.11, (November 2001), pp. 1309-1313

Scarpignato, C., & Hunt, R.H. (2010). Nonsteroidal antiinflammatory drug-related injury to the gastrointestinal tract: clinical picture, pathogenesis, and prevention. *Gastroenterol Clin North Am*, Vol.39, No.3, (September 2010), pp. 433-464

Schmassmann, A., et al. (1995). Influence of acid and angiogenesis on kinetics of gastric ulcer healing in rats: interaction with indomethacin. *Am J Physiol Gastrointest Liver Physiol*, Vol.268, No.2 pt 1, (February 1995), pp. G276-G285

Schmassmann, A. (1998). Mechanisms of ulcer healing and effects of nonsteroidal anti-inflammatory drugs. *Am J Med*, Vol.104, No.2 pt 1, (February 1998), pp. 43S-51S

Schmassmann, A., & Reubi, J.C. (2000). Cholecystokinin-B/gastrin receptors enhance wound healing in the rat gastric mucosa. *J Clin Invest*, Vol.106, No.8, (October 2000), pp. 1021-1029

Schmassmann, A., et al. (2006). Role of the different isoforms cyclooxygenase and nitric oxide synthase during gastric ulcer healing in cyclooxygenase-1 and -2 knockout mice. Am J Physiol Gastrointest Liver Physiol, Vol.290, No.4, (April 2006), pp. G747-G756

Schneeberger, E.E., & Lynch, R.D. (2004). The tight junction: a multifunctional complex. *Am J Physiol Cell Physiol*, Vol.286, No.6, (June 2004), pp. C1213–C1228

Shahin, M., et al. (1997). Gastric ulcer healing in the rat: kinetics and localization of de novo procollagen synthesis. *Gut*, Vol.41, No.2, (August 1997), pp. 187-194

Shahin M., et al. (2001). Remodelling of extracellular matrix in gastric ulceration. *Microsc Res Tech*, Vol.53, No.6, (June 2001), pp. 396-408

Simon, W.A., et al. (2006). Hydroxyl radical scavenging reactivity of proton pump inhibitors. *Biochem Pharmacol*, Vol.71, No.9, (April 2006), pp. 1337-1341

Soncin, F., & Calderwood, S.K. (1996). Reciprocal effects of pro-inflammatory stimuli and anti-inflammatory drugs on the activity of heat shock factor-1 in human monocytes. *Biochem Biophys Res Commun*, Vol.229, No.2, (December 1996), pp. 479-484

Stadelmann, W., et al. (1998). Physiology and healing dynamics of chronic cutaneous wounds. *Am J Surgery*, Vol.176, No.suppl 2A, (August 1998), pp. 26S-38S

Suzuki, M., et al. (1995). Lansoprazole inhibits oxygen-derived free radical production from neutrophils activated by Helicobacter pylori. *J Clin Gastroenterol*, Vol.20, No.suppl 2, (February 1995), pp. S93-S96

Suzuki, M., et al. (1999). Omeprazole attenuates neutrophil-endothelial cell adhesive interaction induced by extracts of Helicobacter pylori. *J Gastroenterol Hepatol*, Vol.14, No.1, (January 1999), pp. 27-31

Szabo, I.L., et al. (2001). NSAIDs inhibit the activation of egr-1 gene in microvascular endothelial cells. A key to inhibition of angiogenesis? *J Physiol (Paris)*, Vol.95, No.1-6, (January-December 2001), pp. 379-383

Takeuchi, K., et al. (1997). Roles of prostaglandin E-receptor subtypes in gastric and duodenal bicarbonate secretion in rats. *Gastroenterology*, Vol.113, No.5, (November 1997), pp. 1553-1559

Takeuchi, K., et al. (2002). Gastric mucosal ulcerogenic responses following barrier disruption in knockout mice lacking prostaglandin $EP_1$ receptors. *Aliment Pharmacol Ther*, Vol.16, No.suppl 2, (April 2002), pp. 74- 82

Tamura, M., et al. (2002). Vascular endothelial growth factor up-regulates cyclooxygenase-2 expression in human endothelial cells. *J Clin Endocrinol Metab*, Vol.87, No.7, (July 2002), pp. 3504-3507

Tanaka, D., et al. (2007). Genetic evidence for a protective role of heat shock factor 1 against irritant-induced gastric lesions. *Mol Pharmacol*, Vol.71, No.4, (April 2007), pp. 985-993

Tarnawski, A.S., & Jones, M.K. (2003). Inhibition of angiogenesis by NSAIDs: molecular mechanisms and clinical implications. *J Mol Med*, Vol.81, No.10, (October 2003), pp. 627-636

Tarnawski, A. (2005). Cellular and molecular mechanisms of gastrointestinal ulcer healing. *Dig Dis Sci*, Vol.50, No.suppl 1, (October 2005), pp. S24-S33

Taupin, D., & Podolsky, D.K. (2003). Trefoil factors initiators of mucosal healing. *Nat Rev Mol Cell Biol*, Vol.4, No.9, (September 2003), pp. 721-732

Thim, L., et al. (2002). Effect of trefoil factors on the viscoelastic properties of mucus gels. *Eur J Clin Invest*, Vol.32, No.7, (July 2002), pp. 519-527

Tsuji, S., et al. (1995). Gastric ulcer healing and basic fibroblast growth factor: effects of lansoprazole and famotidine. *J Clin Gastroenterol*, Vol.20, No.Suppl 2, (March 1995), pp. S1-S4

Tsuji, S., et al. (2002). Lansoprazole induces mucosal protection through gastrin receptor-dependent up-regulation of cyclooxygenase-2 in rats. *J Pharmacol Exp Ther*, Vol.303, No.3, (December 2002), pp. 1301-1308

Tsujii, M., et al. (1998). Cyclooxygenases regulates angiogenesis induced by colon cancer cells. *Cell*, Vol.93, No.5, (May 1998), pp. 705-716

Tsukimi, Y., & Okabe, S. (2001). Recent advances in gastrointestinal pathophysiology: role of heat shock proteins in mucosal defense and ulcer healing. *Biol Pharm Bull*, Vol.24, No.1, (January 2001), pp. 1-9

Vane, J.R., et al. (1998). Cyclooxygenases 1 and 2. *Annu Rev Pharmacol Toxicol*, Vol.38, No.1, (April 1998), pp. 97–120

Villegas, I., et al. (2002). Effects of oxicam inhibitors of cyclooxygenase on oxidative stress generation in rat gastric mucosa. A comparative study. *Free Radic Res*, Vol.36, No.7, (July 2002), pp. 769-777

Walan, A., et al. (1989). Effect of omeprazole and ranitidine on ulcer healing and relapse rates in patients with benign gastric ulcer. *N Engl J Med*, Vol.320, No.2, (January 1989), pp. 69-75

Wallace, J.L., et al. (2000). NSAID-induced gastric damage in rats: requirement for inhibition of both cyclooxygenase 1 and 2. *Gastroenterology*, Vol.119, No.3, (September 2000), pp. 706–714

Wallace, J.L. (2001). Pathogenesis of NSAID-induced gastroduodenal mucosal injury. *Best Pract Res Clin Gastroenterol*, Vol.15, No.5, (October 2001), pp. 691–703

Wallace, J.L. (2005). Recent advances in gastric ulcer therapeutics. *Curr Opin Pharmacol*, Vol.5, No.6, (December 2005), pp. 573-577

Wallace, J.L. (2006). COX-2: a pivotal enzyme in mucosal protection and resolution of inflammation. *Scientific World J*, Vol.6, (May 2006), pp. 577–588

Wallace, J.L. (2007). Hydrogen sulfide-releasing anti-inflammatory drugs. *Trends Pharmacol Sci*, Vol.28, No.10, (October 2007), pp. 501-505

Wandall, J.H. (1992). Effects of omeprazole on neutrophil chemotaxis, super oxide production, degranulation, and translocation of cytochrome b-245. *Gut*, Vol.33, No.5, (May 1992), pp. 617-621

Wang JY., & Johnson LR. (1994). Expression of proto-oncogenes c-fos and c-myc in healing of gastric mucosal stress ulcers. *Am J Physiol*, Vol. 266, No.5 pt 1, (May 1994), pp. G878-G886

Whittle, B.J. (2002). Gastrointestinal effects of nonsteroidal anti-inflammatory drugs. *Fundam Clin Pharmacol*, Vol.17, No.3, (June 2002), pp. 301–313

Wilder-Smith, C.H., et al. (2006). Dose-effect comparisons of the CINOD AZD3582 and naproxen on upper gastrointestinal tract mucosal injury in healthy subjects. *Scand J Gastroenterol*, Vol.41, No.3, (March 2006), pp. 264-273

Wong, W.M., et al. (2000). Peptide gene expression in gastrointestinal mucosal ulceration: ordered sequence or redundancy? *Gut*, Vol.46, No.2, (February 2000), pp. 286-292

Yang, Y.H., et al. (2006). The cationic host defense peptide rCRAMP promotes gastric ulcer healing in rats. *J Pharmacol Exp Ther*, Vol.318, No.2, (August 2006), pp. 547–554

Yeomans, N.D., et al. (1998). A comparison of omeprazole with ranitidine for ulcers associated with nonsteroidal anti-inflammatory drugs. Acid Suppression Trial: Ranitidine Versus Omeprazole for NSAID-Associated Ulcer Treatment (ASTRONAUT) Study Group. *N Engl J Med*, Vol.338, No.11, (March 1998), pp. 719-726

Zedtwitz-Liebenstein, K., et al. (2002). Omeprazole treatment diminishes intra- and extracellular neutrophil  reactive oxygen production and bactericidal activity. *Crit Care Med,* Vol.30, No.5, (May 2002), pp. 1118-1122

Zimmermann, K.C., et al. (1998). Constitutive cyclooxygenase-2 expression in healthy human and rabbit gastric mucosa. *Mol Pharmacol,* Vol.54, No.3, (September 1998), pp. 536–540

# 8

# Gastric Ulcer Healing –
# Role of Serum Response Factor

Jianyuan Chai
*VA Long Beach Healthcare System, Long Beach and the*
*University of California, Irvine,*
*USA*

## 1. Introduction

Histologically, a gastric ulcer is viewed as a necrotic lesion penetrating through the entire mucosal thickness of the stomach. Because of its great similarities with ulcers in other parts of the digestive tract, gastric ulcer is often reviewed with esophageal and duodenal ulcers together as peptic ulcer disease (PUD). Although it is not as common as duodenal ulcers, gastric ulcers are more often to develop malignancy.

PUD can be found in any part of the world and is probably the most common chronic infection in human population. It causes considerable loss of life year and creates a great economic burden (Figure 1). It had a tremendous effect on morbidity and mortality until the last few decades of the last century when epidemiological trends started to point to an impressive fall in its incidence, particularly in the Western countries. The reason why the rates of PUD decreased is thought to be the development of new effective medication, and of course, the discovery of the pathogen – *Helicobacter pylori*. It is now commonly accepted that the main cause of PUD is *H. pylori*, a helix-shaped Gram-negative bacterium, which infects more than 50% of world population and can be transmitted by contaminated food, groundwater, and even through human saliva (such as from kissing or sharing food utensils). For this reason, higher incidence of PUD is found in the third world countries and low socioeconomic groups. In the developed countries, on the other hand, although *H. pylori* infection is under controlled, thanks to the easy access to advanced treatment and better living condition, extensive use of non-steroidal anti-inflammatory drugs (NSAIDs) keeps the incidence of complicated gastric ulcer and hospitalization stable (Feinstein et al, 2010).

Treatment of PUD usually involves a combination of antibiotics (e.g. metronidazole, clarithromycin, tetracycline, amoxicillin), acid suppressors (e.g. cimetidine, ranitidine, omeprazole, lansoprazole), and mucosa protectors (e.g. bismuth subsalicylate). Unfortunately, patients have to take as many as 20 pills a day and often end up with multiple side effects including nausea, vomiting, diarrhea, dizziness, and headache. Perforated ulcers require surgical repair, while bleeding ulcers have to be taken care by endoscopic cautery, injection or clipping. In any case, healing of an ulcer normally requires multiple molecular and cellular processes to achieve. This chapter will dissect molecular and cellular mechanisms of gastric ulcer healing and focus on an important molecule – Serum Response Factor (SRF) and its role in this event.

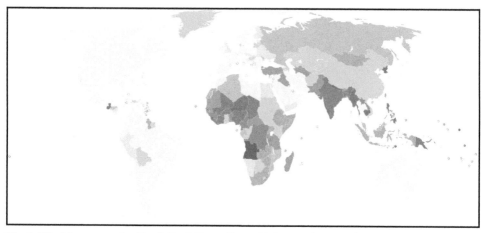

Fig. 1. World age-standardized disability-adjusted life year (DALY) for peptic ulcer disease per 100,000 inhabitants (Wikimedia Commons, based on WHO data in 2004). DALY is a term used by WHO to measure overall disease burden and is expressed as the number of years lost due to illness, disability or early death. It is calculated by summation of the years of life lost and years lived with disability. (☐ no data ☐ less than 20 ☐ 20-40 ☐ 40-60 ☐ 60-80 ☐ 80-100 ☐ 100-120 ☐ 120-140 ☐ 140-160 ☐ 160-180 ☐ 180-200 ☐ 200-220 ☐ more than 220)

## 2. Prevalence of gastric ulcers

Our body function relies on two sources of energy, oxygen and food. Oxygen is taken into our biological system through breath and is directly utilized in the biochemical reaction, while food has to be processed in a very long and complicated structure to become useful to our body. That structure is called digestive system, which includes mouth, esophagus, stomach, small intestine, colon, liver, gall bladder, and pancreas. Any illness in these organs can cause the entire body suffering, often collapse. According to the World Health Organization (WHO), each year, more than 6 million people on earth die of various digestive disorders, making it the second most common cause of death in the world, after heart disease (~7 million). Among all the digestive fatalities, one third is caused by diarrhea, which kills 1.5 million children each year, more than AIDS, malaria and measles combined. For instance, in India, diarrhea causes 386,600 child deaths annually; and in Angola, it contributes to more than 17% of the overall death. Similar to diarrhea, PUD is also most prevalent in the third world countries, responsible for 4% of the total death toll caused by all kinds of digestive diseases combined (Figure 2). The top 15 most affected countries by PUD are listed in Table 1. Philippines is on the top of the list. In this country the PUD death rate is close to 16%, making it the third most deadly gastrointestinal disorder of the country, after diarrhea (37.4%) and liver diseases (23.6%). In the developed countries, on the other hand, the situation is totally different. Take the United States as an example, among eight major categories of digestive diseases, PUD (2%) is the least cause of death, next to diarrhea (2.4%). Instead, colorectal cancer (32.9%), liver disease (25.4%) and pancreas cancer (17.5%) become the top three deadly gastrointestinal problems (Figure 2). According to National Institute of Diabetes and Digestive and Kidney Diseases (NIDDK), PUD affects 14.5 million Americans and about 350,000 new cases are diagnosed each year. Among them, duodenal ulcers are four times as many as gastric ulcers. The annual mortality is approximately 3,000.

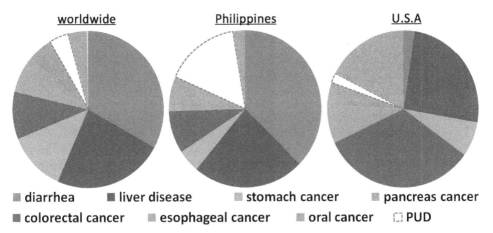

diarrhea ■ liver disease stomach cancer pancreas cancer
■ colorectal cancer esophageal cancer oral cancer PUD

Fig. 2. Death caused by major digestive diseases. Diarrhea is the No.1 cause of death worldwide; however, in the developed countries such as the U.S.A, it becomes the least concern. So is PUD. (Data are extracted from WHO documents).

## 3. Causes of gastric ulcers

For decades, the causes of gastric ulcers were believed to be spicy food, stress, and excessive acid secretion. As the German Protestant theologian Karl Schwarz said "Ohne sauren Magensaft kein peptisches Geschwür", meaning no acid, no ulcer. Therefore, treatment options were confined to acid suppression medications and surgical operation. The successful rate of PUD treatment by acid suppressive operations was reported in the literature repeatedly. At the time, people did not believe that bacteria could survive in the human stomach, as the stomach produces extensive amounts of acid of strength similar to the acid found in a car battery.

By 1875, German scientists Bottcher and Letulle had examined the base of ulcers and found bacteria growing on the floors as well as on the margins of ulcers (Kidd & Modlin, 1998). They postulated, but never proved, that bacteria play a role in the development of PUD. Further effort had been made to dig the issue. In 1886, a Polish clinical researcher Jaworski found the same bacteria in the sediments of stomach washings from human and published his work in the *Handbook of Gastric diseases* in 1899, but the work had little impact because it was written in Polish (Konturek, 2003). The same bacteria were also found in the stomachs of animals including dogs (Bizzozero, 1892), cats and mice (Salomon, 1896). In 1938, Doenges discovered that 43% of 242 stomachs that he examined contained spirochete-like bacteria (Doenges, 1938); and in 1947, Freedburg and Barron confirmed this discovery in 37% of 35 specimens that they examined and they also noticed these bacteria appearing more frequently near ulcers than ulcer inside (Freedburg & Barron, 1940). Based on their observations, they concluded that the bacteria were opportunistic infections rather than the cause of PUD. However, interest in the role of bacteria in gastric diseases faded when Palmer, a pathologist at Walter Reed Army Medical Center in Washington DC, found no bacteria at all in 1,180 biopsies taken from living individuals and he was very confident to claim that other people's discovery of bacteria in PUD was simply contamination (Palmer, 1954).

| Rank | Country | Population | PUD Death Rate |
|------|---------|------------|----------------|
| 1 | PHILIPPINES | 94,013,200 | 16.8 |
| 2 | CAMBODIA | 13,395,682 | 16.7 |
| 3 | KIRIBATI | 100,000 | 15.3 |
| 4 | GUATEMALA | 14,361,666 | 15.2 |
| 5 | NEW GUINEA | 10,324,000 | 14.7 |
| 6 | NORTH KOREA | 23,991,000 | 14.5 |
| 7 | MYANMAR | 50,496,000 | 14.5 |
| 8 | NEPAL | 28,584,975 | 14.3 |
| 9 | TIMOR-LESTE | 1,171,000 | 12.5 |
| 10 | ANGOLA | 18,993,000 | 10.5 |
| 11 | BANGLADESH | 149,804,000 | 10.4 |
| 12 | SIERRA LEONE | 5,836,000 | 9.9 |
| 13 | NIGER | 15,203,822 | 9.5 |
| 14 | INDONESIA | 237,556,363 | 9.0 |
| 15 | LAOS | 6,436,000 | 9.0 |

Table 1. Top 15 countries are mostly affected by PUD. Death rate is calculated by dividing the number of deaths caused by PUD with the total number of deaths. (Data are extracted from WHO documents).

Eager to understand the role of bacteria in gastric diseases was revived in the 1970s when Steer showed an image of the bacterium in the ultra-structure of gastric epithelia from PUD patients (Steer, 1975). Meantime, an Australian pathologist Warren and his clinical fellow Marshall were trying to isolate the bacteria and culture them *in vitro*. After numerous unsuccessful attempts, finally they succeeded in 1982 when they found colonies on their petri dishes that they accidentally left in the incubator for the Easter weekend. Marshall wanted to prove that the bacterium was a gastric pathogen, so he decided to use himself to do an experiment. He swallowed the bacteria isolated from a 66-year-old man with known dyspepsia. Two weeks later, he found the bacteria colonized in his stomach in association with gastritis, proving his speculation (Marshall, 2002).

The bacterium was later identified as a new species named *Helicobacter pylori*, which infects upper gastrointestinal tract of more than half of the world's population, and in some regions of Africa and Asia, the prevalence can be as high as 80-90% of the local residents. In the developed countries, the rate is around 25% (Pounder & Ng, 1995). The ability of *H. pylori* surviving in the stomach comes from an enzyme – urease, which can break down urea into carbon dioxide and ammonia. The ammonia is converted into ammonium by taking a proton (H+), which leaves only hydroxyl ion. Hydroxyl ions then react with carbon dioxide, producing carbonate, which neutralizes gastric acid. Urease activity is low at neutral pH but can increase 10- to 20-fold as the external pH falls between 6.5 and 5.5, and remains high at pH 2.5 (Scott et al, 1998). *H. pylori* also expresses another protein – urel, which is a urea transporter that brings urea into the cytoplasm of the bacteria for urease to digest. About 50-70% of *H. pylori* strains in Western countries carry the *cag* pathogenicity island (*cag* PAI), a 40kb DNA segment containing more than 30 genes (Peek & Crabtree, 2006). Patients infected with this strain have a stronger inflammatory response in the stomach and are at a greater risk of developing peptic ulcers or stomach cancer than those infected with strains lacking the island (Kusters et al, 2006). The bacterium produces many different molecules that allow it to adhere to the mucosal surface. Following attachment of *H. pylori* to stomach epithelial cells, the type IV secretion system expressed by the *cag* PAI "injects" the inflammation-inducing agent, peptidoglycan, from their own cell wall into the epithelial cells. The injected peptidoglycan is recognized by the cytoplasmic pattern recognition receptor (immune sensor) Nod1, which then stimulates expression of cytokines that promote inflammatory response, such as gastritis, from the host (Viala et al, 2004). This inflammation leads to mucosal atrophy in the host, which predisposes to formation of ulcers. Therefore, eradication of the bacterium from the host has been proven to efficiently eliminate ulcer reoccurrence.

However, gastric ulcers are also found in people without *H. pylori* infection. Studies have associated this group of patients with overly use of NSAIDs. Most NSAIDs are non-selective inhibitors of cyclooxygenases (Cox-1, Cox-2), which convert arachidonic acid to prostaglandins (Pai et al, 2001). Prostaglandins are mediators of inflammation. Inhibition of prostaglandin synthesis in the stomach causes increased gastric acid secretion and decreased mucus secretion, thereby weakening gastric mucosa protection and allowing the acid to come into close contact with the mucosal epithelium.

It is currently believed that 70-90% of gastric ulcers are caused by *Helicobacter pylori* infection, and utilization of NSAIDs is responsible for the remainder. However, in both conditions, doctors have noticed that adding acid-suppressive drugs to the treatment regimen can greatly help ulcer healing and prevent ulcer reoccurrence. Some even argue that *H. pylori* itself cannot cause ulcers at all; even Dr. Robin Warren, the Noble laureate for the discovery of *H. pylori* as the pathogen of gastric ulcers, admitted that the bacteria cannot be responsible for so many ulcers without acid. Therefore, acid is still a factor. It is my belief that no matter *H. pylori* or NSAIDs, their actions lead to removal of mucosal protection, which allows the acid to come into a direct contact with the mucosal epithelium and that causes ulcer development. Zollinger-Ellison syndrome is an example, in which gastric acid is over-secreted due to high level of hormone gastrin. Gastrin induces parietal cells to produce more acid and also stimulates parietal cell hyperplasia, which leads to severe gastric ulceration. One might conclude that the dictum "no acid, no ulcer" still holds true.

## 4. Molecular and cellular mechanisms of gastric ulcer healing

A gastric ulcer is a deep wound in the stomach wall that involves epithelium, endothelium, connective tissue, and smooth muscle. Therefore, healing of a gastric ulcer means a restoration of all these tissue components that have been damaged during ulceration. At the cellular level, this process requires participation of all the cell types that originally make these tissues, including epithelial cells, endothelial cells, fibroblasts, myofibroblasts, smooth muscle cells, and immune cells. All these cells are activated to move towards the ulcer to fill in the positions that had been vacant due to damage and loss. Some of these cells (e.g. epithelial cells) need to divide to make up the number, while others (e.g. immune cells) need to be differentiated from progenitor stem cells. In addition to cell proliferation and differentiation, there is a third source to get the cell supply needed to re-build the tissue, that is, cell transformation. Some of these cells, if not all, can transform from one cell type to another (Chai et al, 2010a). For example, epithelial cells can start to express mesenchymal molecules (e.g. vimentin, N-cadherin, smooth muscle α-actin) to become fibroblasts or even myofibroblasts, while fibroblasts or myofibroblasts can express epithelial markers (e.g. E-cadherin, ZO-1, γ-catenin) to connect with each other and form cellular sheets like epithelium. The former event is called epithelial-mesenchymal transition (EMT), and the later, of course, is mesenchymal-epithelial transition (MET). In a normal individual, all these events take place in a well synchronized spatial and temporal manner so that the damaged tissue is eventually replaced by new tissue precisely like the old tissue before ulceration. This job is done at the molecular level.

Like any other wounds, ulcer healing starts with a process of coagulation and hemostasis immediately after ulceration is initiated. The principal of this process is to prevent exsaguination and to provide a matrix for the cells coming into the ulcer in the later phase of healing. A dynamic balance between endothelial cells, platelets, coagulation, and fibrinolysis regulates hemostasis and determines the amount of fibrin deposited at the wound site, thereby influencing the progress of healing. Normally, endothelial cells produce heparin-like molecules and thrombomodulin to prevent blood coagulation and also nitric oxide and prostacyclin to inhibit platelet aggregation; however, when a vascular injury occurs during ulceration, these cells stop making these molecules, instead, start to secrete von Willebrand factor and thromboplastin to adhere platelets to the exposed collagen and to convert prothrombin to thrombin. Thrombin then converts fibrinogen to fibril to strengthen platelet plug. Once platelets come in contact with collagen, they become activated to release growth factors and cytokines, such as platelet derived growth factor (PDGF), transforming growth factor-β (TGF-β), epidermal growth factor (EGF), insulin-like growth factor (IGF), basic fibroblast growth factor (bFGF), vascular endothelial growth factor (VEGF), Tumor necrosis factor-α (TNF-α), interleukin-1 (IL-1), and interleukin-6 (IL-6). These molecules act as promoters in the ulcer healing cascade by activating and attracting neutrophils and later, macrophages, endothelial cells, fibroblasts, and myofibroblasts to the ulcer area, and move the healing process to the next phase – inflammation. The main function of neutrophils is to prevent infection. These cells can destroy and remove bacteria and damaged tissue by phagocytosis. Once this task is completed, neutrophils are eliminated by apoptosis. Then macrophages move in to clean up the cell remnants and apoptotic bodies of neutrophils. Macrophages are key regulatory cells during ulcer healing because they not only continue neutrophil's job, but also produce an abundant reservoir of potent growth factors to activate additional endothelial cells and fibroblasts.

The inflammatory phase is ended when lymphocytes attracted to the ulcer by IL-1, an important regulator of collagenase activity that is later needed for extracellular matrix (ECM) remodeling. Fibroblasts synthesize ECM to replace the provisional network of fibrin and fibronectin and form granulation tissue under the ulcer bed. Fibroblasts are attracted to the ulcer by TGF-β and PDGF that are produced by inflammatory cells and platelets. Once in the ulcer, fibroblasts proliferate rapidly and produce abundant ECM proteins, such as fibronectin, proteoglycans and procollagen, whose accumulation in the ulcer provides further support for cell migration and tissue repair. Thereafter, fibroblasts transform into myofibroblasts with thick actin bundles underneath the cell membrane which generate powerful forces to pull the wound edges together to close the ulcer. Granulation tissue is a reflection of active angiogenesis. A number of molecules released during hemostasis are angiogenic factors, such as VEGF, PDGF, bFGF, and TGF-β, which can stimulate resident endothelial cells to proliferate. The activated endothelial cells produce proteases (matrix metalloproteinases or MMPs) to digest the basal lamina in the parental vessels in order to crawl through the ECM and to re-gather to form new blood vessels in the wound center, giving bumpy appearance to the ulcer bed. Angiogenesis is essential for ulcer healing, because it provides nutrients for the healing process to move forward.

Meantime, mucosal epithelial cells at the ulcer margin are stimulated by ulceration to form a contractile actomyosin ring around the ulcer. Actomyosin ring is made of filamentous actin (F-actin) and myosin-II in association with radially organized microtubules (Mandato & Bement, 2003). F-actin cable in each epithelial cell at the ulcer margin links to neighboring cells through adherens junctions and is operated by the motor protein myosin-II, jointly like a purse string provides the force necessary to draw the wound edges together to achieve re-epithelialization (Figure 3). The whole process is regulated by the small GTPases including RhoA, Rac and Cdc42. RhoA activates the assembly of F-actin stress fibers by cortical flow, Rac is required for the rapid actin polymerization to form lamellipodia, and Cdc42 is essential for myosin-II organization and actin assembly/disassembly (Garcia-Fernandez et al, 2009; Darenfed & Mandato, 2005). The cells directly bordering the ulcer are connected by a continuous actomyosin cable, anchored at cell-cell junctions, and form lamellipodia at their leading edge (Figure 3). At the final stage of wound closure, opposing leading edge cells make contact through lamellipodia and seal the gap.

Epithelial cell migration stops once the gap is sealed. However, healing process still continues into the next phase – tissue remodeling within the ulcer. A new basement membrane starts to build underneath the epithelium. Granulation tissue is gradually replaced by regenerated tissue that more closely resembles the original tissue before ulceration. The main players in this phase are MMPs and their antagonists TIMPs. They keep in a very delicate dynamic balance and work together in a coordinated fashion to allow tissue synthesis and breakdown to take place simultaneously.

## 5. Serum Response Factor in gastric ulcer healing

During ulcer healing, epithelial cells proliferate and migrate from nearby to close the wound; smooth muscle cells and myofibroblasts multiply to restore the musculature; endothelial cells are motivated to generate vessels to make sure the newly generated tissue has an adequate nutrient supply; and immune cells stand by to guard the wounded area and protect from invasions of pathogens. All these cellular activities are directed and regulated by dozens of molecules including growth factors, cytokines, chemokines, and more importantly, transcription factors, because every one of these molecules has to be transcribed from its gene fundamentally and transcription factors are the ones for this job. Among many transcription factors involved in ulcer healing, Serum response factor (SRF) is the master regulator. SRF is ubiquitously expressed in every type of tissue and its targeted genes take up nearly 1% of our entire genome (Sun et al, 2006; Miano, 2010). SRF can be activated by growth factors, cytokines and chemokines, and in return, activated SRF can direct expressions of these molecules to heal ulcers in a precisely organized manner. Moreover, CagA, one of the main products of *H. pylori*, can increase SRF binding capacity by 40 fold (Hirata et al, 2002). SRF is involved in every stage of the healing process including re-epithelialization, angiogenesis and granulation tissue remodeling.

### 5.1 Story of SRF

SRF was first identified by a British scientist Richard Treisman in 1986 (Treisman, 1986), for which he was awarded the EMBO Medal in 1995. Treisman's discovery was built on a prior observation by Michael Greenberg, a postdoctoral research fellow at the time in Edward Ziff' lab at New York University. Greenberg's work showed that resting fibroblasts responded to serum addition with a rapid activation of *c-fos* (Greenberg & Ziff, 1984). Since its activation does not require new protein synthesis, *c-fos* was classified as an immediate early gene. Later, it was found that in addition to serum, other mitogenic agents such as growth factors have the same effect on *c-fos* activation (Rollins & Stiles, 1989). During that time, Treisman was a struggling postdoctoral research fellow at Harvard University who was interested in *c-myc* regulation (Treisman, 1995). In the summer of 1984, he met Edward Ziff and heard about Greenberg's discovery. Treisman immediately forsook *c-myc* and switched to *c-fos*. After he returned to England, Treisman rapidly proceeded with *c-fos* study by focusing on 5' regulatory region. Several regulatory DNA elements were identified in the promoter region of *c-fos* gene, but a particular attention was given to a short sequence located about 300bp upstream of the transcription initiation site. For convenience, Treisman named this sequence Serum Response Element (SRE) and the protein that identifies this sequence Serum Response Factor (Treisman, 1986). SRE is an A/T rich core flanked by an inverted repeat, $CC(A/T)_6GG$, and for this reason, SRE is also referred to as CArG box. Treisman demonstrated that *c-fos* activation by serum requires SRF binding to SRE. By that time, several other labs also identified the existence of SRF (Gilman et al, 1986; Prywes & Roeder, 1986; Greenberg et al, 1987). Since then, SRE has been identified in many genes across our entire genome (Sun et al, 2006). The list of SRE-containing genes is still growing.

In 1986, Greenberg moved to Boston and became a faculty of Harvard Medical School with his own lab. His initial observation stimulated many researchers to look in that direction and led to a series of important discoveries in the area of gene transcriptional regulation. His colleagues wrote a song to portrait him and his work around c-fos:

"He was a bald headed man
He was brutally handsome
And they were terminally busy
They held him up
And he held them for ransom
In a lab in a cold, cold city
He had a nasty reputation
As a cru-el dude
They said he was ruthless,
Said he was crude
They had one thing in common
They were always uptight
He'd say "Faster, faster,
Let's publish by tonight"
Life in the fos lane
Surely make you lose your mind
Life in the fos lane
Eager for action
Hot for the game
The Sephadex fraction
The quest for the fame
They read all the right journals
They paid gigantic bills
They threw outrageous parties
They had infamous spills
There were bands on the Northern
But no counts could be traced
He pretended not to notice
He was caught up in the race
In every evening, until it was light
They were so tired, they faked it
He was too tired to fight about it

Life in the fos lane
Surely make you lose your mind
Life in the fos lane
Life in the fos lane
Everything, all the time
Life in the fos lane
Rapid and transient
Transcribed in a burst
In all cell responses
c-fos turns on first
He said listen Bernie
We need space to work in
We've been up and down this
hallway
And never seen Ed Lin
He said call Howard Hughes
I think I'm gonna crash
Six post-docs are coming
And I'm almost out of cash
He kept pushing them to publish
"Go for Cell" he would shout
They didn't care
They were just dying to get out
And it was
Life in the fos lane
Surely make you lose your mind
Life in the fos lane
Life in the fos lane
Everything all the time
Life in the fos lane"

## 5.2 Biology of SRF

The human SRF gene is 10607bp long containing 7 exons and is mapped to the chromosome 6p21.1. The full length of SRF transcript is 4201bp including exon 1 (1-871), exon 2 (872-1138), exon 3 (1139-1400), exon 4 (1401-1520), exon 5 (1521-1712), exon 6 (1713-1789), and exon 7 (1790-4201). SRF can be expressed in different isoforms due to alternative splicing and some of them appear to display tissue specificity. For instance, SRF-S, which lacks both exon 4 and 5 ($\Delta$4, 5), has only been detected in the aorta, while SRF-I, which is the shortest isoform (missing exon 3, 4 and 5), is specific to embryonic tissues. On the other hand, SRF-M, which lacks only exon 5, has been shown as a dominant negative mutant. SRF expression is self regulated, because SRF gene promoter contains four SRE sites. Full length SRF protein (~67 kDa) contains three distinct domains: a SRE DNA binding domain, a transactivation domain and multiple phosphorylation sites. The DNA binding domain, which also serves for dimerization and interaction with accessory factors, has been highly conserved throughout evolution, showing a 93% homology between fruit flies and humans. Phosphorylation at Serine 103, which is immediately adjacent to the DNA binding domain, was shown to greatly enhance SRF activity (Chai & Tarnawski, 2002; Modak & Chai, 2010).

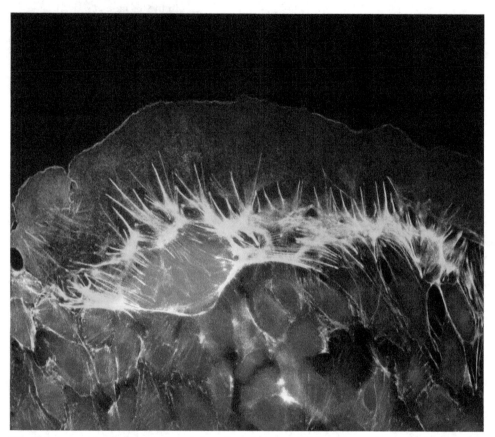

Fig. 3. Actomyosin ring formation at the edge of a wound. Monolayer of rat gastric mucosal epithelial cells (RGM1) was wounded by scratch with a pipette tip. Two hours later, cells were fixed in 3.7% formaldehyde, permeabilized with acetone, and stained for F-actin (green) with Oregon Green-conjugated phalloidin and for G-actin (red) with Texas Red-conjugated DNase I. The image shows a part of the ring and lamellipodia.

### 5.3 Functions of SRF

What is SRF? A few years ago, the **Medical News Today** conducted an interview with Joseph Miano from University of Rochester, one of the prominent SRF researchers, and described that "SRF is one of nature's oldest proteins and is essential for life because it supports the basic internal structure of all living cells. Its function is to carefully turn on 300 of our 30,000 genes" (Orr, 2004). In another word, about 1% of the total human genes carries

SRF target – SRE. These genes fall into a broad spectrum and some of them have multiple SRE sites, for example, EGR1 has six and CCN1 has five, even SRF itself has four SRE sequences (Sun et al, 2006). In addition to the well-known immediate early genes (e.g. FOS and EGR1), SRF also controls a long list of muscle-related genes (ACTA2, MYH6, MYH11, SM22α, TNNT1, ATP2A1, etc). In fact, most of the published SRF studies focus on its role in muscular structures including cardiac muscle, smooth muscle and skeletal muscle. Ten years ago, I was a postdoctoral research fellow at Harvard University, walking behind the giants like Greenberg and Treisman and trying to find new meanings for SRF. We created transgenic mice with cardiac-specific overexpression of SRF. The mice died within 6 months after birth due to heart failure. Histological examination revealed severe cardiomyocyte hypotrophy and interstitial fibrosis (Zhang et al, 2001a). The image made to the cover of the **American Journal of Physiology**. From this study, we have learned that too much SRF can drive overexpression of numerous cardiac genes (MYH7, ACTA1, NPPA, etc.) and end up with a bigger and heavier heart than in normal individuals. The heart-to-body weight ratio was almost 4 times greater in transgenic mice compared to non-transgenic littermates. To look at the other side of the coin, we also produced transgenic mice that express a dominant mutant SRF in heart. The mutated SRF gene generated a protein product that was incapable to bind to SRE, and therefore, cardiac genes never had a chance to fully express during embryogenesis. As a result, most embryos died before born, and a few survivors barely made to the second week of their age. Histological examination displayed serious cardiac ventricle dilation and myofiber degeneration (Zhang et al, 2001b). These studies demonstrate that properly functional SRF is essential for both embryonic development and post-natal development. This concept is also supported by the earlier transgenic study showing that complete knockout of SRF was lethal (Arsenian et al, 1998). Similar consequences have been also observed in transgenics of skeletal muscle (Li et al, 2005; Chavret et al, 2006; Lahoute et al, 2008) and smooth muscle (Miano et al, 2004; Werth et al, 2010).

SRE has also been identified in cytoskeletal genes (ACTB, CFL1, DES, DSTN, TTN, KRT17, etc.), another major category with more than 1,000 members, whose protein products form an intracellular network connecting membranous subcellular structures to the cell membrane and the nucleus. Some of these genes are expressed in all types of cells, suggesting that SRF is essential for maintenance of cell shape and locomotion in everywhere of our body. SRF regulates cytoskeletal organization; on the other hand, SRF itself is regulated by the dynamics of actin cytoskeleton. For instance, every time G-actin polymerizes into F-actin, SRF gets activated.

The remaining SRE-containing gene products fall into many diversified categories, such as growth factors (e.g. IGF2, FGF10, FGFR3, TGFB1i1, etc.), ECM proteins (e.g. CCN1, CTGF, etc.), cell adhesion molecules (e.g. ITGA1, ITGA5, ITGB1, etc.), intercellular junctional molecules (e.g. TJP1, CDH5, CDH11, etc.), neuronal receptors (e.g. NR4A1, NR4A2, etc.), and apoptosis regulators (BCL2).

In addition to the hundreds of genes that SRF directly regulates, a growing number of genes that do not contain SRE have been found to respond to SRF activity (Khachigian & Collins, 1997; Miano et al, 2007). From this, one can imagine the influence of SRF on life.

### 5.4 SRF in ulcer healing

Like any other human diseases, gastric ulcer and gastric ulcer healing have been studied both clinically as well as experimentally. Since the rules and regulations on clinical studies are extremely strict, most of the mechanistic studies have to be done in animal models complemented by *in vitro* cell culture. Researchers have developed several animal models for gastric ulcer study, which generally can be classified as chemical-induced and surgical-induced. Comparison of all these models reveals striking similarities in the morphological evolution as well as molecular dynamics involved in healing process. Therefore, it is generally accepted that ulcer undergoes common stages of healing, as discussed above, once it develops, regardless the cause (Tarnawski, 2005). Figure 4A shows a typical gastric ulcer developed in rat by topical application of acetic acid on the serosal side of the stomach. This model was initially developed by Japanese researchers and modified and validated by others (Okabe & Pfeiffer, 1972). Briefly, the animal needs to be fasted 12 hours before operation, otherwise, the food in the stomach would interfere ulcer induction. Laparotomy is performed under anesthesia to expose the stomach. Hold the stomach tightly with one hand and apply 50μl of acetic acid to the wall of the glandular stomach with the other hand, through a pipette tip (Ø 4.00mm). Hold for 90 seconds and then clean up the area with saline. In this way, a gastric ulcer can develop within 3-5 days after induction (Chai et al, 2004a; Nguyen et al, 2007).

Immunohistological examination shows that SRF is highly activated in the ulcerated mucosa as well as in underneath connective tissue (Figure 4B). Figure 4C shows a higher magnification of regenerating gastric mucosal glands in the ulcer, and the bright red nuclear stain indicates SRF activation. The similar result can be seen in human gastric ulcer as well (Figure 4D).

To determine what role SRF plays in gastric ulcer healing, we injected SRF expressing plasmid around the ulcer induction site to boost the local level of SRF. As a result, ulcer healing was significantly accelerated by the treatment (Chai et al, 2004a). In particular, re-epithelialization process was speeded up. In addition, a massive amount of smooth muscle α-actin expressing cells were found in the granulation tissue under the ulcer bed, indicating an increase of smooth muscle cells and/or myofibroblasts. *In vitro* overexpression of SRF in gastric mucosal epithelial cells (RGM1) and smooth muscle cells (A7R5) all proved promotions in cell migration and proliferation, as reflected by increased actin polymerization and activations of *c-fos* and *egr-1*, suggesting that the acceleration of ulcer healing by SRF gene therapy is due to SRF-driven cell migration and proliferation.

As we discussed above, no matter re-epithelialization or smooth muscle structure restoration, they all require blood supply provided by angiogenesis, a process that makes sure the newly generated structures during ulcer healing will survive. In order to test what influence SRF has on angiogenesis during ulcer healing, we did same injection around the ulcer, but this time the SRF cDNA in the plasmid was flipped over to become an antisense generator. The idea was to interfere with local SRF expression and to create a local SRF deficiency. As a result, less number of micro-vessels was found in the granulation tissue, indicating that SRF deficiency impairs angiogenesis (Chai et al, 2004b).

This conclusion was also supported by *in vitro* study, which showed that SRF deficiency impaired endothelial cells migration and proliferation capability so that even the most powerful angiogenic factor like VEGF could not stimulate tube formation in Matrigel or collagen gel matrix (Figure 5), a phenomenon called *in vitro* angiogenesis normally observed in the presence of an angiogenic factor (Jones et al, 2001). Further dissection of the mechanisms revealed that VEGF activates SRF through MEK-ERK and Rho signaling, and blocking these pathways interrupts SRF mediated endothelial cell migration and proliferation, and eventually causes failure of angiogenesis.

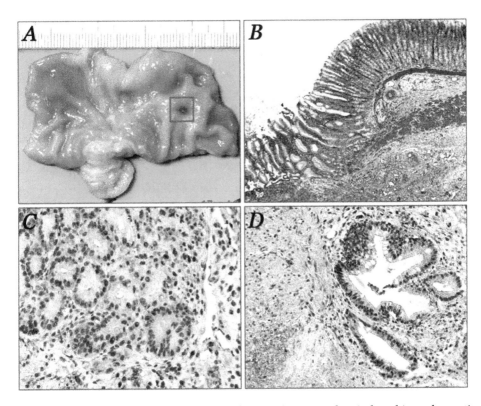

Fig. 4. SRF activation during gastric ulcer healing. *A*. A gastric ulcer induced in rat by acetic acid experimentally. *B*. Immunohistochemistry shows SRF activation in the ulcer region. *C*. SRF activation in the regenerating mucosal glands. *D*. SRF activation in the human gastric ulcer.

In addition to epithelial cells, endothelial cells, and smooth muscle cells, we have also examined another type of cell – myofibroblast. As we discussed above, myofibroblasts play an important role in ulcer healing by producing many growth factors and ECM molecules to mediate the healing process and also by providing contractive force to close the ulcer. We found that ulceration can trigger myofibroblast differentiation from the epithelial cells adjacent to the wound and from the fibroblasts within the ulcer bed (Chai et al, 2007). These cells can be distinguished from their ancestors by their expression of smooth muscle α-actin, and from smooth muscle cells by the absence of smoothelin. Many myofibroblasts were a transient phenotype, once the ulcer was healed, they disappeared. Local increase of SRF level by injecting SRF expressing plasmid into the ulcer greatly boosted the number of cells that express smooth muscle α-actin but not smoothelin, indicating that SRF promotes myofibroblast differentiation. This conclusion was also supported by *in vitro* experiments, which demonstrated that overexpression of SRF in both epithelial cells and fibroblasts induced expression of smooth muscle α-actin (Figure 6).

The involvement of SRF in gastric ulcer healing was also strengthened by the finding of its association with *H. pylori*. In 2001, Japanese researchers found that when gastric cells were co-cultured with *H. pylori* strain that possesses the cag PAI, SRE promoter activity was increased by 3-6 fold (Mitsuno et al, 2001). Their further investigation showed that when cells were transfected with CagA expressing vector, SRE promoter activity can be increased by 40 fold (Hirata et al, 2002). CagA is one of the cag PAI encoded genes. Upon attaching to the mucosal epithelial cells, cag PAI secretion system transports CagA into the host cells, causing actin cytoskeleton rearrangement into "Hummingbird" phenotype (Backert et al, 2001). These studies link SRF to the main cause of peptic ulcer.

In addition to peptic ulcer, SRF has also been associated with other digestive functions and abnormalities, which has been reviewed elsewhere (Modak & Chai, 2010; Miano, 2010).

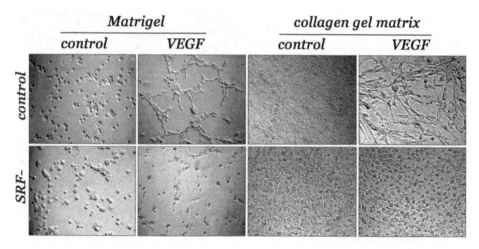

Fig. 5. SRF is required for angiogenesis. Rat gastric microvascular endothelial cells were transfected with either a plasmid expressing antisense SRF (SRF-) or the plasmid vehicle (control). Cells were seeded on Matrigel and collagen gel matrix and treated with either recombinant VEGF at 50ng/ml or vehicle (control). Loss of SRF impaired VEGF-induced tube formation and cell sprouting. Matrigel assay and collagen gel matrix assay are also called 2- and 3-dimensional *in vitro* angiogenesis assay respectively.

## 6. Serum Response Factor regulated genes in gastric ulcer healing

As we discussed above, hundreds of genes are directly or indirectly regulated by SRF. During ulcer healing, all the damaged parts by ulceration, including mucosal epithelium, muscularis mucosa, connective tissue and microvascular structure, must be repaired or regenerated. Needless to say, molecules constituting these components are definitely involved in the ulcer healing process. For instance, smooth muscle α-actin, smooth muscle γ-actin, smooth muscle myosin heavy chain, smooth muscle calponin, smoothelin, and SM22α are basic molecules of muscularis mucosa; Endothelin 1 and VE-cadherin are essential components of blood vessels; Tight Junction protein 1 and cytokeratins such as CK7, CK8, CK14, CK17, CK18 and CK19 make up epithelium. All of these molecules are direct targets of SRF. In addition to structure molecules, SRF-regulated adhesive and locomotive molecules such as integrin-α1, -α5, -α9, and -β1 and vinculin are involved in cell migration;

Bcl-2 regulates apoptosis; SRF-regulated secreted molecules such as connective tissue growth factor and insulin growth factor 2 are mediators of the healing process. Here we will present a couple of SRF targets that have been studied in detail.

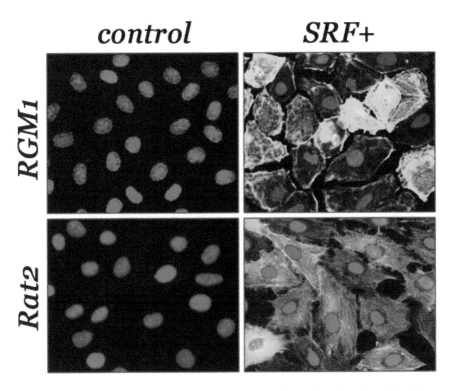

Fig. 6. Overexpression of SRF (SRF+) in rat gastric epithelial cells (RGM1) or fibroblasts (Rat2) can induce myofibroblast phenotype. Cells were stained for smooth muscle α-actin which was identified with a FITC-conjugated secondary antibody. The nuclei were counterstained with propidium iodide.

### 6.1 Egr-1

Egr-1 is an immediate early gene coded transcription factor that is activated in the early phase of ulceration (Khomenko et al, 2006; Szabo et al, 2000). The fact that its activation requires SRF was first noticed in 1993 when leukemia cells were treated with an anti-leukemia drug called 1-(beta-D-arabinofuranosyl)cytosine (Kharbanda et al, 1993). Egr-1 was found transiently activated by the treatment, but deletion of certain region of the Egr-1 promoter, about 95bp upstream from the initiation site, impaired this activation. Further analysis of this region found six SRE sequences, making Egr-1 a close target of SRF. On the other hand, SRF gene promoter contains Egr-1 binding element, 5'-GCGGGGGCG-3', suggesting that SRF itself is also regulated by Egr-1 (Spencer et al, 1999). Microarray analysis screened 12,000 gene promoters and found that at least 283 genes have Egr-1 binding sites (Arora et al, 2008). Many of these genes encode proteins (e.g. TGFβ1, bFGF, PDGF, p53, p73,

PTEN, EGFR, BMP4, MMP9, ITGA5, CK16, Egr-2, etc.) that are known to contribute to ulcer or other wound healing. Through regulation of these genes, Egr-1 greatly extends SRF power.

## 6.2 CCN1

CCN1 (formerly known as Cyr61 or IGFBP10) is another important gene directly regulated by SRF and contains five SRE sites located about 3751bp upstream in the gene promoter. It encodes a matricellular protein that is best known for its angiogenic activity because it stimulates neovascularization in rat corneas and *cyr61*-null mice suffer embryonic death due to vascular defects (Mo et al, 2002). One study demonstrated that intramuscular injection of a CCN1-expression adenovirus in rabbits with ischemic hindlimb improves tissue perfusion even greater than injection of VEGF (Fataccioli et al, 2002). The involvement of CCN1 in wound healing was first known ten years ago in a cutaneous wound model (Chen et al, 2001; Lantinkic et al, 2001). During the experiment, CCN1 was found highly up-regulated in the granulation tissue five days after wounding and remained high for a week till the re-epithelialization was completed. It was shown that CCN1 promotes angiogenesis not only directly but also indirectly through induction of VEGF.

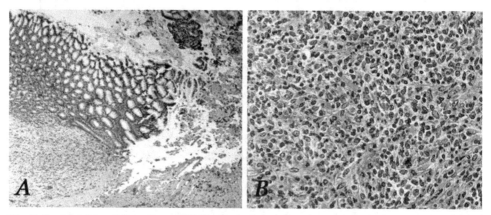

Fig. 7. Gastric ulceration induces CCN1 expression at the ulcer margin (A) and granulation tissue (B).

As a matricellular protein, CCN1 has features intermediate between conventional growth factors and structural ECM molecules; therefore, it can influence tissue remodeling without being an integral element of the structural ECM. In addition to being an angiogenic factor, CCN1 also supports cell adhesion, migration, proliferation, differentiation and survival. Recently, we have found that CCN1 is highly up-regulated in the gastric epithelial cells adjacent to the ulcer and remains high until the wound is healed (Figure 7; Chai et al, 2010b). This was demonstrated by epithelial injury both *in vivo* (gastric ulcer margin) and *in vitro* (gastric epithelial cell culture). Its elevation induces a transient phenotypic change in the mucosal epithelial cells at the ulcer margin and drives the wound closure. These cells lose their epithelial identities and become mesenchymal-like cells. At the molecular level, it shows down-regulation of epithelial markers such as E-cadherin, Occludin and cytokeratins, and up-regulation of mesenchymal markers such as vimentin, N-cadherin and metalloproteinases. Once the wound is healed, these cells and their progeny can resume their original epithelial phenotype as evidenced both *in vitro* and *in vivo*. However, when CCN1 is knocked down in gastric mucosal epithelial cells, injury-induced EMT is disrupted and wound closure is delayed. We have further dissected the molecular mechanisms of this process and found that CCN1-induced E-cadherin loss is not due to transcriptional repression, which is the main mechanism of E-cadherin loss in many other systems (Zhou et al, 2004; Hayashida et al, 2006; Kang & Massague, 2004), but rather protein degradation caused by the collapse of adherens junctions, which is ignited by β-catenin nuclear translocation. CCN1-activated integrin-linked kinase mediates this event. In addition, our *in vivo* study demonstrated that local injection of recombinant CCN1 protein into gastric ulcers can induce expression of vimentin and smooth muscle α-actin in the mucosal epithelial cells and promote re-epithelialization during ulcer healing, and that local injection of CCN1 antibody neutralizes the effect and delays healing process. We have also found that TGFβ1 up-regulates CCN1 expression in gastric epithelial cells through SRF and it fails to do so when SRF is inhibited by shRNA.

## 7. Conclusions

SRF is a ubiquitously expressed transcription factor that targets genes containing SRE (Or CArG box). SRE has been found in nearly 1% of total number of human genes and the list is still growing. Some of these genes encode transcription factors (e.g. FOS, FOSB, EGR1, EGR2, EGR4, ELK1, etc.) which have their own specific gene targets. For example, transcription factor Egr-1 has six SRF binding sites in its gene promoter region, indicating a tight control by SRF. It has been shown that Egr-1 is capable to bind to 283 genes, which double the number of genes directly regulated by SRF and extend SRF power to 2% of the human genome. Some other members of SRF targets encode growth factors (e.g. IGF2, TGFB1I1, FGF10, etc.), integrins (e.g. ITGA1, ITGA5, ITGA9, ITGB1, etc.), and matricellular proteins (e.g. CTGF, CCN1, etc.) and all these molecules can transduce signals to influence many other genes. Taken together, SRF influence, including both direct and indirect, can probably reach a quarter of the entire human genome. By now, one can imagine how powerful SRF is.

Ulcer healing is just one of the things SRF does. One can easily find SRF contributions in each phase of ulcer healing: it promotes the production of growth factors and cytokines to mediate inflammation; it regulates formation of actomyosin ring and lamellipodia to promote re-epithelialization; it regulates apoptosis to remove the dead tissue and unnecessary cells; it supports angiogenesis through regulating endothelial cell migration and proliferation; it coordinates tissue remodeling by synchronizing proteases with their antagonists; and much, much more...

## 8. Acknowledgement

This work is supported by the Department of Veterans Affairs of the United States.

## 9. References

Arora, S., Wang, Y., Jia, Z., Vardar-Sengul, S., Munawar, A., Doctor, K.S., Birrer, M., McClelland, M., Adamson, E., & Mercola, D. (2008). Egr1 regulates the coordinated expression of numerous EGF receptor target genes as identified by ChIP-on-chip. *Genome Biol*, 9(11): R166.

Arsenian, S., Weinhold, B., Oelgeschläger, M., Rüther, U., & Nordheim, A. (1998). Serum response factor is essential for mesoderm formation during mouse embryogenesis. *EMBO J*, 17(21): 6289-99.

Backert, S., Moese, S., Selbach, M., Brinkmann, V., & Meyer, T.F. (2001). Phosphorylation of tyrosine 972 of the *Helicobacter pylori* CagA protein is essential for induction of a scattering phenotype in gastric epithelial cells. *Mol Microbiol*, 42(3): 631-44.

Bizzozero, G. (1893). Ueber die schlauchförmigen Drüsen des Magendarmkanals und die Beziehungen ihres Epitheles zu dem Oberflächenepithel der Schleimhaut. *Archiv für mikroskopische Anatomie*, 42: 82–152.

Chai, J., Baatar, D., & Tarnawski, A. (2004a). Serum response factor promotes re-epithelialization and muscular structure restoration during gastric ulcer healing. *Gastroenterology*, 126(7): 1809-18.

Chai, J., Jones, M.K., & Tarnawski, A.S. (2004b). Serum response factor is a critical requirement for VEGF signaling in endothelial cells and VEGF-induced angiogenesis. *FASEB J*, 18(11): 1264-6.

Chai, J., Modak, C., Mouazzen, W., Narvaez, R., & Pham, J. (2010a). Epithelial or mesenchymal: Where to draw the line? *Biosci Trends*, 4(3): 130-42.

Chai, J., Norng, M., Modak, C., Reavis, K.M., Mouazzen, W., & Pham, J. (2010b). CCN1 induces a reversible epithelial-mesenchymal transition in gastric epithelial cells. *Lab Invest*, 90(8): 1140-51.

Chai, J., Norng, M., Tarnawski, A.S., & Chow, J. (2007). A critical role of serum response factor in myofibroblast differentiation during experimental oesophageal ulcer healing in rats. *Gut*, 56(5): 621-30.

Chai J, Tarnawski AS. (2002). Serum response factor: discovery, biochemistry, biological roles and implications for tissue injury healing. *J Physiol Pharmacol*, 53(2): 147-57.

Charvet, C., Houbron, C., Parlakian, A., Giordani, J., Lahoute, C., Bertrand, A., Sotiropoulos, A., Renou, L., Schmitt, A., Melki, J., Li, Z., Daegelen, D., & Tuil, D. (2006). New role for serum response factor in postnatal skeletal muscle growth and regeneration via the interleukin 4 and insulin-like growth factor 1 pathways. *Mol Cell Biol*, 26(17): 6664-74.

Darenfed, H. & Mandato, C.A. (2005). Wound-induced contractile ring: a model for cytokinesis. *Biochem Cell Biol*, 83(6): 711-20.

Doenges, J.L. (1938). Spirochaetei in gastric glands of macaccus rhesus and humans without definite history of related disease. *Proc Soc Exp Biol Med*, 38: 536-538.

Fataccioli, V., Abergel, V., Wingertsmann, L., Neuville, P., Spitz, E., Adnot, S., Calenda, V., & Teiger, E. (2002). Stimulation of angiogenesis by Cyr61 gene: a new therapeutic candidate. *Hum Gene Ther*, 13(12): 1461-70.

Feinstein LB, Holman RC, Yorita CKL, Steiner CA, Swerdlow DL. (2010). Trends in hospitalizations for peptic ulcer disease, United States, 1998-2005. *Emerg Infect Dis*, 16(9): 1410-1418.

Freedberg, A.S & Barron, L.E. (1940).The presence of spirochaetes in human gastric mucosa. *Am J Dig Dis,* 38: 443-445.

Garcia-Fernandez, B., Campos, I., Geiger, J., Santos, A.C., & Jacinto, A. (2009). Epithelial resealing. *Int J Dev Biol,* 53(8-10): 1549-56.

Gilman, M.Z., Wilson, R.N., & Weinberg, R.A. (1986). Multiple protein-binding sites in the 5'-flanking region regulate c-fos expression. *Mol Cell Biol,* 6(12): 4305-16.

Greenberg, M.E, Siegfried, Z., & Ziff, E.B. (1987). Mutation of the c-fos gene dyad symmetry element inhibits serum inducibility of transcription *in vivo* and the nuclear regulatory factor binding *in vitro. Mol Cell Biol,* 7(3): 1217-25.

Greenberg, M.E & Ziff, E.B. (1984). Stimulation of 3T3 cells induces transcription of the c-fos proto-oncogene. *Nature,* 311(5985): 433-8.

Hayashida, Y., Urata, Y., Muroi, E., Kono, T., Miyata, Y., Nomata, K., Kanetake, H., Kondo, T., & Ihara, Y. (2006). Calreticulin represses E-cadherin gene expression in Madin-Darby canine kidney cells via Slug. *J Biol Chem,* 281: 32469-84.

Hirata, Y., Maeda, S., Mitsuno, Y., Tateishi, K., Yanai, A., Akanuma, M., Yoshida, H., Kawabe, T., Shiratori, Y., & Omata, M. (2002). *Helicobacter pylori* CagA protein activates serum response element-driven transcription independently of tyrosine phosphorylation. *Gastroenterology,* 123(6): 1962-71.

Jones, M.K., Kawanaka, H., Baatar, D., Szabó, I.L., Tsugawa, K., Pai, R., Koh, G.Y., Kim, I., Sarfeh, I.J., & Tarnawski, A.S. (2001). Gene therapy for gastric ulcers with single local injection of naked DNA encoding VEGF and angiopoietin-1. *Gastroenterology,* 121(5): 1040-7.

Kang, Y. & Massague, J. (2004). Epithelial-mesenchymal transitions: twist in development and metastasis. *Cell,* 118: 277-9.

Khachigian, L.M. & Collins, T. (1997). Inducible expression of Egr-1-dependent genes. A paradigm of transcriptional activation in vascular endothelium. *Circ Res,* 81(4): 457-61.

Kharbanda, S., Saleem, A., Rubin, E., Sukhatme, V., Blenis, J., & Kufe, D. (1993). Activation of the early growth response 1 gene and nuclear pp90rsk in human myeloid leukemia cells by 1-(beta-D-arabinofuranosyl)cytosine. *Biochemistry,* 32(35): 9137-42.

Khomenko, T., Szabo, S., Deng, X., Jadus, M.R., Ishikawa, H., Osapay, K., Sandor, Z., & Chen, L. (2006). Suppression of early growth response factor-1 with egr-1 antisense oligodeoxynucleotide aggravates experimental duodenal ulcers. *Am J Physiol Gastrointest Liver Physiol,* 290(6): G1211-8.

Kidd, M. & Modlin, I.M. (1998). A century of Helicobacter pylori: paradigms lost-paradigms regained. *Digestion,* 59(1): 1-15.

Konturek, J.W. (2003). Discovery by Jaworski of Helicobacter pylori and its pathogenetic role in peptic ulcer, gastritis and gastric cancer. *J Physiol Pharmacol,* 54 Suppl 3: 23-41.

Kusters, J.G., van Vliet, A.H., & Kuipers, E.J. (2006). Pathogenesis of *Helicobacter pylori* infection. *Clin Microbiol Rev,* 19(3): 449-90.

Lahoute, C., Sotiropoulos, A., Favier, M., Guillet-Deniau, I., Charvet, C., Ferry, A., Butler-Browne, G., Metzger, D., Tuil, D., & Daegelen, D. (2008). Premature aging in skeletal muscle lacking serum response factor. *PLoS One*, 3(12): e3910.

Li, S., Czubryt, M.P., McAnally, J., Bassel-Duby, R., Richardson, J.A., Wiebel, F.F., Nordheim, A., & Olson, E.N. (2005). Requirement for serum response factor for skeletal muscle growth and maturation revealed by tissue-specific gene deletion in mice. *Proc Natl Acad Sci U S A*, 102(4): 1082-7.

Mandato, C.A. & Bement, W.M. (2003). Actomyosin transports microtubules and microtubules control actomyosin recruitment during *Xenopus* oocyte wound healing. *Curr Biol*, 13(13): 1096-105.

Marshall, B.J. (2002). The Discovery that *Helicobacter pylori*, a spiral bacterium, caused peptic ulcer disease. In: B. Marshall (ed.), *Helicobacter Pioneers*. Singapore: Blackwell Science Asia. pp. 165–202.

Miano, J.M. (2010). Role of serum response factor in the pathogenesis of disease. *Laboratory Investigation*, 90: 1274-1284.

Miano, J.M., Long, X., & Fujiwara, K. (2007). Serum response factor: master regulator of the actin cytoskeleton and contractile apparatus. *Am J Physiol Cell Physiol*, 292(1): C70-81.

Miano, J.M., Ramanan, N., Georger, M.A., de Mesy, Bentley K.L, Emerson, R.L, Balza, R.O. Jr, Xiao, Q., Weiler, H., Ginty, D.D., & Misra, R.P. (2004). Restricted inactivation of serum response factor to the cardiovascular system. *Proc Natl Acad Sci U S A*, 101(49): 17132-7.

Mitsuno, Y., Yoshida, H., Maeda, S., Ogura, K., Hirata, Y., Kawabe, T., Shiratori, Y., & Omata, M. (2001). *Helicobacter pylori* induced transactivation of SRE and AP-1 through the ERK signalling pathway in gastric cancer cells. *Gut*, 49(1): 18-22.

Mo, F.E., Muntean, A.G., Chen, C.C., Stolz, D.B., Watkins, S.C., & Lau, L.F. (2002). CYR61 (CCN1) is essential for placental development and vascular integrity. *Mol Cell Biol*, 22(24): 8709-20.

Modak, C. & Chai, J. (2010). Serum response factor: look into the gut. *World J Gastroenterol*, 16(18): 2195-201.

Nguyen, T., Chai, J., Li, A., Akahoshi, T., Tanigawa, T., & Tarnawski, A.S. (2007). Novel roles of local insulin-like growth factor-1 activation in gastric ulcer healing: promotes actin polymerization, cell proliferation, re-epithelialization, and induces cyclooxygenase-2 in a phosphatidylinositol 3-kinase-dependent manner. *Am J Pathol*,170(4): 1219-28.

Okabe, S & Pfeiffer, C.J. (1972). Chronicity of acetic acid ulcer in the rat stomach. *Am J Dig Dis*, 17(7): 619-29.

Orr, L. (2004). Scientists align billion-year-old protein with embryonic heart defects. *Medical News Today*.

Pai, R., Szabo, I.L., Giap, A.Q., Kawanaka, H., & Tarnawski, A.S. (2001). Nonsteroidal anti-inflammatory drugs inhibit re-epithelialization of wounded gastric monolayers by interfering with actin, Src, FAK, and tensin signaling. *Life Sci*, 69(25-26): 3055-71.

Palmer, E.D. (1954). Investigation of the gastric mucosa spirochaetes of the humans. *Gastroenterology*, 27: 218-220.

Peek, R.M Jr & Crabtree, J.E. (2006). *Helicobacter* infection and gastric neoplasia. J Pathol, 208(2): 233-48.

Pounder, R.E & Ng, D. (1995). The prevalence of *Helicobacter pylori* infection in different countries. *Aliment Pharmacol Ther*. 9: Suppl 2: 33-9.

Prywes, R & Roeder, R.G. (1986). Inducible binding of a factor to the c-fos enhancer. *Cell*, 47(5): 777-84.

Rollins, B.J & Stiles, C.D. (1989). Serum-inducible genes. *Adv Cancer Res*, 53:1-32.

Salomon, H. (1896). Über das Spirillum des Säugetiermagens und sein Verhalten zu den Belegzellen. *Zentrallbl Bakteriol*, 19: 433-442.

Scott, D.R, Weeks, D., Hong, C., Postius, S., Melchers, K., & Sachs, G. (1998). The role of internal urease in acid resistance of *Helicobacter pylori*. *Gastroenterology*, 114(1): 58-70.

Spencer, J.A., Major, M.L., & Misra, R.P. (1999). Basic fibroblast growth factor activates serum response factor gene expression by multiple distinct signaling mechanisms. *Mol Cell Biol*, 19(6): 3977-88.

Steer, H.W. (1975). Ultrastucture of cell migration through the gastric epithelium and its relation to bacteria. *J Clin Pathol*, 28: 639-646.

Sun, Q., Chen, G., Streb, J.W., Long, X., Yang, Y., Stoeckert, C.J. Jr, & Miano, J.M. (2006). Defining the mammalian CArGome. *Genome Res*, 16(2): 197-207.

Szabo, S., Khomenko, T., Gombos, Z., Deng, X.M., Jadus, M.R., & Yoshida, M. (2000). Review article: transcription factors and growth factors in ulcer healing. *Alimnet Pharmacol Ther*, 14(suppl. 1): 33-43.

Tarnawski, A.S. (2005). Cellular and molecular mechanisms of gastrointestinal ulcer healing. *Digestive Diseases and Sciences*, 50: Suppl. S24-S33.

Treisman, R. (1986). Identification of a protein-binding site that mediates transcriptional response of the c-fos gene to serum factors. *Cell*, 46(4): 567-74.

Treisman, R. (1995). Journey to the surface of the cell: Fos regulation and the SRE. *The EMBO Journal*, 14(20): 4905-4913.

Viala, J., Chaput, C., Boneca, I.G., Cardona, A., Girardin, S.E., Moran, A.P., Athman, R., Mémet, S., Huerre, M.R., Coyle, A.J., DiStefano, P.S., Sansonetti, P.J., Labigne, A., Bertin, J., Philpott, D.J., & Ferrero, R.L. (2004). Nod1 responds to peptidoglycan delivered by the *Helicobacter pylori* cag pathogenicity island. *Nat Immunol*, 5(11): 1166-74.

Werth, D., Grassi, G., Konjer, N., Dapas, B., Farra, R., Giansante, C., Kandolf, R., Guarnieri, G., Nordheim, A., & Heidenreich, O. (2010). Proliferation of human primary vascular smooth muscle cells depends on serum response factor. *Eur J Cell Biol*. 89(2-3): 216-24.

Zhang, X., Azhar, G., Chai, J., Sheridan, P., Nagano, K., Brown, T., Yang, J., Khrapko, K., Borras, A.M., Lawitts, J., Misra, R.P., & Wei, J.Y. (2001a). Cardiomyopathy in transgenic mice with cardiac-specific overexpression of serum response factor. *Am J Physiol Heart Circ Physiol*, 280(4): H1782-92.

Zhang, X., Chai, J., Azhar, G., Sheridan, P., Borras, A.M., Furr, M.C., Khrapko, K., Lawitts, J., Misra, R.P., & Wei, J.Y. (2001b). Early postnatal cardiac changes and premature death in transgenic mice overexpressing a mutant form of serum response factor. *J Biol Chem*, 276(43): 40033-40.

Zhou, B.P., Deng, J., Xia, W., Xu, J., Li, Y.M., Gunduz, M., & Hung, M.C. (2004). Dual regulation of Snail by GSK-3beta-mediated phosphorylation in control of epithelial-mesenchymal transition. *Nat Cell Biol*, 6: 931-40.

# 9

# Role of New Appetite Hormones Ghrelin, Orexin-A and Obestatin in the Mechanism of Healing of Chronic Gastric Ulcers

Thomas Brzozowski Aleksandra Szlachcic[1], Robert Pajdo[1], Zbigniew Sliwowski[1], Danuta Drozdowicz[1], Jolanta Majka[1], Wladyslaw Bielanski[1], Peter. C. Konturek[2], Stanislaw J. Konturek[1] and Wieslaw W. Pawlik[1]

*[1]Department of Physiology, Jagiellonian University Medical College, Cracow*
*[2]Thuringia-Clinic Saalfeld Georgiou's Agricola GmbH Teaching*
*Hospital of the University of Jena,*
*[1]Poland*
*[2]Germany*

## 1. Introduction

The regulation of appetite is regulated by complex mechanism involving brain-gut axis and hormonal and non-hormonal factors acting through the activity of satiety and hunger centers located in the hypothalamus [Wren & Bloom, 2007]. Among hormones controlling appetite are gastrointestinal hormones such as cholecystokinin, PYY, pancreatic polypeptide, glucagon-like peptide 1, oxyntomedulin, the endocrine pancreatic hormones including insulin and glucagon and endocannabinoids [Wren &Bloom, 2007]. Recent discoveries of ghrelin and orexin-A gave a new insight into the understanding of mechanism of appetite control, satiety and obesity. Ghrelin is a novel 28-amino acid peptide that has recently been discovered in rat and human gastrointestinal tract, particularly in gastric mucosa, as an endogenous ligand for growth hormone (GH) secretagogue receptor (GHS-R) [Kojima et al., 1999]. Ghrelin stimulates food intake and body weight gain exerting a modulating effect on energy expenditure acting through afferent nerves and directly on hypothalamic feeding centers [Kojima et al., 1999; Tomasetto et al., 2000]. This peptide was also shown to enhance the gastric motility and gastric secretion [Tschop et al., 2000; Date et al., 2001]. Ghrelin is considered as an orexigenic peptide produced by the stomach, acting as a meal initiator [Masuda et al., 2000; Ariyasu et al., 2001]. Little is known about other factors that might affect ghrelin secretion in the stomach and its influence on gastrointestinal integrity has not been fully elucidated. A recent study in humans revealed that stomach is a major source of circulating ghrelin and that gastrectomy produced dramatic fall in the plasma ghrelin levels, whereas fasting and *anorexia nervosa* was accompanied by elevated plasma ghrelin levels [Ariyasu et al., 2001].

The orexins also called hypocretins, are neuropeptides novel originally discovered in a small group of neurons in the hypothalamic area (LHA) [Sakurai et al., 1998; de Lecea et al., 1998]. identified two peptides that were endogenous ligands to orphan receptor HFGAN72 [Sakurai et al., 1998]. They found that these peptides after i.c.v. injection stimulated food intake and their expression was upregulated upon fasting. Therefore, the group of these peptides has been named "orexins" after the Greek word "orexis" meaning appetite [Komaki et al., 2001]. The orexin group of peptides was originally identified as regulators of food intake and of sleep behavior and act at one or the other of 2 G protein-coupled receptors, the orexin-1 (OX-R1) and orexin-2 (OX-R2) receptors [Sakurai et al., 1998; Mondal et al., 1999]. OX-A is a 33-residue peptide possessing the identical sequence in humans and rodents, whereas human and rat OX-B differ by two residues. OX-A and OX-B activate two G protein-coupled receptors known as OX-1 and OX-2, the OX-1 receptor having a greater affinity for OX-A over OX-B, whereas the OX-2 receptor has similar affinity for both ligands [Sakurai, 2003]. Besides the presence in the brain, orexin-like immunoreactivity was found in the ENS of different species including guinea pig, rat, mouse and humans [Kirchgessner & Liu, 1999]. Interestingly, the prepro-orexin, orexin A and orexin receptor mRNA expression were demonstrated in the myenteric plexus and afferent nerves co-localizing with VIP-ergic nerves and in the gastrin-producing cells of the rat stomach [Kirchgessner & Liu, 1999]. Orexin-A has been linked with the peripheral energy balance and central nervous system mechanisms that coordinate sleep-wakefulness and motivated behaviors such as food seeking, especially in physiological state of fasting stress [Mondal et al., 1999; Sakurai, 2003]. Recent studies in humans revealed that the plasma orexin-A concentrations are increased during fasting in humans [Komaki et al., 2001].

The question remains as to whether these newly discovered peptides could play a role in the mechanism of gastric integrity and gastric mucosal defense has not been fully explored. Both, ghrelin and orexin-A were implicated in the mechanism of gastroprotection but their role in the healing process of chronic gastric ulcers has been little investigated. Previous studies by [Sibilia et al., 2003] and our group [Brzozowski et al., 2004; Brzozowski et al., 2006 b.; Konturek et al., 2004] revealed that that central and peripheral administration of ghrelin reduced the formation of acute gastric lesions induced by ethanol and cold stress. It was proposed that NO and sensory neuropeptides mediate these gastroprotective effects of ghrelin because the blockade of NO-synthase (NOS) activity with L-NAME and the functional ablation of sensory afferent nerves with capsaicin attenuated the protection and gastric hyperemia induced by ghrelin [Brzozowski et al., 2004; Brzozowski et al., 2006a.; Dimitrova et al., 2010]. In contrast to prevention of acute damage to the mucosal structure, the healing of chronic gastric ulcers lasts days and weeks and may involve restoration of gland architecture, angiogenesis and scar formation and it remains unknown whether appetite hormones may influence these processes.

Recently, endogenous prostaglandins (PG) have been implicated in the control of food intake and appetite [Lugarini et al., 2002; Scholz, 2003] but the possibility that these arachidonate metabolites may play any important role in the mechanism of ghrelin or orexin-A affecting ulcer healing has not been explored. This prompted our interest in endogenous PG because these arachidonate metabolites play an essential role in the mechanism of gastric defense and ulcer healing [Brzozowski et al., 2001] but the importance of PG derived from cyclooxygenase (COX-1) and COX-2 in the possible ulcer healing effects of orexigenic peptides has not been so far determined.

This study was designed to compare the effects of daily intraperitoneal (i.p.) administration of vehicle, ghrelin, orexin-A and obestatin on healing of preexisting gastric ulcers and accompanying changes in the gastric blood flow (GBF) at ulcer margin and the generation of $PGE_2$ in the gastric mucosa. An attempt was made to examine the effect of antagonism of

GHS-R1a and OX-A1 receptors with D-lys³GHRP-6 and SB334867 [Peeters, 2005; Smart et al., 2001] respectively, on spontaneous ulcer healing and the alteration in ulcer size induced by ghrelin and orexin-A. We also determined the effects of PG inhibition with a non-selective (indomethacin) and selective cyclooxygenase (COX)-1 (SC-560) and COX-2 (rofecoxib) inhibitors and blockade with L-NNA, the NO-synthase inhibitor on healing of these ulcers and accompanying changes in the GBF in rats without and with ghrelin or orexin-A administration. In addition, the expression of ghrelin mRNA at the ulcer margin and that in non-ulcerated gastric mucosa was assessed in rats with gastric ulcer. Finally, ghrelin rats were concomitantly treated with obestatin to check whether obestatin, recently considered as physiological opponent of ghrelin regarding food intake and appetite control [Zhang et al., 2005], could influence the ulcer healing itself and affect the healing and hyperemic effects of ghrelin.

## 2. Material and methods

Male Wistar rats, weighing 200-250 g and fasted for 24 h were used in all studies. All experimental procedures were run according to Helsinki Declaration and approved by the Jagiellonian University Institutional Animal Care and Use Committee.

### 2.1 Production of gastric ulcers

Gastric ulcers were produced in rats using our modification (19) of acetic acid method originally proposed by Okabe et al. (1971) with our group modification [Konturek et al., 1987]. Animals were anesthetized with ether, the stomach was exposed and 75 µl of acetic acid was poured through the plastic mold (6 mm diameter) onto serosal surface of anterior wall of the stomach just proximal to the antral gland area for 25 s. This produced an immediate necrosis of the entire mucosa and submucosa (but not serosa) within the area where the acetic acid was applied, i.e., about 28 mm². The excess of acetic acid was then removed and the serosa was gently washed out with saline. Our previous studies documented that these ulcers became chronic within 2-3 days and healed completely within 2-3 weeks without perforation or penetration to the surrounding organs as described in original technique [Konturek et al., 1987; Okabe et al., 1971]. After the application of acetic acid the animals were allowed to recover from anesthesia and received only water at the day of operation (day 0). Then, they were divided into various groups and received normal chow and water *ad libitum* for the next 9 days and then were sacrificed.

### 2.2 Effect of orexin-A, ghrelin without and with the antagonists of ghrelin and orexin-A receptors on ulcer healing and the alterations in GBF at ulcer margin

Several groups of rats with gastric ulcers, each consisting of 6-8 animals, were treated daily either with 1) vehicle (saline), 2) ghrelin or orexin-A (2.5-30 µg/kg-d i.p.), 3) D-Lys³-GHRP-6 (200 µg/kg i.p.), the ghrelin receptor antagonist (Peeters, 2005), or SB 334867 which is a selective non-peptide OX-R1 receptor antagonist [Smart, et al., 2001; Holland, et al., 2006] administered alone or in the combination with ghrelin and orexin-A (standard dose of 30 µg/kg-d i.p.), respectively. SB 334867 was dissolved in DMSO and kept in a 20 mM solution as recommended by manufacturer [Tocris Cookson Ltd., Bristol, UK]. The dose of OX-R1 antagonist used in this study was selected on the basis of our earlier studies (unpublished observation) with dose-dependent inhibition of orexin-A protection against WRS damage obtained with this orexin-A antagonist.

In another group of animals with gastric ulcers and treated with COX-1 and COX-2 inhibitors with or without ghrelin, orexin-A and obestatin administration, the effect of prostaglandin replacement therapy using 16,16 dimethyl $PGE_2$ [Upjohn, Kalamazoo, MI, USA] applied i.g. in a dose of 5 μg/kg-d was examined. This dose of dimethyl $PGE_2$ was found in our preliminary study to be without any influence on ulcer healing and accompanying fall in GBF at ulcer margin. For this reason, synthetic $PGE_2$ analog was administered together with each COX-1 or COX-2 inhibitor with or without ghrelin, orexin-A and obestatin administration.

Upon the termination of experiment, the animals were anesthetized with pentobarbital, their abdomen was opened by midline incision and the stomach exposed for measurement of GBF by means of the $H_2$-gas clearance technique as described previously [Brzozowski et al., 2000 a]. For this purpose two electrodes of an electrolytic regional blood flow meter (Biotechnical Science, Model RBF-2, Osaka, Japan) were inserted into the gastric mucosa. The measurements were made in three areas of the oxyntic mucosa at ulcer margin and the mean values were calculated and expressed as percent changes of those recorded in the control animals. After GBF measurement, the stomach was removed, rinsed with saline and pinned open for macroscopic examination. The area of gastric lesions was determined by computerized planimetry (Morphomat, Carl Zeiss, FRG) [Brzozowski et al., 2000 b] by a researcher blind to the experimental grouping.

Samples of the oxyntic gland area from the ulcer margin were taken by biopsy (about 100 mg) immediately after the animals were sacrificed to determine the mucosal generation of $PGE_2$ by specific radioimmunoassay (RIA) as described previously [Konturek et al., 1995; Brzozowski et al., 2000]. $PGE_2$ was measured in duplicate using RIA kits (New England Nuclear, Munich, Germany). The mucosal generation of $PGE_2$ was expressed in nanograms per gram of wet tissue weight.

## 2.3 Effect of ghrelin and orexin-A on the healing of acetic acid ulcers and accompanying changes in the GBF at ulcer margin. Involvement of the COX-PG and NO-NOS systems in ghrelin-induced acceleration of ulcer healing

The involvement of the COX-PG system in the ulcer healing effects of ghrelin was studied in rats treated with (or without) indomethacin, a non-selective COX-1 and COX-2 inhibitor, and with SC-560, a selective COX-1 inhibitor or rofecoxib, a specific COX-2 inhibitor [Brzozowski et.al., 1999]. In the experimental protocol, the following groups of rats, each consisting of 6-8 animals, were used: 1) vehicle (saline 1 ml i.p.); 2) ghrelin, orexin-A or obestatin, each applied in a standard dose of 30 μg/kg-d i.p.; 2) indomethacin (5 mg/kg i.p.), SC-560 (5 mg/kg-d i.g.) and rofecoxib (10 mg/kg-d i.g.), each applied alone or co-administered with ghrelin, orexin-A or obestatin (30 μg/kg-d i.p.). The doses of SC-560 and rofecoxib were selected on the basis of previous studies showing that these agents almost completely suppress $PGE_2$ generation in exudates of air-pouch inflammation and inhibit gastric $PGE_2$ production in mucosa with preexisting gastric ulcer [Futaki et al., 1993; Lesch et al., 1998]. SC-560 (Cayman Chemical Co., Ann Arbor, Michigan, USA) was first dissolved in absolute ethanol to obtain a stock solution of 50 mg/ml and then diluted to the desired concentration with isotonic saline. Rofecoxib [Sharp & Dhome, Warsaw, Poland] was first dissolved in methanol to obtain a stock solution 75 mg/ml and then diluted to the desired concentration with isotonic saline. Control rats received the corresponding vehicle. Our preliminary studies (data not included) showed that none of the COX inhibitors used in this study produced by itself any gastric lesions at the doses tested. At the dose used in the present study, indomethacin has been shown previously to inhibit gastric $PGE_2$ generation by ~ 90 % without itself causing any mucosal damage [Konturek et al., 1987].

In another group of animals with gastric ulcers and treated with COX-1 and COX-2 inhibitors with or without ghrelin, orexin-A and obestatin administration, the effect of prostaglandin replacement therapy using 16, 16 dimethyl $PGE_2$ (Upjohn, Kalamazoo, MI, USA) applied i.g. in a dose of 5 µg/kg-d was examined. This dose of dimethyl $PGE_2$ was found in our preliminary study to be without any influence on ulcer healing and accompanying fall in GBF at ulcer margin. For this reason, synthetic $PGE_2$ analog was administered together with each COX-1 or COX-2 inhibitor with or without ghrelin, orexin-A and obestatin administration.

Upon the termination of experiment, the animals were anesthetized with pentobarbital, their abdomen was opened by midline incision and the stomach exposed for measurement of GBF by means of the $H_2$-gas clearance technique as described previously [Brzozowski et al., 2000 a]. For this purpose two electrodes of an electrolytic regional blood flow meter (Biotechnical Science, Model RBF-2, Osaka, Japan) were inserted into the gastric mucosa. The measurements were made in three areas of the oxyntic mucosa at ulcer margin and the mean values were calculated and expressed as percent changes of those recorded in the control animals. After GBF measurement, the stomach was removed, rinsed with saline and pinned open for macroscopic examination. The area of gastric lesions was determined by computerized planimetry (Morphomat, Carl Zeiss, FRG) [Brzozowski et al., 2000b] by a researcher blind to the experimental grouping.

Samples of the oxyntic gland area from the ulcer margin were taken by biopsy (about 100 mg) immediately after the animals were sacrificed to determine the mucosal generation of $PGE_2$ by specific radioimmunoassay (RIA) as described previously [Konturek et al., 1995]. $PGE_2$ was measured in duplicate using RIA kits (New England Nuclear, Munich, Germany). The mucosal generation of $PGE_2$ was expressed in nanograms per gram of wet tissue weight.

## 2.4 Determination of plasma ghrelin, orexin-A and obestatin levels by radioimmunoassay

At the termination of some experiments with obestatin applied i.p. alone or co-administered with ghrelin, the rats were anesthetized with pentobarbital and blood samples (about 3 ml) taken from the *vena cava* for the measurement of plasma ghrelin, orexin-A and obestatin levels by RIA. Intact rats fasted overnight and given only vehicle (saline) i.p. were measured similarly in order to determine control values for plasma ghrelin, orexin-A and obestatin concentration. Blood samples were collected in heparin coated polypropylene tubes and centrifuged at 3000 rpm for 20 minutes at 4°C. The supernatant was then stored at -80°C until measurement of plasma ghrelin, orexin-A and obestatin levels using an RIA-kit for rat ghrelin, orexin-A and obestatin (Phoenix Peptide, Belmont, CA, USA) [Brzozowski et al., 2004; Brzozowski et. al., 2006 b]. Briefly, the ghrelin, orexin-A and obestatin RIA involved the competition of each rat peptide sample with [125]I-rat ghrelin, orexin-A and obestatin tracers for binding to a specific rabbit anti-ghrelin-, anti-orexin-A- and anti-obestatin polyclonal antibody. The limit of assay sensitivity for ghrelin, orexin-A and obestatin were 3 pg, 6pg and 5 pg per tube, the intra-assay variation was less than 8%,7% and 9%, and the interassay variation less than 5%, 4% and 7%, respectively.

## 2.5 Reverse-transcriptase-polymerase chain reaction (RT-PCR) for detection of messenger RNA (mRNA) for ghrelin and proinflammatory cytokines IL-1β and TNF-α in rats without and with gastric ulcers

The stomachs were removed from vehicle (control) rats for the determination of ghrelin mRNA expression using specific primers by RT-PCR. Gastric mucosal specimens were scraped off from oxyntic mucosa using a slide glass and immediately snap frozen in liquid nitrogen and stored at -80°C until analysis. Total RNA was extracted from mucosal samples by a guanidium isothiocyanate/phenol chloroform method using a kit from Stratagene® (Heidelberg, Germany). Single stranded cDNA was generated from 5 μg of total cellular RNA using StrataScript reverse transcriptase and oligo-(dT)-primers (Stratagene, Heidelberg, Germany). The polymerase chain reaction mixture was amplified in a DNA thermal cycler (Perkin-Elmer-Cetus, Norwalk, CT) in an area set aside for performing the PCR reaction. The nucleotide sequences of the primers for ghrelin and β-actin were selected on the basis of the published cDNA encoding ghrelin and β-actin, respectively [Konturek et al., 2004; Brzozowski et al., 2006 b]. The sense primer for ghrelin was 5'-TTGAGCCCAGAGCACCAGAAA-3', and the antisense primer was 5'-AGTTGCAGAGGAGGCAGAAGCT-3'. The IL-1β primer sequences were designed according to the published cDNA sequence for primer sequences and were as follows: up-stream, 5' GCT ACC TAT GTC TTG CCC GT; downstream, 3' GAC CAT TGC TGT TTC CTA GG. The expected length product was 543 bp. The TNF-α primer sequences were as follows: up-stream, 5'TAC TGA ACT TCG GGG TGA TTG GTC C; downstream, 3' CAG CCT TGT CCC TTG AAG AGA ACC. The expected length product was 295 bp [Konturek et al., 2010]. The oligonucleotide sequences for β-actin were TTG TAA CCA ACT GGG ACG ATA TGG (sense) and GAT CTT GAT CTT CAT GGT GCT AGG (antisense). The primers were synthesized by GIBCO BRL/Life Technologies, Eggenstein, Germany. The signals for ghrelin mRNA was standardized against the β-actin signal for each sample and results were expressed as the ratio of ghrelin mRNA to β-actin mRNA.

## 3. Results

### 3.1 Effect of treatment with orexin-A, ghrelin and obestatin on ulcer healing and the accompanying changes in the GBF at ulcer margin

The effect of i.p. administration of orexin-A applied in graded doses ranging from 1 μg/kg-d up to 30 μg/kg-d and ghrelin administered in a dose of 30 μg/kg-d (i.p.) on acetic acid-induced gastric ulcers are shown in Fig.1. Orexin-A dose-dependently reduced the ulcer area, the dose inhibiting this area by 50% ($ED_{50}$) was 15 μg/kg.

Almost double reduction of the ulcer area was obtained with orexin-A administered at the dose 30 μg/kg as compared with control rats injected i.p. with vehicle (saline). This reduction in ulcer area achieved with orexin-A was accompanied by the dose-dependent increase in GBF. Ghrelin administered in a dose of 30 μg/kg-d i.p. significantly reduced the ulcer area and significantly increased GBF with the extent similar to that observed with orexin-A applied in the highest dose. Eight days of i.p. administration of obestatin applied in graded doses ranging from 2.5 μg/kg up to 30 μg/kg-d, dose-dependently reduced the

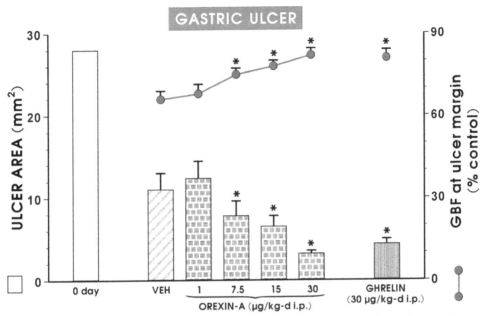

Fig. 1. The area of gastric ulcer induced by acetic acid and gastric blood flow (GBF) at ulcer
margin at 8 day upon ulcer induction in rats treated with vehicle (saline) or with various
doses of orexin-A (1 - 30 µg/kg-d i.p.) or ghrelin (30 µg/kg-d i.p.). Means ± SEM of 6-8 rats.
Asterisk indicates a significant change (p<0.05) as compared to the vehicle-control values.

area of gastric ulcer and significantly increased the GBF at ulcer margin starting from the
dose of 5 µg/kg (Fig. 2). The maximal reduction of ulcer area accompanied by a significant
rise in the GBF at ulcer margin was recorded at the dose of 30 µg/kg of obestatin where 35%
reduction of ulcer area and an increase by about 19% of GBF at ulcer margin were observed
as compared to the respective values in vehicle-treated animals.

### 3.2 Role of cyclooxygenase (COX)-1 and COX-2 inhibition and the blockade of nitric oxide (NO) synthase on ulcer healing activity and alterations in the GBF at ulcer margin in rats treated with ghrelin, orexin-A and obestatin

As shown in Fig. 3, ghrelin and orexin-A given i.p. in dose 30 µg/kg-d significantly
decreased ulcer area and enhanced GBF as compared to those observed in vehicle.
Treatment with D-Lys³-GHRS-6 (200 µg/kg i.p.), the ghrelin GHS-R1a receptor antagonist,
by itself failed to affect the area of gastric ulcers and GBF at ulcer margin at day 8 upon ulcer
induction. The decrease in the area of these ulcers and accompanying rise in the GBF at
ulcer margin induced by ghrelin and orexin-A were significantly attenuated by concurrent
treatment with ghrelin and orexin-A receptor antagonists, D-Lys³-GHRS-6 and SB334867.
The administration of D-lys³GHRP, which is a specific ghrelin receptor antagonist or
SB334867, an antagonist of orexin-A OXR-1 receptors when applied alone, failed to affect the
area of gastric ulcer and the GBF at ulcer margin as compared to those measured in vehicle-
treated rats. Treatment with D-lys³GHRP significantly attenuated ghrelin-induced
acceleration of ulcer healing and the accompanying increase in GBF at ulcer margin.

Concomitant treatment of orexin-A with its receptor antagonist, SB334867 (5 mg/kg-d s.c.), completely abolished the reduction in ulcer area induced by orexin-A. This antagonist of orexin-A receptors reversed also an increase in GBF at ulcer margin caused by orexin-A.

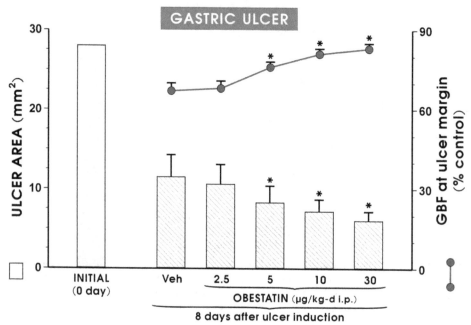

Fig. 2. The area of gastric ulcers and the alterations in the GBF at ulcer margin in rats treated for 8 days with vehicle (Veh; control) or obestatin applied i.p. in graded doses ranging from 2.5 µg/kg-d up to 30 µg/kg-d. Mean ± SEM of 6-8 rats. Asterisk indicates a significant change (p<0.05) compared to the vehicle-pretreated controls.

As shown in Fig. 4, treatment with ghrelin, orexin-A and obestatin (30 µg/kg-d i.p.) resulted in a similar attenuation in the area of gastric ulcer and a similar rise in GBF as that shown in Figs. 1 and 2. The mucosal generation of $PGE_2$ was significantly increased at ulcer margin as compared to the respective value in the non-ulcerated control (128±9 vs. 189±12 ng/g wet tissue weight, p<0.05). Ghrelin, orexin-A and obestatin applied i.p. resulted in a significant increase in the $PGE_2$ generation at ulcer margin as compared to vehicle-treated animals with gastric ulcer (189±12 vs 234±19 ng/g, 189±12 vs 228±9 ng/g and 189±12 vs 219±8 ng/g, respectively, p<0.05). Indomethacin (5 mg/kg i.p.), which by itself significantly increased the ulcer area, suppressed the generation of $PGE_2$ by about 85% (p<0.02) and produced a significant fall in GBF as compared to vehicle-pretreated animals (Fig. 4). Treatment with this non-selective COX-1 and COX-2 inhibitor completely abolished the reduction in the area of gastric ulcers and the accompanying rise in GBF evoked by ghrelin, orexin-A and obestatin. The decrease in the area of ulcer and accompanying increase in GBF caused by ghrelin, orexin-A and obestatin as well as the rise in the $PGE_2$ generation they induced were also significantly attenuated by pretreatment with rofecoxib, the selective COX-2 inhibitor (Fig. 4). SC-560 (5 mg/kg-d i.g.), which by itself significantly reduced the $PGE_2$ generation (not shown), significantly attenuated the ghrelin-, orexin-A- and obestatin-induced decrease in ulcer area

and the accompanying rise in GBF at ulcer margin (Fig. 4). Concurrent treatment with a
minute amount of synthetic dimethyl analog of PGE$_2$ (5 µg/kg-d i.g.) in addition to ghrelin,
orexin-A and obestatin restored the decrease in the ulcer area and the increase in GBF at ulcer
margin in rats treated with indomethacin, SC-560 or rofecoxib (Fig. 4).

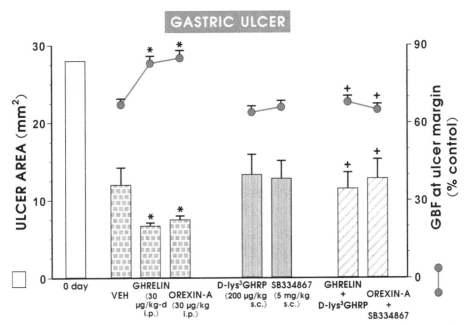

Fig. 3. The area of gastric ulcers and the accompanying changes in the GBF at ulcer margin
in rats with or without ghrelin or orexin-A (both at a dose of 30 µg/kg-d i.p.) applied
without or with the ghrelin receptor antagonist D-Lys3-GHSR-6 (200 µg/kg-d i.p.) or orexin-
A receptor antagonist SB334867 (200 µg/kg-d i.p.). Mean ± SEM of 6-8 rats. Asterisk
indicates a significant change (p<0.05) compared to the vehicle-pretreated controls. Cross
indicates a significant change (p<0.05) compared to the values obtained in rats treated with
ghrelin and orexin-A without the concurrent treatment with GHS-R1a receptor or OXR-1
receptor antagonists.

### 3.3 Expression of ghrelin and proinflammatory cytokines in ulcer area during ulcer healing without and with ghrelin treatment

The effect of eight day administration of L-NNA (20 mg/kg-d i.p.), the NO-synthase
inhibitor on ulcer area  and the changes in GBF at ulcer margin in rats treated without and
with vehicle, ghrelin, orexin-A and obestatin, each applied in a dose of  30 µg/kg-d i.p. is
presented in Fig. 5. Treatment with ghrelin, orexin-A and obestatin significantly reduced the
ulcer area and increased the GBF at ulcer margin as shown in Fig. 4. Treatment with L-
NNA, which by itself significantly enhanced ulcer area also significantly decreased GBF at
ulcer margin as compared to respective values in vehicle-control. Concurrent treatment with
L-NNA together with ghrelin, orexin-A and obestatin reversed the ghrelin-, orexin-A- and
obestatin-induced decrease in ulcer area and the accompanying rise in the GBF at ulcer
margin.

Fig. 6 shows that ghrelin was expressed in intact non-ulcerated gastric mucosa and that with gastric ulcer. Ghrelin mRNA expression was detected as the strong signal in intact gastric mucosa and vehicle-treated gastric mucosa with gastric ulcer. Ratio of mRNA for ghrelin over β-actin revealed that this ratio was significantly higher in ulcerated gastric mucosa as in case of that in intact animals without an ulcer (Fig. 6, left panel).

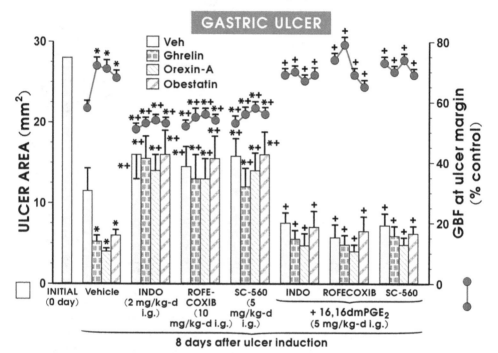

**8 days after ulcer induction**

Fig. 4. The area of gastric ulcers and the accompanying changes in the GBF at ulcer margin in rats treated for a period of 8 days with vehicle (saline) and ghrelin, orexin-A and obestatin (each given in a dose of 30 µg/kg-d i.p.) with or without the concurrent treatment with indomethacin (5 mg/kg-d i.p.), rofecoxib (10 mg/kg-d i.g.) or SC-560 (5 mg/kg-d i.g.) applied alone or combined with synthetic 16,16 dimethyl (dm) PGE₂ analog (5 µg/kg-d i.g.). Mean ± SEM of 6-8 rats. Asterisk indicates a significant decrease (p<0.05) as compared to the value obtained in vehicle-controls. Asterisk and cross indicate a significant increase (p<0.05) as compared to vehicle-treated controls administered without or with ghrelin, orexin-A or obestatin. Cross indicate a significant change (p<0.02) as compared to respective values obtained in animals treated with indomethacin, SC-560 or rofecoxib without the concurrent treatment with PGE₂ analog.

As shown in Fig. 7, the signal of mRNA for IL-1β and TNF-α mRNAs was faintly expressed in intact gastric mucosa but it was observed as strong signal in vehicle-control mucosa of animals with gastric ulcer. Ratio of mRNA for ghrelin over β-actin indicated that expression of mRNA for IL-1β and TNF-α was significantly increased in vehicle-treated rats with gastric ulcer over that recorded in intact gastric mucosa. In contrast, in rats treated with ghrelin applied i.p. at the doses of 15 µg/kg and 30 µg/kg, the signal for IL-1β and TNF-α

mRNAs was significantly decreased in gastric mucosa with gastric ulcer as compared to that
in vehicle-control animals. Ratio of mRNA for IL-1β and TNF-α mRNA over β-actin mRNA
revealed that this ratio was significantly decreased in gastric mucosa of rats treated with
ghrelin administered at the dose of 15 μg/kg. The ratio of IL-1β and TNF-α was significantly
decreased in animals treated with ghrelin applied i.p in a higher dose of 30 μg/kg than in
those treated with ghrelin administered in a lower dose of 15 μg/kg of this peptide (Fig. 7).

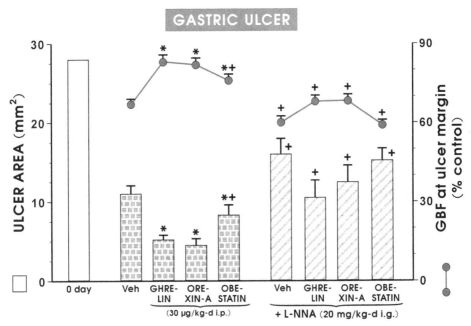

Fig. 5. The area of gastric ulcers and the accompanying changes in the GBF at ulcer margin
in rats treated with vehicle (Veh; saline-control), ghrelin, orexin-A and obestatin (each
administered in a dose of 30 μg/kg-d i.p.) applied without or with the NO-synthase
inhibitor L-NNA (20 mg/kg-d i.p.). Mean ± SEM of 6-8 rats. Asterisk indicates a significant
change (p<0.05) compared to the vehicle-treated controls. Asterisk and cross indicate a
significant change (p<0.05) compared to the values obtained in rats treated with vehicle.
Cross indicates the significant change (p<0.02) compared to the values obtained in ghrelin,
orexin-A and obestatin without the concurrent treatment with L-NNA.

### 3.4 Effect of treatment with obestatin on ulcer healing in rats with of ghrelin administration

Fig. 8 shows the effects of eight day of concomitant administration of ghrelin, the appetite
stimulating peptide, and obestatin which is opponent of ghrelin acting as the natural ligand
of the GPR39 receptor, on the alterations in area of gastric ulcer and accompanying changes
in GBF at ulcer area and plasma ghrelin and obestatin levels. Ghrelin and obestatin given
i.p. in the same comparable dose of 30 μg/kg-d significantly reduced the area of gastric
ulcer, however the significantly greater reduction in ulcer area was observed in ghrelin-

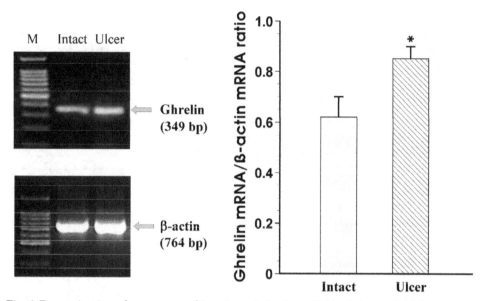

Fig. 6. Determination of expression of β-actin and ghrelin mRNAs (left panel) by RT-PCR and the ratio of ghrelin to β-actin mRNA (right panel) in non-ulcerated (intact) gastric mucosa (lane Intact) and in gastric mucosa at ulcer margin (lane Ulcer), M - DNA size marker. Mean ± SEM of 4-6 rats. Asterisk indicates a significant change (p<0.05) as compared to the value obtained in non-ulcerated gastric mucosa.

treated rats as compared with those treated with obestatin. Plasma ghrelin level increased after i.p. administration of exogenous ghrelin but remained unchanged after combined treatment of ghrelin with obestatin as compared with those treated with ghrelin alone. The plasma obestatin concentration which was significantly increased in obestatin-treated rats with gastric ulcer was not significantly affected by the concurrent ghrelin administration as compared to vehicle-treated rats. The combined treatment of obestatin co-administered with ghrelin failed to significantly the affect the ghrelin-induced attenuation of ulcer area and the accompanying rise in plasma ghrelin level which reached similar values, as in case of ghrelin administered alone.

## 4. Discussion

This study shows that appetite hormones such as ghrelin, orexin-A and obestatin besides their well recognized action in the control of food intake and energy expenditure, exhibit ulcer healing and hyperemic activities as documented by an acceleration of ulcer healing by these peptides accompanied by an increase in the GBF at ulcer margin. These healing and hyperemic effects of ghrelin and orexin A seem to be very specific because both hormones induced acceleration of the healing and hyperemia at ulcer margin were reversed by ghrelin receptor antagonist D-Lys3-GHRP-6, and orexin-A receptor antagonist SB 334867, respectively, indicating that ghrelin- and orexin A-induced ulcer healing promoting and hyperemic effects are mediated by the functionally active form of GHS-R1a receptor and orexin (OX-R1) receptors. These receptors GHS-R1a and OX-R1 have been shown to bind

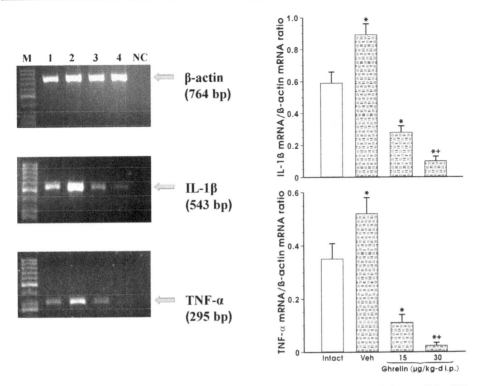

Fig. 7. Determination of expression of β-actin, IL-1β and TNF-α mRNAs (left panel) by RT-
PCR and the ratio of mRNA for ghrelin, orexin-A and obestatin (each administered at the
dose of 30 μg/kg-d i.p.) to β-actin mRNA (right panel) in intact non-ulcerated gastric
mucosa and in those with acetic acid-induced gastric ulcer treated with vehicle (saline) or
ghrelin applied i.p. in a dose of 15 μg/kg or 30 μg/kg, M - DNA size marker. Mean ± SEM
of 4-6 rats. Asterisk indicates a significant change (p<0.05) as compared to the value
obtained in intact non-ulcerated gastric mucosa. Asterisk and cross indicate a significant
change (p<0.05) as compared to the value obtained in animals treated eight days with
ghrelin administered daily i.p. at the dose of 15 μg/kg-d.

acylated ghrelin and orexin A, respectively. Moreover, we found that ghrelin, orexin A and
to lesser extent also obestatin increased the $PGE_2$ generation at ulcer margin and that these
peptides ulcer healing promoting and hyperemic effects and an increase in $PGE_2$ generated
at ulcer margin were significantly attenuated by non-selective (indomethacin), selective
COX-1 (SC-560) and selective COX-2 inhibitors (rofecoxib). These findings indicate that
endogenous PG derived from both COX-1 and COX-2 enzymatic pathways are involved in
the mechanism of ulcer healing by these hormones. Obestatin which was originally claimed
to act as ghrelin opponent in the regulation of appetite behaviour [Zhang et. al., 2005], also
accelerated ulcer healing and increased the GBF at ulcer margin in our study though these
effects were less pronounced as compared with those of ghrelin and orexin-A.
Ghrelin is a recently described 28-amino acid peptide that has been discovered in rat and
human gastrointestinal tract, particularly in gastric mucosa, as an endogenous ligand for

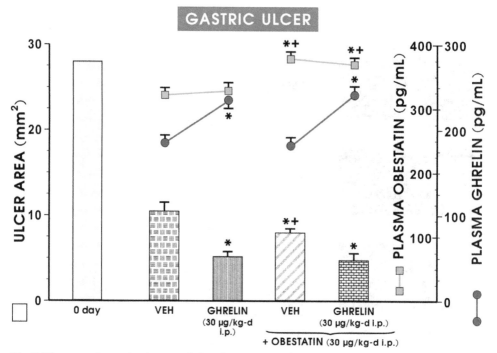

Fig. 8. The area of gastric ulcers and the alterations in the GBF at ulcer margin in rats treated for 8 days with vehicle (Veh, saline) or ghrelin (30 µg/kg-d i.p.) without or with concurrent treatment with obestatin (30 µg/kg-d i.p.). Mean ± SEM of 6-8 rats. Asterisk indicates a significant change (p<0.05) compared to vehicle-control- or obestatin-treated rats. Asterisk and cross indicate a significant change (p<0.05) compared to rats treated with ghrelin.

growth hormone secretagogue receptor (GHS-R) [Kojima et al., 1999, Hosoda et. al., 2000]. Previous studies revealed that two GHS-R subtypes are generated by alternative splicing of a single gene: the full-length type 1a receptor (GHS-R1a) and a carboxyl-terminally truncated GHS-R type 1b (GHS-R1b) [Peeters , 2005; Brzozowski et al., 1999]. The GHS-R1a is the functionally active, signal transducing form of the GHS-R, while the GHS-R1b is devoid of high-affinity ligand binding and signal transduction activity. Ghrelin molecules, produced by endocrine cells of gastric glands exist in two major molecular forms, ghrelin and des-n-octanoyl ghrelin (des-acyl ghrelin) [Hosoda et al., 2000; Fukuhara et al., 2005]. The acylation by n-octanoic acid of the hydroxyl group of their third residue, which is either serine or threonine, is essential for binding of ghrelin to the GHS-R1a [Hosoda et al., 2000]. We attempted in this study to determine whether the expected ulcer healing activity of ghrelin and orexin A is due to a direct activation of GHS-1a and orexin A receptors or involves other mediators or receptors, as yet uncharacterized and distinct from the GHS-R and orexin A. We have found that the acceleration of healing and the functional features of this healing such as an improvement in the GBF at ulcer area, the crucial mechanism involved in the healing of gastric ulcer, were mediated by specific ghrelin and orexin-A receptors.

Ghrelin was originally reported to exhibit gastroprotective activity against mucosal lesions induced by corrosive substances such as ethanol as well as against damage induced by stress and ischemia-reperfusion [Sibilia et al., 2003; Brzozowski et al., 2004; Konturek et al., 2004; Brzozowski et al., 2006]. These effects were associated with a significant increase in plasma ghrelin concentration as well as marked attenuation of the fall in GBF provoked by stress and I/R but remained independent on gastric acid secretory activity of this peptide [Brzozowski et al., 2006]. This study attempted to determine the effects of graded doses of exogenous orexin-A and obestatin compared with ghrelin on healing of acetic acid ulcers and GBF at ulcer margin and $PGE_2$ generation in the gastric mucosa. We found that peripherally administered orexin-A dose-dependently accelerated ulcer healing, elevated mucosal generation of $PGE_2$ and raised GBF at ulcer margin. Ghrelin and obestatin also accelerated ulcer healing with the magnitude similar to orexin-A while causing an increase in GBF and $PGE_2$ generation in the ulcerated gastric mucosa. The key finding of this study is the demonstration that ghrelin mRNA is upregulated in the margin of gastric ulcer suggesting that endogenous ghrelin might reduce the size of the ulcer and improve the microcirculation around the ulcer bed. Interestingly, ghrelin mRNA was also increased in the gastric mucosa exposed to ischemia-reperfusion suggesting that enhanced expression of transcripts of ghrelin may limit the extent of gastric damage provoked by I/R. Thus, our study is in partial agreement with previous observations that plasma ghrelin is increased following stress-induced gastric lesions, and that its enhanced immunoreactivity is associated with duodenal ulcerations induced by cysteamine in rats [Brzozowski et al., 2006; Fukuhara et al., 2005].

Since endogenous prostaglandins (PGs) have been implicated in the control of food intake and appetite [Eberhart, E.C, 1995; Scholz, H, 2003] we hypothesized that these cytoprotective arachidonate metabolites could play an important role in the healing effect of ghrelin. This prompted our interest in endogenous PGs because their role as well as the importance of expression of cyclooxygenase (COX-1) and COX-2 at ulcer margin in the possible ulcer activity of appetite hormones such as ghrelin, orexin-A and obestatin have not been studied. The present study supports the notion that the ulcer healing and hyperemic activities of ghrelin, orexin-A and obestatin during the time-course of ulcer healing involve an increase in mucosal generation of endogenous PGs. Previous studies have established that PG synthesis depends upon the activity of cyclooxygenase (COX), a rate limiting enzyme in the synthesis of eicosanoids from arachidonic acid [Eberhart CE & Dubois RN, 1995]. In contrast to COX-1, COX-2 is not constitutively expressed in most of tissues, but is dramatically upregulated during inflammation and ulcer healing [Takeuchi et al., 2004; Brzozowski et al., 2006] and following inhibition of mucosal COX-1 activity [Davies et al., 1997; Tanaka et al., 2002; Takeuchi et al., 2004]. First, we found that all hormones tested that is mean ghrelin, orexin A and obestatin enhance the $PGE_2$ generation at ulcer margin as compared with that of vehicle-control at day 8 upon ulcer induction. Second, indomethacin almost completely abolished, while SC-560, the selective COX-1 inhibitor and rofecoxib, the selective COX-2 inhibitor, greatly attenuated the ulcer healing and hyperemic effects of ghrelin, orexin A and obestatin, indicating that endogenous PGs, potentially derived from the activities of both COX-1 and COX-2, are responsible for the putative beneficial effects of this peptide on ulcer healing. It is of interest that COX-1 and COX-2 inhibitors by themselves delayed ulcer healing and abolished the ulcer healing promoting activity of ghrelin, orexin A and obestatin and counteracted their accompanying rise in GBF at ulcer margin suggesting that endogenous PG might be considered as primary mediators involved in the mechanism of ulcer healing by these peptides.

It is not excluded that the beneficial effect of these hormones depend also upon the activation of NO/NOS system by these hormones, which is an important metabolic pathway involved in the mechanism of mucosal defense and ulcer healing. The involvement of cNOS/iNOS-NO system in ulcer healing and the possible role of ghrelin in ulcer healing are not quite clear from this and other studies [Sibillia et al., 2009]. Although the non-specific suppression of cNOS/iNOS-NO system by L-NNA was found in our study to delay ulcer healing, little is known whether appetite hormones could affect the expression and activity of cNOS or iNOS or both. Indeed, the concurrent treatment with L-NNA not only markedly reduced the acceleration of ulcer healing but also the accompanying hyperemia at ulcer margin caused by these hormones. This finding suggests that NO could be considered as one of the essential mediator of both, the ulcer healing and the hyperemic activity of ghrelin, orexin A and obestatin. Thus we propose that NO possibly derived from constitutive cNOS rather than inducible iNOS expression and activity, plays an important role in the ghrelin-, orexin A and obestatin induced acceleration of the ulcer healing process. However, factors other than endogenous PGs and NO, possibly also sensory neuropeptides such as CGRP could also contribute to this effect, and therefore, their involvement in ulcer healing activity of ghrelin, orexin A and obestatin should be addressed in future studies. The finding that COX-1 and COX-2 inhibitors greatly attenuated the ulcer healing activity of ghrelin, is in keeping with the observation that ghrelin is ineffective in the protection against indomethacin-induced gastric ulcers [Sibillia et al., 2004], where the mucosal generation of $PGE_2$ is greatly suppressed.

Interestingly, the overexpression of TNF-$\alpha$a and IL-1$\beta$ was detected in vehicle treated control rats with gastric ulcer comparing to intact gastric mucosa , and this effect was probably caused by severe tissue ischemia, resulting from the application of acetic acid. This overexpression of proinflammatory cytokines such as TNF-$\alpha$ and IL-1$\beta$, likely contributed to early tissue damage and formation of ulceration. As reported by our group recently [Brzozowski et al., 2006] vascular injury leading to ischemia is the major factor associated with early induction of acute mucosal damage and also involved in the time-course of chronic ulceration in the stomach, where the acetic acid was applied. [Guo et al., 2003] reported an early rise in the expression of iNOS, suggesting that this expression accompanied by excessive generation of NO possibly forming peroxynitrate, was probably responsible for the enlargement of ulcer crater observed at early first days upon ulcer induction by acetic acid in rats. Our results seem to support this notion by overexpression of mRNA for proinflammatory cytokines, TNF-$\alpha$ and IL-1$\beta$, that could be responsible for the formation of focal tissue damage caused by acetic acid application. Treatment with ghrelin markedly attenuated the expression of IL-1$\beta$ and TNF-$\alpha$ in gastric mucosa around the ulcer suggesting that the acceleration of ulcer healing by ghrelin could be, at least in part, due to the potent anti-inflammatory activity of this hormone.

We reported before that the induction of gastric ulcer by serosal application of acetic acid is accompanied by the co-expression of gastroprotective COX-2-PG system with the increased expression and release of vasoactive, proliferative and trophic gastric hormones such as gastrin and ghrelin [Konturek et al., 2008]. Ghrelin was shown to exhibit gastroprotective activity and our present study confirming that this hormone can accelerate ulcer healing, suggests that the upregulation in the ghrelin gene expression could play the central event in the mechanism of gastric ulcer healing. These protective and trophic hormonal responses of gastric mucosa to ulceration, as manifested by increased expression of ghrelin co-expressed with COX-2 [Konturek et al., 2008] possibly triggered by an overexpression of IL-1β and TNF-α, seem to play a crucial role in the restoration cellular and glandular structure of the mucosa and the quality of ulcer healing.

Interestingly, obestatin, which is encoded by the same gene as ghrelin has recently been reported to counteract physiological effects of ghrelin [Zhang et al., 2005]. Intraperitoneal and intracerebroventricular treatment with obestatin suppressed food intake in a time-dependent and dose-dependent manner. This was supported by observation that obestatin effectively blunted the hunger caused by short-term starvation and inhibited feeding or body weight in rats [Sibillia et al., 2009] and food consumption in mice [Lagaut et al., 2007]. However, the vast majority of studies indicates that obestatin exerts little or no effects on food intake and body weight and failed to modify the CCK-induced decrease in food intake [Moechrs et al., 2006; Nogueiras et al., 2007; Tremblay et al., 2007]. Our present findings are in keeping with these latter observations because obestatin by itself accelerated ulcer healing but when administered together with ghrelin, remained without influence on ghrelin induced promotion of the ulcer healing and an increase in the GBF at ulcer margin and plasma ghrelin levels. This suggests that obestatin might not be considered as physiological opponent of ghrelin with the respect to ulcer healing activity which clearly was enhanced by this peptide.

## 5. Conclusion

In summary, these results demonstrate for the first time, that administration of exogenous ghrelin dose-dependently accelerates healing of chronic gastric ulcers and that other hormones involved in the control of appetite and food intake such as orexin-A and obestatin can also exert beneficial effect on the speed of ulcer healing. An evidence was provided that these ulcer healing effects of orexin-A, ghrelin and obestatin may depend upon endogenous PGs derived from COX-1 and COX-2 activity and an enhancement of gastric microcirculation around the ulcer area, possibly mediated by NO. Our finding that ghrelin is expressed in gastric mucosa, particularly at ulcer margin during ulcer healing suggests that this hormone may act locally by paracrine pathway to activate the vasoactive compounds such as PG and NO that may lead to an acceleration of the ulcer healing and the suppression of the mucosal expression and the release of proinflammatory cytokines TNF-α and IL-1β.

## 6. References

Ariyasu, H.; Takaya, K.; Tagami, T.; Ogawa, Y.; Hosoda, K; Akamizu, T.; Suda, M.; Koh, T.; Natsui, K.; Toyooka, S.; Shirakami, G.; Usui, T.; Shimatsu, A.; Doi, K.; Hosoda, H.; Kojima, M.; Kangawa, K. & Nakao, K. (2001). Stomach is a major source of circulating ghrelin, and feeding state determines plasma ghrelin-like immunoreactivity levels in humans. *Journal Clinical Endocrinology and Metabolism*, Vol.86, No.10, pp.4753-4758, ISSN 0021-972X

Brzozowski, T.; Konturek, P.C.; Konturek, S.J; Sliwowski, Z.; Drozdowicz, D.; Stachura, J.; Pajdo, R. & Hahn, E.G. (1999). Role of prostaglandins generated by cyclooxygenase-1 and cyclooxygenase-2 in healing of ischemia-reperfusion-induced gastric lesions. *European Journal Pharmacology*, Vol.385, No.1, pp. 47-61, ISSN 0014-2999.

Brzozowski, T.; Konturek, P.C.; Konturek, S.J.; Drozdowicz, D.; Kwiecien, S.; Pajdo, R.; Bielanski, W. & Hahn, E.G. (2000a). Role of gastric acid secretion in progression of acute gastric erosions induced by ischemia-reperfusion into gastric ulcers. *European Journal of Pharmacology*, Vol.398, No.1, pp.147-158, ISSN 0014-2999.

Brzozowski, T.; Konturek, P.C.; Konturek, S.J.; Pierzchalski, P.; Bielanski, W.; Pajdo, R.; Drozdowicz, D.; Kwiecien, S. & Hahn, E.G. (2000b). Central leptin and cholecystokinin in gastroprotection against ethanol-induced damage. *Digestion*, Vol.62, No.2-3, pp.126-142, ISSN 0012-2823.

Brzozowski, T.; Konturek, P.C.; Konturek, S.J.; Sliwowski, Z.; Pajdo, R.; Drozdowicz, D.; Ptak, A. & Hahn, E.G. (2001). Classic NSAID and selective cyclooxygenase (COX)-1 and COX-2 inhibitors in healing of chronic gastric ulcers. *Microscopy Research and Technique*, Vol.53, No.5, pp. 343-353, ISSN:1059-910X.

Brzozowski, T.; Konturek, P.C.; Konturek, S.J.; Kwiecien, S.; Drozdowicz, D.; Bielanski, W.; Pajdo, R.; Ptak, A.; Nikiforuk, A.; Pawlik, W.W. & Hahn, E.G. (2004). Exogenous and endogenous ghrelin in gastroprotection against stress-induced gastric damage. *Regulatory Peptides*, Vol.120, No.1-3, pp.39-51, ISSN 0167-0115.

Brzozowski, T.; Konturek, P.C.; Sliwowski, Z.; Drozdowicz, D.; Kwiecien, S.; Pawlik, M.; Pajdo, R.; Konturek, S.J.; Pawlik, W.W. & Hahn EG. (2006a). Neural aspects of ghrelin-induced gastroprotection against mucosal injury induced by noxious agents. *Journal Physiology and Pharmacology*, Vol.57, Suppl.6, pp.63-76, ISSN 0867-5910.

Brzozowski, T.; Konturek, P.C.; Sliwowski, Z.; Pajdo, R.; Drozdowicz, D.; Kwiecien, S. (2006b). Prostaglandin/cyclooxygenase pathway in ghrelin-induced gastroprotection against ischemia-reperfusion injury. *Journal of Pharmacology and Experimental Therapeutics*, Vol.319, No.1, pp.447-487, ISSN 0022-3565.

Date, Y.; Nakazato, M.; Murakami, N.; Kojima, M.; Kangawa, K. & Matsukura, S. (2001). Ghrelin acts in the central nervous system to stimulate gastric acid secretion. *Biochemical and Biophysical Research Communication*, Vol.280, No.3, pp.904-907, ISSN 0006-291X.

Davies, N.M.; Sharkley, K.A.; Asfaha, S.; MacNaughton, W.K. & Wallace, J.L. (1997). Aspirin causes rapid up-regulation of cyclooxygenase-2 expression in the stomach of rats. *Alimentary Pharmacology & Therapeutics*, Vol.11, No.6, pp.1101-1108, ISSN 0269-2813.

de Lecea, L.; Kilduff, T.S.; Peyron, C.; Gao, X.B.; Foye, P.E.; Danielson, P.E. ; Fukuhara, C.; Battenberg, E.L.; Gautvik, V.T.; Bartlett, F.S.; Frankel, W.N.; van den Pol, A.N.; Bloom, F.E.; Gautvik, K.M & Sutcliffe, J.G. (1998) The hypocretins: hypothalamus-specific peptides with neuroexcitatory activity. *Proceedings of the National Academy of Sciences of the USA*, Vol.95, No.1, pp.322-327, ISSN 0027-8424.

Dimitrova, D.Z.; Dimitrov, S.D.; Iliev, I.; Mladenov, MI.; Hristov, K.L.; Mihov, DN.; Duridanova, D.B. & Gagov, H.S. (2010). Ghrelin signaling in human mesenteric arteries. *Journal Physiology and Pharmacology*. Vol. 61, No 4, pp. 383-390, ISSN 0867-5910.

Eberhart, C.E. & Dubois RN. (1995). Eicosanoids and the gastrointestinal tract. *Gastroenterology*, Vol.109, No.1, pp.285-301, ISSN 0016-5085.

Fukuhara, S.; Suzuki, H.; Masaoka, T.; Arakawa, M.; Hosoda, H.; Minegishi, Y.; Kanagawa, K.; Ishii, H.; Kitajima, M. & Hibi T. (2005). Enhanced ghrelin secretion in rats with cysteamine-induced duodenal ulcers. *American Journal of Physiology*, Vol.289, No.1, pp.G139-G145, ISSN 0002-9513.

Futaki, N.; Yoshikawa, K.; Hamasaka, Y.; Arai, I.; Higuchi, S.; Izuka, H. & Otomo, S. (1993). NS-398, a novel non-steroidal anti-inflammatory drug with potent analgesic and antipyretic effects which causes minimal stomach lesions. *General Pharmacology*. Vol. 24, No.1, pp.105-110, ISSN 0306-3623.

Guo, J.S., Cho, C.H., Wang, W.P., Shen, X.Z., Cheng, C.L., Koo, M.W. (2003). Expression and activities of three inducible enzymes in the healing of gastric ulcers in rats. *World J Gastroenterol*. Vol. 9, No. 8, pp.1767-71, ISSN 1007-9327.

Holland, P.R.; Akerman, S. & Goadsby, P.J. (2006). Modulation of nociceptive dural intput to the trigeminal nucleus caudalis via activation of the orexin 1 receptor in the rat. *European Journal of Neuroscience*, Vol.24, No.10, pp.2825-2833, ISSN 0953-816X.

Hosoda, H.; Kojima, M.; Matsuo, H. & Kangawa, K. (2000). Ghrelin and des-acyl ghrelin: two major forms of rat ghrelin peptide in gastrointestinal tissue. *Biochemical and Biophysical Research Communications*, Vol.279, No.3, pp.909-913, ISSN 0006-291X.

Kirchgessner, A.L. & Liu, M.T. (1999). Orexin synthesis and response in the gut. *Neuron*, Vol.24, No.4, pp.941-951, ISSN 0896-6273.

Kojima, M.; Hosoda, H.; Date, Y.; Nakazo, M.; Matsuo, H. & Kangawa, K. (1999). Ghrelin is a growth-hormone-releasing acylated peptide from stomach. *Nature*, Vol.402, No.6762, pp.656-660, ISSN 00228-0836.

Komaki, G.; Matsumoto, Y.; Nishikata, H.; Kawai, K.; Nozaki, T.; Takii, M.; Sogawa, H. & Kubo, C. (2001). Orexin-A and leptin change inversely in fasting non-obese subjects. *European Journal of Endocrinology*, Vol.144, No.6, pp.645-651, ISSN 0804-4643.

Konturek, P.C.; Brzozowski, T.; Pajdo, R.; Nikiforuk, A.; Kwiecień, S.; Harsch, I.; Drozdowicz, D.; Hahn, E.G. & Konturek, S.J. (2004). Ghrelin - a new gastroprotective factor in gastric mucosa. *Journal Physiology and Pharmacology*, Vol.55, No.2, pp.325-336, ISSN 0867-5910.

Konturek, P.C.; Brzozowski, T.; Burnat, G.; Szlachcic, A.; Koziel, J.; Kwiecien, S.; Konturek, S.J. & Harsch, IA. (2010). Gastric ulcer healing and stress-lesion preventive properties of pioglitazone are attenuated in diabetic rats. *Journal Physiology and Pharmacology* Vol.61, No 4, pp.429-36, ISSN 0867-5910.

Konturek, P.C., Konturek, S.J., Burnat, G., Brzozowski, T., Brzozowska, I., Reiter, R.J. (2008). Dynamic physiological and molecular changes in gastric ulcer healing achieved by melatonin and its precursor L-tryptophan in rats. Journal of Pineal Research. Sep;45(2), pp.180-90, ISSN 1600-079X.

Konturek, S.J.; Stachura, J.; Radecki, T.; Drozdowicz, D. & Brzozowski, T. (1987). Cytoprotective and ulcer healing properties of prostaglandin $E_2$, colloidal bismuth and sucralfate in rats. *Digestion*, Vol.38, No.2, pp.103-113, ISSN 0012-2823.

Konturek, S.J; Brzozowski, T.; Bielanski, W. & Schally, A.V. (1995). Role of endogenous gastrin in gastroprotection. *European Journal of Pharmacology*, Vol.278, No.3, pp.203-212, ISSN 0014-2999.

Lagaud, G.J.; Young, A.; Ascena, A.; Morton, M.F.; Barrett, T.D. & Shankley, N.P. (2007). Obestatin reduces food intake and suppresses body weight gain in rodents. *Biochemical and Biophysical Research Communications*, Vol.357, No.1, pp.264-269, ISSN 0006-291X.

Lesch, C.A.; Gilbertsen, R.B.; Song, Y.; Dyer, R.D.; Sehrier, D.; Kraus, E.R.. & Sanchez, B.; Guglietta A. (1998). Effect of novel anti-inflammatory compounds on healing of acetic acid-induced gastric ulcer in rats. *Journal of Pharmacology and Experimental Therapeutics*, Vol.287, No.1, pp.301-306, ISSN 0022-3565.

Lugarini, F.; Hrupka, B.J.; Schwartz, G.J.; Plata-Salaman, C.R.; Langhans W. (2002). A role for cyclooxygenase-2 in lipopolysaccharide-induced anorexia nervosa in rats. *American Journal Physiology*, Vol.283, No.4, pp.R862-R868, ISSN 0002-9513.

Masuda Y, Tanaka T, Inomata N, Ohnuma N, Tanaka S, Itoh Z, Hosoda H, Kojima M, Kangawa K. (2000). Ghrelin stimulates gastric acid secretion and motility in rats. *Biochemical and Biophysical Research Communications*, Vol.267, No.3, pp.905-958, ISSN 0006-291X.

Moechars, D.; Depoortere, I.; Moreaux, B.; de Smet, B.; Goris, I. & Hoskens, L.; Daneels, G.; Kass, S.; Ver Donck, L.; Peeters, T. & Coulie B. (2006). Altered gastrointestinal and metabolic function in the GPR39-obestatin receptor-knockout mouse. *Gastroenterology*, Vol.131, No.4, pp.1131-1141, ISSN 0016-5085.

Mondal, M.S.; Nakazato, M.; Date, Y.; Murakami, N.; Yanagisawa, M.& Matsukura, S. (1999). Widespread distribution of orexin in rat brain and its regulation upon fasting. *Biochemical and Biophysical Research Communications*, Vol.256, No.3, pp. 495-499, ISSN 0006-291X.

Nogueiras, R.; Pfluger, P.; Tovar, S.; Arnold, M.; Mitchell, S.; Morris, A.; Perez-Tilve, D.; Vázquez, M.J.; Wiedmer, P.; Castañeda, T.R.; DiMarchi, R.; Tschöp, M.; Schurmann, A.; Joost, H.G.; Williams, L.M.; Langhans, W. & Diéguez, C. (2007). Effects of obestatin on energy balance and growth hormone secretion in rodents. *Endocrinology*, Vol.148, No.1, pp.21-26. ISSN 0013-7227.

Okabe, S.; Roth, J.L. & Pfeiffer, C.J.(1971). A method for experimental penetrating gastric and duodenal ulcers in rats. *American Journal of Digestive Diseases*, Vol.16, No.3, pp.277-284, ISSN 0002-9211.

Peeters, T.L. (2005). Ghrelin: a new player in the control of gastrointestinal functions. *Gut*, Vol.54, No.11, pp.1638-1649, ISSN: 0017-5749.

Sakurai, T. (2003). Orexin. A link between energy homeostasis and adaptive behaviour. *Current Opinion in Clinical Nutrition Metabolic Care*, Vol.6, No.4, pp.353-360, ISSN 1363-1950.

Sakurai, T.; Amemiya.; A.; Ishii, M.; Matsuzaki, I.; Chemelli, RM, Tanaka, H.; Williams, S.C.; Richarson, J.A.; Kozlowski, G.P.; Wilson, S.; Arch, J.R.; Buckingham, R.E.; Haynes, A.C.; Carr, S.A.; Annan, R.S.; McNulty, D.E.; Liu, W.S.; Terrett, J.A.; Elshourbagy, N.A.; Bergsma, D.J. & Yanagisawa, M. (1998). Orexins and orexin receptors: a family of hypothalamic neuropeptides and G protein-coupled receptors that regulate feeding behaviour. *Cell*, Vol.92, No.4, pp.573-585, ISSN 0092-8674.

Scholz H. (2003). Prostaglandins. *American Journal Physiology*, Vol.285, No.3, pp.R512-R514, ISSN 0002-9513.

Shujaa, N.; Zadori, Z.S.; Ronai, A.Z.; Barna, I.; Mergl; Z.; Mozes M.M. & Gyires, K. (2009). Analysis of the effect of neuropeptides and cannabinoids in gastric mucosal defense initiated centrally in the rat. *Journal Physiology and Pharmacology*, Vol.60, Suppl.7, pp.93-100, ISSN 0867-5910.

Sibilia, V.; Rindi, G.; Pagani, F.; Rapetti, D.; Locatelli, V.; Torsello, A.; Campanini, N.; Deghenghi, R. & Netti, C. (2003). Ghrelin protects against ethanol-induced gastric ulcers in rats: studies on the mechanisms of action. *Endocrinology*, Vol.144, No.4, pp.353-359, ISSN 0013-7227.

Sibilia, V.; Torsello, A.; Pagani, F.; Rapetti, D.; Lattuada, N.; Bocatelli, V.; Bulgarelli, I.; Guidobono, F. & Netti C. (2004). Effects of hexarelin against acid-independent and acid-dependent ulcerogens in the rat. *Peptides*, Vol.25, No.12, pp.2163-2170, ISSN 0196-9781.

Sibillia, V.; Bresciani, E.; Lattuada, N.; Lattuada, N.; Rapetti, D.; Locatelli, V.; De Luca, V.; Donà, F.; Netti, C.; Torsello, A. & Guidobono, F. (2006). Intracerebroventricular acute and chronic administration of obestatin minimally affect food intake but not weight gain in the rat. *Journal of Endocrinological Investigation*, Vol.29, No.11, pp.RC31-RC34, ISSN 0391-4097.

Smart, D.; Sabido-David, C.; Brough, S.J.; Jewitt, F.; Johns, A.; Porter, R.A. & Jerman, J.C. (2001). SB-334867: the first selective orexin-1 receptor antagonist. *British Journal of Pharmacology*, Vol.132, No.6, pp.1179-1189, ISSN 0007-1188.

Takeuchi, K.; Tanaka, A.; Hayashi, Y. & Kubo, Y. (2004). Functional mechanism underlying COX-2 expression following administration of indomethacin in rat stomachs: importance of gastric hypermotility. *Digestive Diseases and Sciences*, Vol.49, No.2, pp.180-187, ISSN 0163-2116.

Tanaka, A.; Araki, H.; Hase, S.; Komoike, Y. & Takeuchi, K. (2002). Up-regulation of COX-2 by inhibition of COX-1 in the rat: a key to NSAID-induced gastric injury. *Alimentary Pharmacology & Therapeutics*, Vol.16, Supl.2, pp.90-101, ISSN 0269-2813.

Tomasetto, C.; Karam S.M.; Ribieras S.; Masson R.; Lefebvre O.; Staub A.; Alexander G.; Chenard M.P.& Rio M.C. (2000). Identification and characterization of a novel gastric peptide hormone; the motilin-related peptide. *Gastroenterology*, Vol.119, No.2, pp.395-405, ISSN 0016-5085.

Tremblay, F.; Perreault, M.; Klaman, L.D.; Tobin, J.F.; Smith, E. & Gimeno, R.E. (2007). Normal food intake and body weight in mice lacking the G protein-coupled receptor GPR39. *Endocrinology*, Vol.148, No.2, pp.501-506. ISSN 0013-7227.

Tschop, M.; Smiley D.L. & Heiman M. (2000). Ghrelin induces adiposity in rodents. *Nature*, Vol.407, No.6806, pp.908-913, ISSN 00228-0836.

Wren, A.M. & Bloom S.R. (2007). Gut hormones and appetite control. *Gastroenterology*, Vol.132, No.6, pp.2116-2130, ISSN 0016-5085.

Zhang, J.V.; Ren, P-G.; Avsian-Kretchner, O.; Luo, C-W.; Rauch, R.; Klein, C. & Hsueh A.J. (2005). Obestatin, a peptide encoded by the ghrelin gene, opposes ghrelin's effects on food intake. *Science*, Vol. 301, No.5750, pp. 996-999, ISSN 0036-8075.

# 10

# *Helicobacter pylori* and Peptic Ulcer – Role of Reactive Oxygen Species and Apoptosis

Trinidad Parra-Cid[1,3], Miryam Calvino-Fernández[1,3]
and Javier P. Gisbert[2,3]
*[1]Unidad de Investigación. Hospital Universitario de Guadalajara*
*[2]Servicio de Aparato Digestivo. Hospital Universitario de La Princesa*
*e Instituto de Investigación Sanitaria Princesa (IP)(Madrid)*
*[3]CIBERehd (Centro de Investigación Biomédica en Red,*
*Enfermedades Hepáticas y Digestivas)*
*Spain*

## 1. Introduction

Peptic ulcers and gastritis are a serious and growing health problem in the whole world. Ulcers affect about 5 million Americans each year, and more than 40,000 people annually have ulcer-related surgery. Each year, approximately 15,000 people in the Unites States die of ulcer-related complications, the worst of which are an internal bleeding and perforation.

A peptic ulcer is an open sore or lesion in the gastrointestinal mucosa (stomach or duodenum) that extends through the muscularis mucosa. Peptic ulcers occur when the mucous lining of the stomach or duodenum is not sufficient to protect them against the corrosive action of stomach hydrochloric acid, pepsin digestive enzyme, or against other aggressive substances. These aggressive factors can have an endogenous or exogenous origin. The endogenous harmful factors apart from hydrochloric acid and pepsin, are: refluxed bile, leukotrienes and Reactive Oxygen Species (ROS). The exogenous damaging factors include lifestyle factors, such as alcohol abuse, stress, tension and smoking; also, consume of steroidal and nonesteroidal anti-inflammatory drugs (NSAIDs) or drugs which stimulate gastric acid and pepsin secretion. Moreover, it is completely accepted that the bacterium called *Helicobacter pylori* (*H. pylori*) is implicated in the development of gastric ulcers and gastritis.

However, many researchers suggest that both the presence of *H. pylori* and the circumstances related to lifestyle and the consumption of certain drugs are risk factors to develop ulcer, but not the underlying causes, consequently, they add severity to the problem but are not able to cause it. Although these factors are almost certainly of pathogenic relevance, there are majority of people with exposure to them who remain ulcer-free and only a small number of them develop ulcers. In fact, considering the acid-peptic environment of the stomach, the noxious agents both the endogenous and the exogenous that are ingested, and the high prevalence of *H. pylori* infection, ulcers are surprisingly uncommon.

To explain this, it is thought that in gastric mucosa is established a balance between these aggressive factors and other cytoprotective factors, and that gastric ulcer appears when the balance is lost. The mucosal defense is constituted by mucus-bicarbonate barrier, surface active phospholipid, prostaglandin, mucosal blood flow, cell renewal and migration, antioxidants and antioxidant enzymes, and some growth factors.

## 2. Free radicals and antioxidant defences

Gastroduodenal disease is associated with a variety of risk factors, including tobacco smoke, hereditary influences, sex, diet, stress and the actions of drugs (NSAIDs) (Marotta & Floch, 1991; Wallace, 1992). There is evidence that free radicals and antioxidants may be important components in the pathophysiology of gastroduodenal disease caused by many of these factors, implicating *H. pylori*. Free radicals have been involved in a wide spectrum of human diseases including other digestive disorders such as inflammatory bowel, toxic liver injury or pancreatic disease (Phull et al., 1995).

ROS can be defined as any chemical species capable of independent existence that contain one or more unpaired electrons in their outer orbital. Considering that the most stable molecular species have the electrons within their outer orbital arranged in pairs, free radicals tend to be unstable and highly reactive.

Oxygen is the most abundant radical in biological systems. The seemingly paradoxical consequences of the beneficial and harmful effects of oxygen ($O_2$) have been shown for several decades. While more than 95% of the $O_2$ consumed by the aerobic organisms is fully reduced to water during the process of mitochondrial respiration, a small percentage (<5%) is converted to semireduced species such as superoxide anion radical ($O_2\cdot^-$), hydrogen peroxide ($H_2O_2$) and hydroxyl radical ($OH\cdot$). These species are collectively named "Reactive Oxygen Species or ROS". ROS are formed continuously as normal byproducts of cellular metabolism and several of their sources are mitochondrial oxidative phosphorylation, prostaglandin synthesis, non-mitochondrial respiratory burst of neutrophils, and possibly the inhibition of mitochondrial electron transport.

**Antioxidant defences:** Free radicals play a number of physiological roles, but due to their high reactivity tend to attack the first biochemical component that they encounter inside cells, including macromolecules such as lipids, proteins or nucleic acids and bring about oxidative damage (Reilly et al., 1991). To avoid the oxidative damage, cells have development defence mechanisms to limit or prevent the toxicity caused by an excessive ROS activity. These defenses include non-enzymatic compounds such as vitamin (Vit) A, E and C, and enzymatic substances such as superoxide dismutase, catalase, glutathione peroxidase, and glutathione S-transferase; the latter two enzymes using glutathione (GSH) as a cofactor. Tissue damage may result from excessive ROS activity, from any deficiency in the defence mechanisms or from both of them.

It is well known that low/moderate concentrations of ROS affect a great number of physiological functions. However, when ROS concentration exceeds the antioxidative capacity of an organism, cells enter a state termed oxidative stress, in which the excess ROS induces oxidative damage on cellular components. So, ROS have been implicated in the pathogenesis of many human sufferings like Parkinson's, Alzheimer, Huntington's diseases and many other neurodegenerative conditions (Halliwell B, 1989). There is ample evidence that free radicals and antioxidants may be important components in the pathophysiology of gastroduodenal disease, in fact, as noted above, an exacerbated synthesis of free radicals has been implicated in inflammatory bowel disease, toxic liver injury or pancreatic disorders.

## 3. Free radicals, antioxidant defences and gastroduodenal diseases

A growing body of experimental and clinical evidence suggests that gastric mucosal damage by ethanol, NSAIDs and by *H. pylori* (Davies et al., 1994) is mediated through ROS (Phull et al., 1995). The cause could be the excessive synthesis, the deficiency of antioxidants defences or the coexistence of both reasons.

Most of the studies in this area have focused on the link between low intakes of fresh fruit and/or vegetables and gastric cancer. Several data show that exist an increased risk of gastric cancer specifically related to low intakes of Vit C and β-carotene or that β-carotene and Vit E levels were significantly lower in subjects with gastric dysplasia, a precursor of gastric cancer (Haenszel et al., 1985). Lower plasma levels of Vit A, C and E in subjects with chronic atrophic gastritis (Jaskiewicz et al., 1990) has been detected in a cross-sectional and prospectives studies showing that an increased risk of gastric cancer is associated with low plasma α-tocoferol (Knekt et al., 1991), Vit C, β-carotene (Stahelin et al., 1991), retinal levels and with low selenium levels (van den Brandt et al., 1993). Respect to the selenium, some evidence suggest that the diet of dyspeptic patients is deficient in the micronutrient selenium, which is an important constituent of the antioxidant enzyme glutathione peroxidase (GSH-Px).

Involvement of ROS in the pathogenesis of gastric ulceration was first evident from the studies of ischemia-reoxygenation-induced gastric mucosal injury. Many of the works in this area have been performed by Davies et al using a chemiluminiscence assay (Davies et al., 1994). They have shown significantly greater free radical production in duodenal mucosal biopsies from patients with duodenal ulceration and severe duodenitis that in patients with mild duodenitis or controls. This increased free radical activity in duodenal ulcer patients is accompanied by reduced levels of plasma glutathione (GSH). Recent studies show the same conclusions: there is an increased ROS production in gastric ulceration compared with gastric antral mucosa (Peng et al., 2008). Gastric ulceration also appears to be associated with increased plasma free radical activity and lower levels of Vit C and E, but not with superoxide dismutase (SOD) or catalase. ROS also decrease the level of endogenous antioxidants such as GSH, α-tocopherol and ascorbate, and make the mucosa more prone to oxidative damage.

Moreover, ROS may play an important role in gastric ulceration induced by several kinds of stress. The pathogenesis of gastric mucosal lesions by water immersion restraint stress and burn shock in rat is associated with increased lipid peroxidation. Furthermore, cold restraint stress has been shown to alter the level of various damaging and cytoprotective factors of rat gastric mucosa to cause gastric ulceration (Das et al., 1997). It was reported (Yoshikawa et al., 1989) that the gastric mucosal injury induced by ischemia-reperfusion is avoided after administration of SOD and catalase, indicating the role of lipid peroxidation and ROS in the origin of the lesion. Similarly, astaxanthin has been shown to provide protection against naproxen-induced and stress-induced gastric ulceration by reducing the level of lipid peroxides and free radicals indicating again the role of ROS in gastric damage (Oh et al., 2005). The inhibitory effect of diacerein on indomethacin-induced gastric ulceration by inhibition of neutrophil activation (Tamura et al., 2001), and consequently the suppression of ROS production by these cells, leads to similar conclusions.

Furthermore, Davies et al. (Davies et al., 1994) also detected higher levels of ROS in antral mucosa infected with *H. pylori* and they affirmed that there is no evidence for ROS participation in gastric mucosal injury in cases not related to *H. pylori* infection. Other works show that ROS levels are directly correlated with the infective load of *H. pylori* (Zhang et al., 2007) and lipid peroxidation has been also shown to be increased in *H. pylori*-positive gastric mucosa.

But although it has been established a clear association between bacteria infection and impaired synthesis of ROS, many other clinical data suggest that other factors inherent to host conditions (stress, diet, tobacco, hygiene, genetics...) contribute to the pathogenesis of this infection (Oh et al., 2005). It should be noted that some of these factors, including ingested food and tobacco smoke, directly influence in mucosal oxidative status, since they expose the gastric epithelium to the ROS that they generate within the gastric lumen in a sustained manner.

## 4. *Helicobacter pylori* and gastroduodenal diseases

### 4.1 Short history

The evolution over time of the peptic ulcer epidemiology reflects a complex and multifactorial etiology. Peptic ulcers were rare before 1800, so the gastric ulcer pathology was not described until 1835 (J. 1835 Cruveilhier maladies de l'estomac In Anatomy of Human Bailliere Pathologique du Corps, Paris ...). During the nineteenth century, the predominant form was gastric ulcer in young women, while duodenal ulcer was rare until the twentieth century. However, duodenal ulcer was gradually more prevalent until become the more frequent condition in the middle of the century. Moreover, in developed countries the mortality from peptic ulcer has been drastically reduced for the cohorts born after the start of the twentieth century (Sonnenberg, 2007).

It is now clear that the epidemiology of the peptic ulcer is mainly due to external environmental factors, among which are include *H. pylori* infection, the use of NSAIDs and smoking. However, these factors do not explain the whole story of the evolution in time and the birth-cohort effect for peptic ulcer. Specifically, *H. pylori* was a prevalent human infection before 1800, so that infection per se cannot explain the increased prevalence of the ulcer after this time nor the shift from gastric ulcer to duodenal ulcer (Graham, 2003). Interest in understanding the role of *H. pylori* in gastroduodenal diseases was started in the 1970s with the visualization of bacteria in the stomach of gastric ulcer patients, although the more important researches about it were carry out by the Australian pathologist Berry Marshal in 1979 in collaboration with J Robin Warren from 1981 (Warren JR, 1983). Almost by accident, successful culture of *H. pylori* in 1982 occurred. Marshall frustrated by not being able to get a good animal model of infection, ingested these bacteria and he became ill, developed inflammation and ulcer of stomach, and he was able to culture the bacteria from his own ulcer, proving *H. pylori* to be the cause of ulcers. They published the results of self-induced infection in 1985 (Marshall et al., 1985) and initially, the isolated bacteria was termed *Campylobacter pyloridis* but it was re-named *Helicobacter pylori* (*H. pylori*) when biochemical and genetic characterization of the organism showed that it was not a member of the *Campylobacter* genus (Tan & Wong, 2011).

### 4.2 Morphological and biochemical characteristics

*H. pylori* is a spiral-shaped, flagellated, microaerophilic Gram-negative bacillus. It inhabits various areas of stomach and duodenum. Stomach is normally a hostile environment to the survival of viruses, bacteria and other micro-organisms due to its low pH. However *H. pylori* has evolved to be uniquely suited to thrive in the harsh stomach environment (Fig. 1).

The bacterium secretes urease, a special enzyme that converts urea to ammonia. Ammonia reduces the acidity of stomach, making it more hospitable home for *H. pylori* (Pandey et al., 2010).

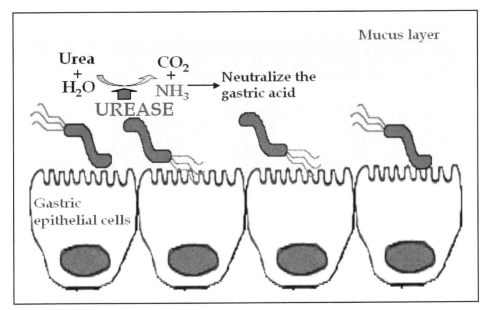

Fig. 1. *H. pylori* localization in the gastric mucosa and ammonia production.

*H. pylori* exerts a trophic influence on the gastric epithelium, but before it can attach to the epithelium surface it has first to cross the thick mucus layer by adhering to the mucosal surface. The presence of unipolar flagella helps to establish the *H.pylori* colonization of the stomach and its attachment to the epithelial surface of mucosa in the stomach despite the host attempts to rid itself of the bacterial infection. It is of interest that mutant *H. pylori* strains that are non-motile are unable to colonize the stomach of gnotobiotic piglets (Eaton et al., 1989).

### 4.3 Time, mode and geographic distribution of infection

*H. pylori* colonizes the gastric mucosa of more than 50% of human population. Infection is usually acquired in childhood while natural acquisition in adults is rare. The major risk factor for *H. pylori* infection are the socio-sanitary conditions lived during childhood, particularly at home, being important factors the level of sanitation, hygiene, and number of people in the household (the overcrowding). Studies in Kazakhstan (Nurgalieva et al., 2002) and Peru (Klein et al., 1991), have confirmed that high *H. pylori* infection prevalence in children in these countries, is related to these factors besides with the use of contaminated water with bacteria. These data determine that the water could be a reservoir and a transmission route for the bacteria.

Moreover, although it has been demonstrated a family association for infection (Nam et al., 2011), the transmission mode of *H. pylori* between individuals and within families remains to be elucidated and several interesting myths related to oral-oral transmission have been debunked when a study of couples without children revealed a low concordance of *H.pylori* infection (Perez-Perez et al., 1991); currently favored mechanisms of transmission appear to be gastro-oral and faecal-oral routes (Xia & Talley, 1997). Genetic susceptibility also appears to be significant in the acquisition of *H.pylori* infection as well as its clearance (Malaty et al., 1994).

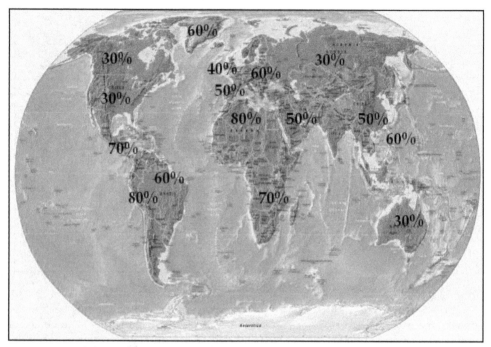

Fig. 2. *H. pylori* world distribution

Although generally speaking a rate of infection worldwide by about 50%, prevalences varying widely within countries (Fig. 2), and even between geographical areas of the same country (Krejs, 2010). Thus, in developing countries such as the eastern regions of Asia and in some parts of Latin America, the infection prevalence is characterized by a rapid rate of acquisition, usually in childhood, so that about 80% of the population is infected by the age of 20 (Graham et al., 1991).

In contrast, in developed countries such as Spain, USA, UK or Australia, the prevalence of *H. pylori* infection in children is low for ages below 10 years, and peaks of 40% aproximately, occur about to 30-40 years of age (Lehours & Yilmaz, 2007).

### 4.4 General features of *Helicobacter pylori* infection

In all infected subjects by *H. pylori*, the basic process that mediates the mucosa damage is the development of gastritis, whose extent and distribution will determine the clinical outcome (Amieva & El-Omar, 2008).

The arrival of lymphocytes and plasma cells in the mucosa signals augmentation of the acute inflammatory response by the production of cytokines and specific anti-*H. pylori*

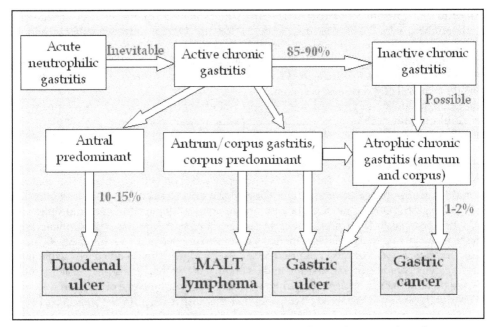

Fig. 3. *H. pylori*, gastritis and disease. During infection with *H. pylori* a number of inflammation patterns are associated with different disease stages.

antibodies. However, this vigorous response fails to eliminate infection, and the continued presence of *H. pylori* leads to the development of a second arm of the immune response more specifically aimed at preventing the damaging effects of intraluminal pathogens.

The initial acute phase of infection is subclinical in the great majority of subjects. This phase is short lived, and histologically results in a neutrophilic gastritis followed by a gradual infiltration of the gastric mucosa by inflammatory cells, and is coupled with a transient hypochlorhydria (Egan et al., 2007).

In a small minority of people, and particularly in childhood, the bacteria may be spontaneously cleared, the cellular infiltrate resolves, and the mucosa return to normal appearance. However, in the majority of subjects although *H. pylori* stimulates a robust inflammatory and immune response, the host fails to eliminate the infection and over the next 3 or 4 weeks there is a gradual accumulation of chronic inflammatory cells that come to dominate the histological picture. An acute neutrophilic gastritis gives way to an active chronic gastritis or "bening gastritis" characterized by mild pangastritis with little disruption of gastric acid secretion. This phenotype is exhibited by the asymptomatic subjects and those who do not develop serious gastrointestinal alterations (Amieva & El-Omar, 2008). In fact, it is commonly accepted that *H. pylori* infection, followed by the induction of inflammatory changes in gastric mucosa, may persist for decades without causing any gastric disturbances (Konturek et al., 2009).

Chronic gastritis is a common denominator linking peptic ulceration, gastric carcinoma, and lymphoma, and the histological picture encompassed chronic inflammation, atrophy, and intestinal metaplasia and finally adenocarcinoma (Dixon, 2001) (Fig. 3). Once chronic gastritis is established, it can progress mainly towards two topographic patterns that are related to different clinical outcomes. The first pattern named "duodenal ulcer" phenotype is an antral predominant gastritis, accounts for up 15% of infected subjects and is characterized by inflammation mostly limited to the antrum. Subjects with this phenotype have high antral inflammatory scores, high gastrin, relatively healthy corpus mucosa, and very high acid output (Graham & Yamaoka, 1998). These subjects also have defective inhibitory control of gastric acid secretion.

This combination of pathophysiologic abnormalities contributes to the development of peptic ulcers, and confers protection against gastric cancer. Conversely, gastric ulcers are thought to be initially associated with a chronic non-atrophic gastritis which progresses to chronic atrophic gastritis involving both corpus and, invariably, the antrum and decreased acid output.

The second pattern, termed "gastric cancer" phenotype, is one of progressive pan-gastritis or multifocal atrophic gastritis, and hypo- or achlorhydria, characterized by active infection of both the gastric corpus and antrum with progressive development of gastric atrophy and intestinal metaplasia. These abnormalities affect at 1% of *H. pylori*-infected individuals who presented an increased risk of development gastric carcinoma (Amieva & El-Omar, 2008).

It is clear that *H. pylori* infection can lead to several divergent clinical outcomes. Explaining this apparent paradox is essential for understanding the pathogenesis of *H. pylori*-related disease because the mechanisms underlying the differences in outcome of *H. pylori* infection are currently poorly understood. It appears that the host reaction to the infection is very complex and it has been hypothesized that many sequential events and several mechanisms of tissue injury participate in the process. Between these pathogenic mechanisms of *H. pylori* are identified the induction of gastric inflammation, the disruption of the gastric mucosal barrier and the altered gastrin-gastric acid homeostasis (Dunn et al., 1997). Also, these different clinical manifestations of the infection are influenced by the host characteristics, the environmental factors and the bacterial genetic. Host factors are mainly related to the recognition of *H. pylori* by the immune system, variations in the level of cytokine response, sex and hereditary influences. Environmental data include tobacco smoke, diet, stress and the action of drugs such as NSAIDs. Bacterial factors may increase the risk of more severe disease, causing increased proinflammatory cytokine release. Strains possessing the "cag pathogenicity island" are more likely to be associated with peptic ulceration or gastric adenocarcinoma than strains lacking it. Another genes and proteins, such as iceA, vacA, OipA, BabA, have been analyzed but different studies were unable to show an association between them and the pattern of gastritis (Egan et al., 2007).

### 4.5 Toxicity of *Helicobacter pylori* on gastric mucosa (ROS)

In the early stages of infection, *H. pylori* induces secretion of chemokines (RANTES, GROα, MIP-1α, ENA-78, MCP-1, and IL-8), as well as of proinflammatory cytokines (IL-1, IL-6 and TNF-α, mainly) (Ibraghimov & Pappo, 2000). These molecules provoke recruitment of cells (macrophages, PMN, mast cells, T and B lymphocytes) to the infected gastric tissue, being neutrophils the initial inflammatory component of the response to the pathogen (Naito & Yoshikawa, 2002). Recruited PMNs, in turn, secrete more inflammatory mediators that amplify the primary signal and mediates directly the influx of more PMN to the gastric mucosa. Furthermore, soluble proteins of *H. pylori* can also function as chemoattractants for neutrophils. PMNs into gastric tissue induce oxidative burst responses in phagocytes being these activities typical in the development of gastric disease. It is demonstrated that *H. pylori* isolates which induce a strong and rapid oxidative burst in neutrophils are associated with higher inflammation scores in gastric ulcer patients and with histological mucosal damage (Louw et al., 1993). Furthermore, IL-8 levels secreted by mucosa cells positively correlate with infiltration of PMN and mononuclear cells, and with higher production of ROS in *H. pylori*-infected antral gastric mucosa (Danese et al., 2001).

ROS production in *H. pylori* infection is catalyzed by nicotinamide adenine dinucleotide phosphate oxidase (NADPH oxidase; Nox) on the cell membrane (Lambeth, 2004). It is also produced superoxide anion ($O_2^-$), a precursor of microbicidal oxidants. This $O_2^-$ is converted to hydrogen peroxide ($H_2O_2$) by superoxide dismutase (SOD) catalysis, or by non-enzymatic dismutation in the phagosome. $H_2O_2$ can passively permeate cell membranes and is converted to hypochlorous acid (HOCl), which is 100 times more toxic than $H_2O_2$. This conversion is mediated by myeloperoxidases (MPO) released by Azur granules in phagocytes in the presence of chloride ions (Cl-). $H_2O_2$ also reacts nonenzymatically with $O_2^-$ to form hydroxyl radicals ($^{\cdot}OH$) in the presence of ferrous (Fe2+) or cuprous (Cu+) ions. In general, these highly reactive ROS (i.e., HOCl and $^{\cdot}OH$) are used by the phagocyte to kill pathogenic bacteria (Fig.4).

However, in *H. pylori*-infected gastric mucosa, these ROS cannot eradicate *H. pylori* and this excessive production is believed to be a major cause of gastric mucosal damage, inducing oxidative stress to the gastric mucosa cells (Handa et al., 2010).

Thus, the role of oxidative stress on gastric mucosa is multi-functional. For neutrophils, it is the result of excessive defense reactions of the body against *H. pylori* intrusion, and for *H. pylori*, it is a convenient tool for invading the human gastric mucosa.

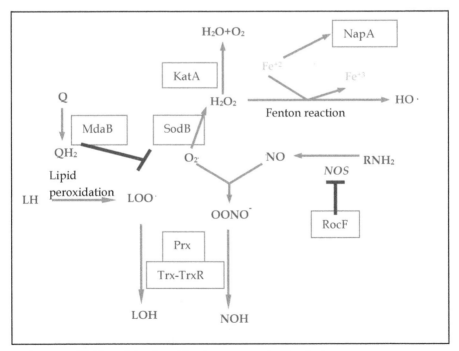

Fig. 4. Sources of ROS and the detoxification systems in *H. pylori*

As noted above, some factors that may further aggravate the pathogenicity caused by *H. pylori* are the genetic characteristics of bacteria. In fact, the possession of "cytotoxin-associated gene (cagA) or pathogenicity island" is associated with a high prevalence of peptic ulcer disease. And also, according to the authors Danese et al (Danese et al., 2001) and others, the gastric mucosa of patients infected by CagA (+) strains are characterized by increased ROS generation and neutrophil counts greater than that observed in CagA (-) subjects.

### 4.6 *Helicobacter pylori*, ROS and cellular apoptosis

Several studies have shown a relationship between *H. pylori* infection and an increased apoptosis rate in gastric lesions such as chronic gastritis, generally accompanied by glandular atrophy, gastric ulcer and intestinal metaplasia. Specifically, studies in patients with gastric ulcer determine a higher apoptotic index in this type of gastric lesion with *H. pylori* infection compared to *H. pylori*-negative normal gastric mucosa (Targa et al., 2007). Results of Satoh et al (Satoh et al., 2003) showed that apoptosis, not only of surface epithelial cells but also of glandular cells in the upper portion of fundic glands, is increased in *H. pylori*-positive patients with gastric ulcers and decreased to normal levels after eradication of *H. pylori*. Recent studies are intended to avoid triggering apoptotic processes caused by *H. pylori* (Hsu et al., 2010). In these experiments, authors use substances capable of inhibiting the activation of caspase cascade (extract solanum lyratum in this study). This could be a new approach for the treatment of infection with *H. pylori*.

It is known that some of the major stimuli that can induce apoptosis are: ionising radiation, viral infection, growth factor depletion, cytoplasmic stress, serum starvation, presence of hormones such as corticosteroids, the damage to genetic material and an excessive presence of free radical. Given that one of the factors that triggers cellular apoptosis is the excess of ROS, it is reasonable to think that the apoptosis observed in gastric mucosal cells infected by *H. pylori* may have this origin.

Apoptosis was first described in 1972 by Currie and colleagues (Kerr et al., 1972). It plays a pivotal part in many physiological settings, including the embryonic and post-embryonic development of multicellular organisms, tissue homeostasis and the removal of damaged and/or infected cells. It is delicately regulated and balanced in a physiological context. Failure of this regulation results in pathological conditions such as developmental defects, autoimmune diseases, neurodegeneration or cancer (Thompson, 1995). Apoptosis is by far the best-characterized mode of programmed cell death that is associated to morphological features that had been repeatedly observed in various tissues and cell types. Apoptotic cells display typical morphological features such as nuclear fragmentation, chromatin condensation and cell shrinkage, and eventually break down into apoptotic bodies. These morphological changes are accompanied by ATP-dependent biochemical changes that lead to the cells to various functional alterations. The results of these changes are reflected in an asymmetry of the cytoplasmic membranes by translocation of phosphatidylserine to the surface, breaking of DNA in multiples fragments (ladder pattern), release of pro-apoptotic proteins (cytochrome c (cyt c), AIF,...) from the mitochondria to cytosol, activation of caspases cascade, and finally, cell death.

Apoptotic cascade appears to have many regulatory "switch points" between proapoptotic and antiapoptotic forces. The imbalance of these forces has led to several key concepts regarding the importance of apoptosis in health and disease. Thus, atrophy of an organ with a decrease in cell numbers could be related to an increase in cellular apoptosis, whereas tissue proliferation may be associated with molecular inhibition of apoptosis; in some diseases, internal or external factors could trigger the proapoptotic machinery within the cell causing cell death and tissue destruction; or cellular malignant transformation may occur because of a failure to activate apoptosis and delete cells with genetic damage (i.e., oncogenic mutations). These concepts suggest the possibility that several treatment strategies are useful in certain clinical conditions. Thus, inhibition of apoptosis could facilitate tissue repair processes by promoting cellular proliferation, and tissue regeneration, and, moreover, induction of apoptosis could be proven useful in treating malignant carcinomas (Que & Gores, 1996).

In relationship with the gastrointestinal tract, apoptosis plays an important role in the regulation of epithelial cell numbers, being the deregulation of the apoptotic pathway implicated in a number of disease processes in the gastrointestine. In *H. pylori*-induced chronic gastritis, cell loss by apoptosis is excessive compared with proliferation, suggesting that infection with the bacteria triggers the acceleration of apoptosis, fact that has been proven in *in vivo* experiments (Hall et al., 1994).

Two distinct, but partially overlapping, pathways are known to lead to apoptosis (Fig.5):
-   the extrinsic (receptor mediated pathway), and
-   the intrinsic (mitochondrial pathway).

The extrinsic pathway is activated by apoptotic stimuli comprising external signals such as the binding of death inducing ligands to cell surface receptors. Among death inducing ligands more studied are Fas, tumor necrosis factor receptor or TRAIL receptors.

Death ligand stimulation results in oligomerization of the receptors and recruitment of the adaptor protein Fas-associated death domain (FADD) and caspase-8, forming a death-inducing signalling complex (DISC). Autoactivation of caspase-8 at the DISC is followed by activation of effector caspases, including caspase-3, -6 and -7, which function as downstream effectors of the cell death program (Ashkenazi & Dixit, 1998). Fas has a central role in the physiological regulation of apoptosis and has been implicated in the pathogenesis of various malignancies as well as in diseases of the immune system. Fas is involved in cytotoxic T-cell mediated killing of cells (for example, CTL-mediated killing of virus-infected cells), destruction of inflammatory and immune cells in immune-privileged sites, deletion of self-reacting B cells and activated T-cells at the end of an immune response (Jin & El-Deiry, 2005).

Some *in vitro* studies reveal that *H. pylori* stimulates apoptosis of gastric epithelial cells in association with the enhanced expression of the Fas receptor, indicating a role for Fas-mediated signaling in the programmed cell death that occurs in response to *H. pylori* infection (Jones et al., 1999). Wang et al. (Wang et al., 2000) also demonstrated that local Th1 cells (cellular subtype that is mainly recruited to the gastric mucosa during the infection) may contribute to the pathogenesis of gastric disease during *H. pylori* infection by increasing the expression of Fas on gastric epithelial cells and inducing apoptosis through Fas/FasL interactions. Moreover, *H. pylori* can sensitize human gastric epithelial cells and enhance susceptibility to TRAIL-mediated apoptosis (Wu et al., 2004).

Intrinsic apoptotic pathway is initiated inside cells. The most important turning point in the course of the intrinsic apoptotic process occurs in the mitochondria. Their structure and compartmentalization are highly related to a perfect performance of their functions, being the most relevant, in eukaryotic cells, energy production in ATP form molecules (Chinnery & Schon, 2003).

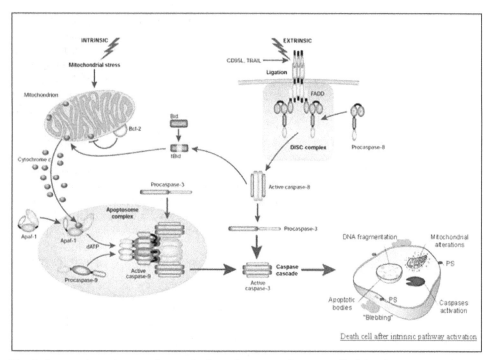

Fig. 5. Apoptotic pathways: the extrinsic pathway involves so-called death receptors, the intrinsic one involves mitochondrial alterations. Both pathways converge at caspase-3 activation, where classic biochemical and morphological changes in association with the apoptotic phenotype are originated

Every mitochondrion has a double lipid envelope that delimites the matrix, located within the inner mitochondrial membrane (IMM) and the intermembrane space located, in turn, between the IMM and the outer mitochondrial membrane (OMM). IMM cristae or invaginations increase the area where specific mitochondrial processes develop (electron transport and oxidative phosphorylation) (Fig. 6). The efficacy of these processes greatly depends on the bilayer's appropriate composition and structure, which relies on the role of the phospholipid cardiolipin (CL). CL is a specific component of IMM and the most abundant in it. On the CL are anchored many proteins such as respiratory chain I-IV complexes and cytochrome c (cyt c) (Calvino Fernandez & Parra Cid, 2010). Particularly relevant is the electrostatic binding between CL and cyt c in the IMM since this limits the amounts of cyt c that can be released during apoptosis (Iverson & Orrenius, 2004; Ott et al., 2002).

The crucial step in mitochondrion regulated apoptosis is the permeabilization of the OMM, often considered as the "point of no return" in apoptosis signalling (Orrenius et al., 2003), accompanied by the loss of mitochondrial membrane potential ($\Delta\Psi$m) and mitochondrial transition pores (MTP) opening. OMM permeabilization is followed by the release of caspase activating proteins such as cyt c and second mitochondrion-derived activator of caspase (SMAC; also known as DIABLO) into the cytosol.

The past 10 years have seen considerable efforts to decipher the molecular pathways leading to permeabilization of the OMM, and it was early recognized that the Bcl-2 family of

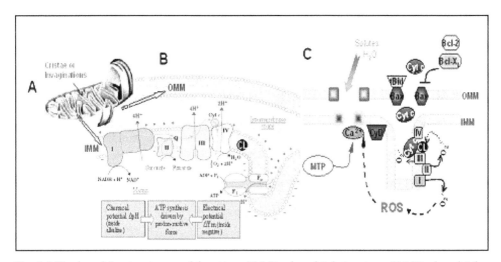

Fig. 6. Mitochondria: structure and function. **A)** Mitochondrial structure. **B)** Mitochondrial membranes: relationship between electron transport chain complexes, cytochrome c, and cardiolipin. **C)** Mitochondrial transition pore formation: ruptured links between protein complexes and cardiolipin, and release of cytochrome c into the cytosol . OMM: outer mitochondrial membrane; IMM: inner mitochondrial membrane; CL: cardiolipin; cyt c: cytochrome c; MTP: mitochondrial transition pores.

proteins play a prominent role in the regulation and execution of this process. As a result of this work, three different types of Bcl-2 family proteins have been identified: (a) the pro-apoptotic mediators, namely Bax and Bak; (b) the anti-apoptotic effectors, notably Bcl-2, Bcl-XL and Mcl-1; and (c) a host of Bcl-2 homology domain 3 (BH3-only) proteins which control either both the pro- and anti-apoptotic family members or only a specific member of one group (Youle & Strasser, 2008). The exact mechanisms of action and interplay of all these proteins are still a matter of vibrant debate. But there is general agreement that Bax and Bak are the terminal mediators of OMM permeabilization. As a result of Bax insertion /oligomerization into the OMM (promoted, i.e., by the cleavage of the BH3-only protein, Bid), pores are formed that mediate the release of pro-apoptotic proteins from the intermembrane space into the cytosol. The molecular nature of such pores, that is whether they are proteinaceous or lipidic, is currently not known (Ott et al., 2009).

Recently, apoptosis by mitochondrial pathway in *H. pylori* infection has been thoroughly studied (Calore et al., 2010; Calvino-Fernandez et al., 2008; Chiozzi et al., 2009; Domanska et al., 2010; Kim et al., 2010; Kim et al., 2007; Matsumoto et al., 2010; Yamasaki et al., 2006; Zhang et al., 2007). Thus, in this research line we can find papers that evidence how VacA, one of the major pathogenic products of *H. pylori* which induces large vacuoles within gastric epithelial cells, stimulates apoptosis via a mitochondria-dependent pathway (Chiozzi et al., 2009; Domanska et al., 2010; Galmiche et al., 2000; Kim et al., 2010). Some authors say that it interferes with mitochondrial permeability and reduces ΔΨm, followed by cyt c release. It is suggested that VacA may not act directly to induce cyt c release from mitochondria, instead Bax and Bcl-2 homologous antagonist/killer (Bak), were activated and relocated to mitochondria, promoting cyt c release (Calore et al., 2010; Matsumoto et al., 2010; Yamasaki et al., 2006).

Not only VacA has been seen to be involved in *H. pylori*-induced mitochondria pathway apoptosis. Apurinic/apyrimidinic endonuclease-1 (APE-1) regulates transcriptional activity of p53, and *H pylori* (and ROS) induce APE-1 expression in human gastric epithelial cells, increasing intracellular calcium ion concentration of these cells which induces APE-1 acetylation. This *H. pylori*-mediated acetylation of APE-1 suppresses Bax expression, preventing p53-mediated apoptosis when *H. pylori* infects gastric epithelial cells (Bhattacharyya et al., 2009; Chattopadhyay et al., 2010).

*In vivo* studies indicate that *H. pylori*-induced apoptosis is associated with an increase in Bak expression in gastric biopsies from patients colonized by the bacterium. Konturek et al. reported induction of apoptosis with evidence of Bax up-regulation and Bcl-2 down-regulation in duodenal ulcer patients with *H. pylori* infection (Konturek et al., 1999).

It is known that mitochondria are one of the possible targets and the major intracellular source of free radicals (ROS), since it is estimated that 1–2% of the oxygen consumed by mitochondria (and they consume 85% of all body oxygen) in the electron transport chain is converted to $O_2{}^-$ (Shigenaga et al., 1994). Elevated amounts of $O_2{}^-$ could have detrimental effects on nearby molecules, modifying several proteins of the mitochondrial membrane, lipids or even mitochondrial DNA (which has limited protection because of its lack of histones). In physiological conditions, mitochondria have several enzymes (manganese-dependent superoxide dismutase, glutathione peroxidase) and non-enzimatic systems (NADPH, Vit C and E) that maintain $O_2{}^-$ concentrations at very low levels. But when some events cause an overproduction of free radicals, these systems are not able to eliminate the excess. Therefore, overproduction of ROS may also reduce the antioxidant defenses.

This oxidative stress may damage cellular components (Fig. 7), including polyunsaturated fatty acids, carbohydrates, structural and regulatory proteins, and DNA (Baik et al., 1996; Calvino-Fernandez et al., 2008; Jacobson, 1996).

It could well play a role in epithelial proliferation, apoptosis, and oxidative DNA damage.

Lipids of cellular membranes, such as CL, are particularly susceptible to oxidation due to the amount of double bonds in their structure, and it is expected that structural changes would be deleterious to normal mitochondrial function (Calvino-Fernandez et al., 2008; Calvino Fernandez & Parra Cid, 2010).

It is widely known that *H. pylori* infection increases epithelial apoptosis in gastric mucosa, which may play an important role in gastric carcinogenesis (Xia & Talley, 2001), and *H. pylori*-induced apoptosis may stimulate compensatory hyperproliferation which results in potential preneoplastic changes in chronic *H. pylori* infection (Moss et al., 1996). Besides, as noted above, higher levels of apoptosis have been detected in ulcer lesions (Satoh et al., 2003; Targa et al., 2007) in patients infected with bacteria, and also, this increased apoptosis disappears when *H. pylori* is eradicated. In both clinical alterations, ulcer and cancer, are also shown that there is an increase of oxidative stress.

With all these data, it is reasonable to assume that whether *H. pylori* causes oxidative stress with an increase of free radicals production, these ROS could directly affect mitochondria and trigger the apoptosis by a similar way shown in Fig.7 (Calvino Fernandez & Parra Cid, 2010).

An indisputable proof that these two processes (ROS and apoptosis) are related to, is the inhibition of apoptosis by treatment with antioxidants. In *in vitro* experiments (Calvino-Fernandez et al., 2008), *H. pylori* caused apoptosis in gastric epithelial cells. Simultaneously alterations in several structural and functional characteristics of mitochondria (high $O_2{}^-$ synthesis, decreased levels of antioxidant enzymes, cardiolipin oxidation, loss of membrane potential, large amounts of cytosolic cit c, higher levels of Bax and caspases,...) were detected. All these changes were eliminated by incubating the cells with Vit E during the period of infection. The antioxidant, also prevented that the cells died by apoptosis.

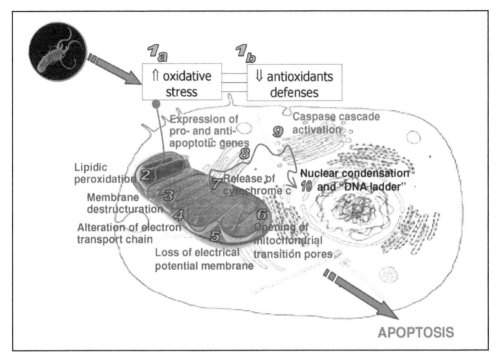

Fig. 7. Morphologic and functional alterations caused by *H. pylori* in epithelial gastric cells. ROS can directly affect mitochondria and trigger apoptotic process.

Solanum lyratum extract (SLE) was also able to suppress *H. pylori*-induced apoptosis (Hsu et al., 2010). SLE inhibited caspase-8 activation, thereby preventing the release of cyt c from mitochondria and activation of the subsequent downstream apoptotic pathway. Thus, SLE may offer a new approach for the treatment of *H. pylori* by down-regulation of apoptosis in the *H. pylori* infected gastric epithelium. As it does not directly target bacteria, SLE treatment might not cause development of resistant strains.

## 5. Conclusions

General knowledge of scientific advances is necessary not only to read and interpret the literature but also to diagnose and treat diseases appropriately. The biological phenomena contributing to oxidative stress and cell death, fundamental processes in many gastrointestinal diseases, are important in the science and practice of gastroenterology. Currently a scientific revolution is ongoing in the understanding of cell death by a process referred to as "apoptosis or programmed cellular death", and the underlying causes of apoptosis are being the subject of many studies.

*H. pylori* infection is associated with chronic gastritis, peptic ulcers, and gastric cancer. Extensive scientific evidence shows that in these alterations are involved oxidative stress (exacerbated synthesis of ROS) caused by the bacteria by different mechanisms. In addition, a common feature of all these pathologies is the activation of apoptosis, either by extrinsic or, as it is more accepted today, for intrinsic pathway.

Novel therapeutic strategies that may be useful in the prevention or treatment of disorders of the stomach and duodenum caused by bacteria, should have as target the inhibition of the synthesis of ROS and/or apoptosis. Whereas the excess of free radicals is the origin of these alterations, the first step to take would be to restore the balance between oxidants and antioxidant systems. This would eliminate the oxidative stress of the gastric mucosa.

With respect to ROS, the actions may be aimed to the inhibition of its exacerbated synthesis, which serve to mitigate the toxic effects caused by the observed deficiencies in the antioxidant levels. Another strategy could be external supplementation of scavengers to remove this excess of free radicals. The antioxidant vitamins are the logical first choice as therapeutic agents, because of the large amount of data available on their role in *H. pylori* infection, gastroduodenal disease and gastric cancer.

Other new approach for the treatment of *H. pylori* could be the down-regulation of apoptosis in infected gastric epithelium. This might be possible by administering substances that inhibit the activation of caspases. Thus, it would prevent the release of cyt c from mitochondria and as a result, the subsequent downstream apoptotic pathway.

These actions are directed against the toxic manifestations caused by infection, while the traditional treatments with antibiotics have as target the bacterium itself. Consequently, these strategies would also prevent the development of resistant strains, an increasingly common problem due to the usual antibiotic treatments.

## 6. Acknowledgment

This chapter was partly funded by a research grant PI-2008134 of Fundación para la Investigación Sanitaria en Castilla La-Mancha (FISCAM). The work of M. Calvino was funded by Instituto de Salud Carlos III through a "Contrato de Apoyo a la Investigación en el SNS" (CA07/00157).

## 7. References

Amieva, M. R., & El-Omar, E. M. (2008). Host-bacterial interactions in Helicobacter pylori infection. *Gastroenterology*, Vol.134, No.1, pp. 306-323, ISSN 1528-0012 (Electronic) 0016-5085 (Linking)

Ashkenazi, A., & Dixit, V. M. (1998). Death receptors: signaling and modulation. *Science*, Vol.281, No.5381, pp. 1305-1308, ISSN 0036-8075 (Print) ISSN 0036-8075 (Linking)

Baik, S. C., Youn, H. S., Chung, M. H., Lee, W. K., Cho, M. J., Ko, G. H., Park, C. K., Kasai, H., & Rhee, K. H. (1996). Increased oxidative DNA damage in Helicobacter pylori-infected human gastric mucosa. *Cancer Res*, Vol.56, No.6, pp. 1279-1282, ISSN 0008-5472 (Print) 0008-5472 (Linking)

Bhattacharyya, A., Chattopadhyay, R., Burnette, B. R., Cross, J. V., Mitra, S., Ernst, P. B., Bhakat, K. K., & Crowe, S. E. (2009). Acetylation of apurinic/apyrimidinic endonuclease-1 regulates Helicobacter pylori-mediated gastric epithelial cell apoptosis. *Gastroenterology*, Vol.136, No.7, pp. 2258-2269, ISSN 1528-0012 (Electronic) 0016-5085 (Linking)

Calore, F., Genisset, C., Casellato, A., Rossato, M., Codolo, G., Esposti, M. D., Scorrano, L., & de Bernard, M. (2010). Endosome-mitochondria juxtaposition during apoptosis induced by H. pylori VacA. *Cell Death Differ*, Vol.17, No.11, pp. 1707-1716, ISSN 1476-5403 (Electronic) 1350-9047 (Linking)

Calvino-Fernandez, M., Benito-Martinez, S., & Parra-Cid, T. (2008). Oxidative stress by Helicobacter pylori causes apoptosis through mitochondrial pathway in gastric epithelial cells. *Apoptosis*, Vol.13, No.10, pp. 1267-1280, ISSN 1573-675X (Electronic) 1360-8185 (Linking)

Calvino Fernandez, M., & Parra Cid, T. (2010). H. pylori and mitochondrial changes in epithelial cells. The role of oxidative stress. *Rev Esp Enferm Dig*, Vol.102, No.1, pp. 41-50, ISSN 1130-0108 (Print) 1130-0108 (Linking)

Chattopadhyay, R., Bhattacharyya, A., & Crowe, S. E. (2010). Dual regulation by apurinic/apyrimidinic endonuclease-1 inhibits gastric epithelial cell apoptosis during Helicobacter pylori infection. *Cancer Res*, Vol.70, No.7, pp. 2799-2808, ISSN 1538-7445 (Electronic) 0008-5472 (Linking)

Chinnery, P. F., & Schon, E. A. (2003). Mitochondria. *J Neurol Neurosurg Psychiatry*, Vol.74, No.9, pp. 1188-1199, ISSN 0022-3050 (Print) 0022-3050 (Linking)

Chiozzi, V., Mazzini, G., Oldani, A., Sciullo, A., Ventura, U., Romano, M., Boquet, P., & Ricci, V. (2009). Relationship between Vac A toxin and ammonia in Helicobacter pylori-induced apoptosis in human gastric epithelial cells. *J Physiol Pharmacol*, Vol.60, No.3, pp. 23-30, ISSN 1899-1505 (Electronic) 0867-5910 (Linking)

Danese, S., Cremonini, F., Armuzzi, A., Candelli, M., Papa, A., Ojetti, V., Pastorelli, A., Di Caro, S., Zannoni, G., De Sole, P., Gasbarrini, G., & Gasbarrini, A. (2001). Helicobacter pylori CagA-positive strains affect oxygen free radicals generation by gastric mucosa. *Scand J Gastroenterol*, Vol.36, No.3, pp. 247-250, ISSN 0036-5521 (Print) 0036-5521 (Linking)

Das, D., Bandyopadhyay, D., Bhattacharjee, M., & Banerjee, R. K. (1997). Hydroxyl radical is the major causative factor in stress-induced gastric ulceration. *Free Radic Biol Med*, Vol.23, No.1, pp. 8-18, ISSN 0891-5849 (Print) 0891-5849 (Linking)

Davies, G. R., Simmonds, N. J., Stevens, T. R., Sheaff, M. T., Banatvala, N., Laurenson, I. F., Blake, D. R., & Rampton, D. S. (1994). Helicobacter pylori stimulates antral mucosal reactive oxygen metabolite production in vivo. *Gut*, Vol.35, No.2, pp. 179-185, ISSN 0017-5749 (Print) 0017-5749 (Linking)

Dixon, M. F. (2001): Pathology of Gastritis and Peptic Ulceration. In M. G. Mobley HLT, Hazell SL (Ed.): *Helicobacter pylori: Physiology and Genetics*, ASM Press, Washington (DC).

Domanska, G., Motz, C., Meinecke, M., Harsman, A., Papatheodorou, P., Reljic, B., Dian-Lothrop, E. A., Galmiche, A., Kepp, O., Becker, L., Gunnewig, K., Wagner, R., & Rassow, J. (2010). Helicobacter pylori VacA toxin/subunit p34: targeting of an anion channel to the inner mitochondrial membrane. *PLoS Pathog*, Vol.6, No.4, pp. e1000878, ISSN 1553-7374 (Electronic) 1553-7366 (Linking)

Dunn, B. E., Cohen, H., & Blaser, M. J. (1997). Helicobacter pylori. *Clin Microbiol Rev*, Vol.10, No.4, pp. 720-741, ISSN 0893-8512 (Print) 0893-8512 (Linking)

Eaton, K. A., Morgan, D. R., & Krakowka, S. (1989). Campylobacter pylori virulence factors in gnotobiotic piglets. *Infect Immun*, Vol.57, No.4, pp. 1119-1125, ISSN 0019-9567 (Print) 0019-9567 (Linking)

Egan, B. J., Holmes, K., O'Connor, H. J., & O'Morain, C. A. (2007). Helicobacter pylori gastritis, the unifying concept for gastric diseases. *Helicobacter*, Vol.12 Suppl 2, pp. 39-44, ISSN 1083-4389 (Print) 1083-4389 (Linking)

Galmiche, A., Rassow, J., Doye, A., Cagnol, S., Chambard, J. C., Contamin, S., de Thillot, V., Just, I., Ricci, V., Solcia, E., Van Obberghen, E., & Boquet, P. (2000). The N-terminal 34 kDa fragment of Helicobacter pylori vacuolating cytotoxin targets mitochondria and induces cytochrome c release. *EMBO J*, Vol.19, No.23, pp. 6361-6370, ISSN 0261-4189 (Print) 0261-4189 (Linking)

Graham, D. Y. (2003). Changing patterns of peptic ulcer, gastro-oesophageal reflux disease and Helicobacter pylori: a unifying hypothesis. *Eur J Gastroenterol Hepatol*, Vol.15, No.5, pp. 571-572, ISSN 0954-691X (Print) 0954-691X (Linking)

Graham, D. Y., Adam, E., Reddy, G. T., Agarwal, J. P., Agarwal, R., Evans, D. J., Jr., Malaty, H. M., & Evans, D. G. (1991). Seroepidemiology of Helicobacter pylori infection in India. Comparison of developing and developed countries. *Dig Dis Sci*, Vol.36, No.8, pp. 1084-1088, ISSN 0163-2116 (Print) 0163-2116 (Linking)

Graham, D. Y., & Yamaoka, Y. (1998). H. pylori and cagA: relationships with gastric cancer, duodenal ulcer, and reflux esophagitis and its complications. *Helicobacter*, Vol.3, No.3, pp. 145-151, ISSN 1083-4389 (Print) 1083-4389 (Linking)

Haenszel, W., Correa, P., Lopez, A., Cuello, C., Zarama, G., Zavala, D., & Fontham, E. (1985). Serum micronutrient levels in relation to gastric pathology. *Int J Cancer*, Vol.36, No.1, pp. 43-48, ISSN 0020-7136 (Print) 0020-7136 (Linking)

Hall, P. A., Coates, P. J., Ansari, B., & Hopwood, D. (1994). Regulation of cell number in the mammalian gastrointestinal tract: the importance of apoptosis. *J Cell Sci*, Vol.107 ( Pt 12), pp. 3569-3577, ISSN 0021-9533 (Print) 0021-9533 (Linking)

Halliwell B, G. J. (1989). Free radicals in biology and Medicine. 2nd edition. *Clarendon Press, Oxford)*, pp. 416

Handa, O., Naito, Y., & Yoshikawa, T. (2010). Helicobacter pylori: a ROS-inducing bacterial species in the stomach. *Inflamm Res*, Vol.59, No.12, pp. 997-1003, ISSN 1420-908X (Electronic) 1023-3830 (Linking)

Hsu, Y. M., Lai, C. H., Su, C. H., Kuo, W. W., Kuo, C. L., Hsu, C. K., Wang, C. K., Chang, C. Y., & Chung, J. G. (2010). Solanum lyratum extract inhibits Helicobacter pylori-mediated apoptosis in human gastric epithelial cells. *Anticancer Res*, Vol.30, No.4, pp. 1189-1193, ISSN 1791-7530 (Electronic) 0250-7005 (Linking)

Ibraghimov, A., & Pappo, J. (2000). The immune response against Helicobacter pylori--a direct linkage to the development of gastroduodenal disease. *Microbes Infect*, Vol.2, No.9, pp. 1073-1077, ISSN 1286-4579 (Print) 1286-4579 (Linking)

Iverson, S. L., & Orrenius, S. (2004). The cardiolipin-cytochrome c interaction and the mitochondrial regulation of apoptosis. *Arch Biochem Biophys*, Vol.423, No.1, pp. 37-46, ISSN 0003-9861 (Print) 0003-9861 (Linking)

Jacobson, M. D. (1996). Reactive oxygen species and programmed cell death. *Trends Biochem Sci*, Vol.21, No.3, pp. 83-86, ISSN 0968-0004 (Print) 0968-0004 (Linking)

Jaskiewicz, K., Van Helden, P. D., Wiid, I. J., Steenkamp, H. J., & Van Wyk, M. J. (1990). Chronic atrophic gastritis, gastric pH, nitrites and micronutrient levels in a population at risk for gastric carcinoma. *Anticancer Res*, Vol.10, No.3, pp. 833-836, ISSN 0250-7005 (Print) 0250-7005 (Linking)

Jin, Z., & El-Deiry, W. S. (2005). Overview of cell death signaling pathways. *Cancer Biol Ther*, Vol.4, No.2, pp. 139-163, ISSN 1538-4047 (Print) 1538-4047 (Linking)

Jones, N. L., Day, A. S., Jennings, H. A., & Sherman, P. M. (1999). Helicobacter pylori induces gastric epithelial cell apoptosis in association with increased Fas receptor expression. *Infect Immun*, Vol.67, No.8, pp. 4237-4242, ISSN 0019-9567 (Print) 0019-9567 (Linking)

Kerr, J. F., Wyllie, A. H., & Currie, A. R. (1972). Apoptosis: a basic biological phenomenon with wide-ranging implications in tissue kinetics. *Br J Cancer*, Vol.26, No.4, pp. 239-257, ISSN 0007-0920 (Print)

Kim, J. M., Kim, J. S., Lee, J. Y., Sim, Y. S., Kim, Y. J., Oh, Y. K., Yoon, H. J., Kang, J. S., Youn, J., Kim, N., Jung, H. C., & Kim, S. (2010). Dual effects of Helicobacter pylori vacuolating cytotoxin on human eosinophil apoptosis in early and late periods of stimulation. *Eur J Immunol*, Vol.40, No.6, pp. 1651-1662, ISSN 1521-4141 (Electronic) 0014-2980 (Linking)

Kim, K. M., Lee, S. G., Park, M. G., Song, J. Y., Kang, H. L., Lee, W. K., Cho, M. J., Rhee, K. H., Youn, H. S., & Baik, S. C. (2007). Gamma-glutamyltranspeptidase of Helicobacter pylori induces mitochondria-mediated apoptosis in AGS cells. *Biochem Biophys Res Commun*, Vol.355, No.2, pp. 562-567, ISSN 0006-291X (Print) 0006-291X (Linking)

Klein, P. D., Graham, D. Y., Gaillour, A., Opekun, A. R., & Smith, E. O. (1991). Water source as risk factor for Helicobacter pylori infection in Peruvian children. Gastrointestinal Physiology Working Group. *Lancet*, Vol.337, No.8756, pp. 1503-1506, ISSN 0140-6736 (Print) 0140-6736 (Linking)

Knekt, P., Aromaa, A., Maatela, J., Aaran, R. K., Nikkari, T., Hakama, M., Hakulinen, T., Peto, R., & Teppo, L. (1991). Vitamin E and cancer prevention. *Am J Clin Nutr*, Vol.53, No.1 Suppl, pp. 283S-286S, ISSN 0002-9165 (Print) 0002-9165 (Linking)

Konturek, P. C., Konturek, S. J., & Brzozowski, T. (2009). Helicobacter pylori infection in gastric cancerogenesis. *J Physiol Pharmacol*, Vol.60, No.3, pp. 3-21, ISSN 1899-1505 (Electronic) 0867-5910 (Linking)

Konturek, P. C., Pierzchalski, P., Konturek, S. J., Meixner, H., Faller, G., Kirchner, T., & Hahn, E. G. (1999). Helicobacter pylori induces apoptosis in gastric mucosa through an upregulation of Bax expression in humans. *Scand J Gastroenterol*, Vol.34, No.4, pp. 375-383, ISSN 0036-5521 (Print) 0036-5521 (Linking)

Krejs, G. J. (2010). Gastric cancer: epidemiology and risk factors. *Dig Dis*, Vol.28, No.4-5, pp. 600-603, ISSN 1421-9875 (Electronic) 0257-2753 (Linking)

Lambeth, J. D. (2004). NOX enzymes and the biology of reactive oxygen. *Nat Rev Immunol*, Vol.4, No.3, pp. 181-189, ISSN 1474-1733 (Print) 1474-1733 (Linking)

Lehours, P., & Yilmaz, O. (2007). Epidemiology of Helicobacter pylori infection. *Helicobacter*, Vol.12 Suppl 1, pp. 1-3, ISSN 1083-4389 (Print) 1083-4389 (Linking)

Louw, J. A., Falck, V., van Rensburg, C., Zak, J., Adams, G., & Marks, I. N. (1993). Distribution of Helicobacter pylori colonisation and associated gastric inflammatory changes: difference between patients with duodenal and gastric ulcers. *J Clin Pathol*, Vol.46, No.8, pp. 754-756, ISSN 0021-9746 (Print) 0021-9746 (Linking)

Malaty, H. M., Engstrand, L., Pedersen, N. L., & Graham, D. Y. (1994). Helicobacter pylori infection: genetic and environmental influences. A study of twins. *Ann Intern Med*, Vol.120, No.12, pp. 982-986, ISSN 0003-4819 (Print) 0003-4819 (Linking)

Marotta, R. B., & Floch, M. H. (1991). Diet and nutrition in ulcer disease. *Med Clin North Am*, Vol.75, No.4, pp. 967-979, ISSN 0025-7125 (Print) 0025-7125 (Linking)

Marshall, B. J., Armstrong, J. A., McGechie, D. B., & Glancy, R. J. (1985). Attempt to fulfil Koch's postulates for pyloric Campylobacter. *Med J Aust*, Vol.142, No.8, pp. 436-439, ISSN 0025-729X (Print)

Matsumoto, A., Isomoto, H., Nakayama, M., Hisatsune, J., Nishi, Y., Nakashima, Y., Matsushima, K., Kurazono, H., Nakao, K., Hirayama, T., & Kohno, S. (2010). Helicobacter pylori VacA Reduces the Cellular Expression of STAT3 and Pro-survival Bcl-2 Family Proteins, Bcl-2 and Bcl-X(L), Leading to Apoptosis in Gastric Epithelial Cells. *Dig Dis Sci*, ISSN 1573-2568 (Electronic) 0163-2116 (Linking)

Moss, S. F., Calam, J., Agarwal, B., Wang, S., & Holt, P. R. (1996). Induction of gastric epithelial apoptosis by Helicobacter pylori. *Gut*, Vol.38, No.4, pp. 498-501, ISSN 0017-5749 (Print) 0017-5749 (Linking)

Naito, Y., & Yoshikawa, T. (2002). Molecular and cellular mechanisms involved in Helicobacter pylori-induced inflammation and oxidative stress. *Free Radic Biol Med*, Vol.33, No.3, pp. 323-336, ISSN 0891-5849 (Print) 0891-5849 (Linking)

Nam, J. H., Choi, I. J., Cho, S. J., Kim, C. G., Lee, J. Y., Nam, S. Y., Park, S. R., Kook, M. C., Nam, B. H., & Kim, Y. W. (2011). Helicobacter pylori infection and histological changes in siblings of young gastric cancer patients. *J Gastroenterol Hepatol*, ISSN 1440-1746 (Electronic) 0815-9319 (Linking)

Nurgalieva, Z. Z., Malaty, H. M., Graham, D. Y., Almuchambetova, R., Machmudova, A., Kapsultanova, D., Osato, M. S., Hollinger, F. B., & Zhangabylov, A. (2002). Helicobacter pylori infection in Kazakhstan: effect of water source and household hygiene. *Am J Trop Med Hyg*, Vol.67, No.2, pp. 201-206, ISSN 0002-9637 (Print) 0002-9637 (Linking)

Oh, T. Y., Yeo, M., Han, S. U., Cho, Y. K., Kim, Y. B., Chung, M. H., Kim, Y. S., Cho, S. W., & Hahm, K. B. (2005). Synergism of Helicobacter pylori infection and stress on the augmentation of gastric mucosal damage and its prevention with alpha-tocopherol. *Free Radic Biol Med*, Vol.38, No.11, pp. 1447-1457, ISSN 0891-5849 (Print) 0891-5849 (Linking)

Orrenius, S., Zhivotovsky, B., & Nicotera, P. (2003). Regulation of cell death: the calcium-apoptosis link. *Nat Rev Mol Cell Biol*, Vol.4, No.7, pp. 552-565, ISSN 1471-0072 (Print) 1471-0072 (Linking)

Ott, M., Norberg, E., Zhivotovsky, B., & Orrenius, S. (2009). Mitochondrial targeting of tBid/Bax: a role for the TOM complex? *Cell Death Differ*, Vol.16, No.8, pp. 1075-1082, ISSN 1476-5403 (Electronic) 1350-9047 (Linking)

Ott, M., Robertson, J. D., Gogvadze, V., Zhivotovsky, B., & Orrenius, S. (2002). Cytochrome c release from mitochondria proceeds by a two-step process. *Proc Natl Acad Sci U S A*, Vol.99, No.3, pp. 1259-1263, ISSN 0027-8424 (Print) 0027-8424 (Linking)

Pandey, R., Misra, V., Misra, S. P., Dwivedi, M., Kumar, A., & Tiwari, B. K. (2010). Helicobacter pylori and gastric cancer. *Asian Pac J Cancer Prev*, Vol.11, No.3, pp. 583-588, ISSN 1513-7368 (Print) 1513-7368 (Linking)

Peng, Y. C., Hsu, C. L., Tung, C. F., Chou, W. K., Huang, L. R., Hung, D. Z., Hu, W. H., & Yang, D. Y. (2008). Chemiluminescence assay of mucosal reactive oxygen species in gastric cancer, ulcer and antral mucosa. *Hepatogastroenterology*, Vol.55, No.82-83, pp. 770-773, ISSN 0172-6390 (Print) 0172-6390 (Linking)

Perez-Perez, G. I., Witkin, S. S., Decker, M. D., & Blaser, M. J. (1991). Seroprevalence of helicobacter pylori infection in couples. *J Clin Microbiol*, Vol.29, No.3, pp. 642-644, ISSN 0095-1137 (Print) 0095-1137 (Linking)

Phull, P. S., Green, C. J., & Jacyna, M. R. (1995). A radical view of the stomach: the role of oxygen-derived free radicals and anti-oxidants in gastroduodenal disease. *Eur J Gastroenterol Hepatol*, Vol.7, No.3, pp. 265-274, ISSN 0954-691X (Print) 0954-691X (Linking)

Que, F. G., & Gores, G. J. (1996). Cell death by apoptosis: basic concepts and disease relevance for the gastroenterologist. *Gastroenterology*, Vol.110, No.4, pp. 1238-1243, ISSN 0016-5085 (Print) 0016-5085 (Linking)

Reilly, P. M., Schiller, H. J., & Bulkley, G. B. (1991). Pharmacologic approach to tissue injury mediated by free radicals and other reactive oxygen metabolites. *Am J Surg*, Vol.161, No.4, pp. 488-503, ISSN 0002-9610 (Print) 0002-9610 (Linking)

Satoh, K., Kawata, H., Tokumaru, K., Kumakura, Y., Ishino, Y., Kawakami, S., Inoue, K., Kojima, T., Satoh, Y., Mutoh, H., Kihira, K., & Sugano, K. (2003). Change in apoptosis in the gastric surface epithelium and glands after eradication of Helicobacter pylori. *Dig Liver Dis*, Vol.35, No.2, pp. 78-84, ISSN 1590-8658 (Print) 1590-8658 (Linking)

Shigenaga, M. K., Hagen, T. M., & Ames, B. N. (1994). Oxidative damage and mitochondrial decay in aging. *Proc Natl Acad Sci U S A*, Vol.91, No.23, pp. 10771-10778, ISSN 0027-8424 (Print) 0027-8424 (Linking)

Sonnenberg, A. (2007). Time trends of ulcer mortality in Europe. *Gastroenterology*, Vol.132, No.7, pp. 2320-2327, ISSN 0016-5085 (Print) 0016-5085 (Linking)

Stahelin, H. B., Gey, K. F., Eichholzer, M., & Ludin, E. (1991). Beta-carotene and cancer prevention: the Basel Study. *Am J Clin Nutr*, Vol.53, No.1 Suppl, pp. 265S-269S, ISSN 0002-9165 (Print) 0002-9165 (Linking)

Tamura, T., Yokoyama, T., & Ohmori, K. (2001). Effects of diacerein on indomethacin-induced gastric ulceration. *Pharmacology*, Vol.63, No.4, pp. 228-233, ISSN 0031-7012 (Print) 0031-7012 (Linking)

Tan, V. P., & Wong, B. C. (2011). Helicobacter pylori and gastritis: Untangling a complex relationship 27 years on. *J Gastroenterol Hepatol*, Vol.26 Suppl 1, pp. 42-45, ISSN 1440-1746 (Electronic) 0815-9319 (Linking)

Targa, A. C., Cesar, A. C., Cury, P. M., & Silva, A. E. (2007). Apoptosis in different gastric lesions and gastric cancer: relationship with Helicobacter pylori, overexpression of p53 and aneuploidy. *Genet Mol Res*, Vol.6, No.3, pp. 554-565, ISSN 1676-5680 (Electronic) 1676-5680 (Linking)

Thompson, C. B. (1995). Apoptosis in the pathogenesis and treatment of disease. *Science*, Vol.267, No.5203, pp. 1456-1462, ISSN 0036-8075 (Print) 0036-8075 (Linking)

van den Brandt, P. A., Goldbohm, R. A., van 't Veer, P., Bode, P., Dorant, E., Hermus, R. J., & Sturmans, F. (1993). A prospective cohort study on toenail selenium levels and risk of gastrointestinal cancer. *J Natl Cancer Inst*, Vol.85, No.3, pp. 224-229, ISSN 0027-8874 (Print) 0027-8874 (Linking)

Wallace, J. L. (1992). Non-steroidal anti-inflammatory drug gastropathy and cytoprotection: pathogenesis and mechanisms re-examined. *Scand J Gastroenterol Suppl*, Vol.192, pp. 3-8, ISSN 0085-5928 (Print) 0085-5928 (Linking)

Wang, J., Fan, X., Lindholm, C., Bennett, M., O'Connoll, J., Shanahan, F., Brooks, E. G., Reyes, V. E., & Ernst, P. B. (2000). Helicobacter pylori modulates lymphoepithelial cell interactions leading to epithelial cell damage through Fas/Fas ligand interactions. *Infect Immun*, Vol.68, No.7, pp. 4303-4311, ISSN 0019-9567 (Print) 0019-9567 (Linking)

Warren JR, M. B. (1983). Unidentified curved bacilli on gastric epithelium in active chronic gastritis. *Lancet*, Vol.1, No.8336, pp. 1273-1275, ISSN 0140-6736 (Print) 0140-6736 (Linking)

Wu, Y. Y., Tsai, H. F., Lin, W. C., Chou, A. H., Chen, H. T., Yang, J. C., Hsu, P. I., & Hsu, P. N. (2004). Helicobacter pylori enhances tumor necrosis factor-related apoptosis-inducing ligand-mediated apoptosis in human gastric epithelial cells. *World J Gastroenterol*, Vol.10, No.16, pp. 2334-2339, ISSN 1007-9327 (Print) 1007-9327 (Linking)

Xia, H. H., & Talley, N. J. (1997). Natural acquisition and spontaneous elimination of Helicobacter pylori infection: clinical implications. *Am J Gastroenterol*, Vol.92, No.10, pp. 1780-1787, ISSN 0002-9270 (Print) 0002-9270 (Linking)

Xia, H. H., & Talley, N. J. (2001). Apoptosis in gastric epithelium induced by Helicobacter pylori infection: implications in gastric carcinogenesis. *Am J Gastroenterol*, Vol.96, No.1, pp. 16-26, ISSN 0002-9270 (Print) 0002-9270 (Linking)

Yamasaki, E., Wada, A., Kumatori, A., Nakagawa, I., Funao, J., Nakayama, M., Hisatsune, J., Kimura, M., Moss, J., & Hirayama, T. (2006). Helicobacter pylori vacuolating cytotoxin induces activation of the proapoptotic proteins Bax and Bak, leading to cytochrome c release and cell death, independent of vacuolation. *J Biol Chem*, Vol.281, No.16, pp. 11250-11259, ISSN 0021-9258 (Print) 0021-9258 (Linking)

Yoshikawa, T., Ueda, S., Naito, Y., Takahashi, S., Oyamada, H., Morita, Y., Yoneta, T., & Kondo, M. (1989). Role of oxygen-derived free radicals in gastric mucosal injury induced by ischemia or ischemia-reperfusion in rats. *Free Radic Res Commun*, Vol.7, No.3-6, pp. 285-291, ISSN 8755-0199 (Print) 8755-0199 (Linking)

Youle, R. J., & Strasser, A. (2008). The BCL-2 protein family: opposing activities that mediate cell death. Nat Rev Mol Cell Biol, Vol.9, No.1, pp. 47-59, ISSN 1471-0080 (Electronic) 1471-0072 (Linking)

Zhang, H., Fang, D. C., Lan, C. H., & Luo, Y. H. (2007). Helicobacter pylori infection induces apoptosis in gastric cancer cells through the mitochondrial pathway. J Gastroenterol Hepatol, Vol.22, No.7, pp. 1051-1056, ISSN 0815-9319 (Print) 0815-9319 (Linking)

# 11

# *Helicobacter pylori* Suppresses Serum Immunoglobulin Levels in Smokers with Peptic Ulcer: Probable Interaction Between Smoking and *H. pylori* Infection in the Induction of Th1 Predominant Immune Response and Peptic Ulceration

Yoshihiro Matsukawa[1] and Kimitoshi Kato[2]
[1]*Division of Hematology and Rheumatology*
[2]*Division of Gastroenterology and Hepatology*
*Department of Medicine*
*Nihon University School of Medicine*
*Japan*

## 1. Introduction

### 1.1 T helper cell subset

*Helicobacter pylori* (*H. pylori*) and smoking are well known risk factors for gastric ulcer, and both are classified as definite carcinogens. Interestingly, the two also reportedly share common immune response features.

With recent advances in immunology, various functions of T lymphocytes (T cells) have been discovered. T cells are divided into suppressor and helper on the basis of immunological functionings, and T helper cells are now known to consist of two distinct groups, as demonstrated using mouse models in the 1980s [Reiner, 2008; Mosman & Coffman, 1989]. Both groups are derived from naïve T cells: interleukin-12 (IL-12) causes naïve T helper cells to differentiate into type 1 (Th1) cells, while augmentation of IL-4 around naïve T cells leads to Th2 differentiation. Th1 cells produce IL-2 and interferon- $\gamma$ (IFN-$\gamma$) to maintain cell mediated immunity against intracellular organisms such as viruses and mycobacteria, and Th2 cells produce IL-4 and IL-13 promoting the differentiation of B cells to plasma cells and the induction of class-switching resulting in IgE production. Differentiated plasma cells produce immunoglobulins which participate in mucosal defense against extracellular organisms including *H. pylori*. Groundbreaking research inspired subsequent studies which finally led to the discovery of Th17 cells [Steinman, 2007] and T regulatory cells (Treg) [Sakaguchi *et al.*, 1995, 2008]. As a consequence of this pioneering research, T helper cells, at present, are sub-grouped into 4 types according to the differences in their cytokine productions (Table 1).

Table 1. T helper subsets

| Inductive, Selective T helper subset | Cytokines | Secreted Cytokines |
|---|---|---|
| Th1* | IL-12, IFN-γ | IL-2, TNF, IFN-γ |
| Th2** | L-4, IL-33 | IL-4, IL-5, IL-6, IL-9, IL-10, IL-13, IL-25 |
| Th17 | TGF-β, IL-6, IL-23 | IL-17, IL-6, IL-22, TNF |
| Treg | TGF- β, IL-10 | TGF- β IL-10, CTLA4 |

Table 1a. Subsets of T helper cells and related cytokines

| T helper subset | Protection | Pathology |
|---|---|---|
| Th1* | Defense against intracellular organisms | Inflammation |
| Th2** | Defense against extracellular bacteria at mucosal and epithelial surface | Allergy |
| Th17 | Defense against extracellular bacteria | Autoimmunity Cancer |
| Treg | Suppression of immune response | Anti-inflammation |

Concept of Th1 and Th2 cells originate from the cytokine production pattern of murine T cells. Therefore attention such differences is necessary when considering human immunity.
*Exert cell mediated immunity
**Exert humoral immunity
CTLA4: Cytotoxic T lymphocyte antigen 4
IFN: Interferon
IL: Interleukin
TGF: Tumor growth factor
TNF: Tumor necrosis factor
Table 1: Table by Reiner modified by authors (ref. 1 p412)

Table 1b. Roles of each T helper subset

Th1 cells produce IL-2, IFN- γ, tumor growth factor-β(TGF- β) and so on, thereby exerting cell mediated immunity mainly through IFN- γ.

Th2 cells produce IL-4, IL-5, IL-6, IL-9, IL-10, IL-13, and so on, thereby up-regulating humoral immunity against extracellular pathogens and inducing allergy mainly through IL-4.

Th17 cells produce IL-17A, IL-17F, IL-22 and so on, thereby eradicating bacterial/fungal infections and might be related to autoimmunity and cancer. Th17 cells produce inflammatory cytokines, and over-expression of such cytokines is associated with autoimmune diseases such as type 1 diabetes, inflammatory bowel disease, rheumatoid arthritis, and multiple sclerosis. IL-6 and TGF- β are key cytokines for differentiation into Th17.

Treg produces TGF- β, IL-10, and cytotoxic T lymphocyte antigen 4 (CTLA4), and suppress activated T cells/dendritic cells. Treg can suppress Th1, Th2, and Th17 to terminate immune responses/inflammation and also plays crucial roles in immune tolerance [Sakaguchi *et al.*, 1995, 2008].

As stated above, Th1 cells can down-regulate immunoglobulin production through secretion/production of IFN-$\gamma$ whereas Th2 cells IL-4-dependently up-regulate immunmoglobulin secretion/production.

## 1.2 Th1 response in patients with peptic ulcer

As to gastric and duodenal ulcers, H. pylori infection has increasingly been reported to exert a Th response on type 1 (Th1 cells) [Hida et al., 1999; Holck et al.; 2003; D'Elios et al., 1997, 2003,2005; Itoh et al., 2005; Goll et al., 2007; Ayada et al., 2009; Mohammadi et al., 1996; Fan et al., 1998; Bamford et al., 1998; sommer et al., 1998; Lindholm et al., 1998; Ihan et al., 2000; Smythies et al., 2000; Akhiani et al., 2002; Guiney et al., 2003; Amedei et al., 2006; Taylor et al, 2006], and peptic ulcer disease has also been increasingly reported to produce Th1 skew [Hida et al., 1999; D'Elios et al., 2007; Goll et al., 2008; Codolo et al., 2008; Del Prete et al., 2008; Shimada et al., 2008; Watanabe et al., 2010; Hosseini et al., 2010]. In addition, a unique study conducted by Itoh et al. suggested Th1 polarization of gastric T cells in the antrum of dyspeptic pateints, irrespective of H. pylori infection [Itoh et al, 1999].

## 1.3 Th1 response in patients with *H. pylori* infection

H. pylori has increasingly been reported to show Th1 predominance [Mohammadi et al., 1996; D'Elios et al., 1997, 2003,2005; Bamford et al., 1998; Fan et al., 1998; Lindholm et al., 1998; Sommer et al., 1998; Hida et al., 1999; Ihan et al., 2000; Smythies et al., 2000; Akhiani et al., 2002; Guiney et al., 2003; Holck et al.; 2003; Itoh et al., 2005;  Amedei et al., 2006; Taylor et al, 2006; Goll et al., 2007; Ayada et al., 2009] with only a few studies obtaining opposing results [Bergman et al., 2004; Campbell et al., 2004; Kayhan et al., 2008; Kido et al., 2010]. Therefore, H. pylori is presumed to down-regulate immunoglobulin production/secretion.

## 1.4 Influence of smoking on serum immunoglobulins and Th response

Smoking has been reported to suppress serum immunoglobulin levels [Andersen et al., 1982; Tollerud et al., 1995; Barbour et al., 1997; Gonzalez-Quintela et al., 2007] and some studies have indicated a Th1 skew in smokers [Hallquist et al., 2000; Whetzel et al., 2007; Kikuchi et al., 2008], although controversial data have also been reported [Hagiwara et al., 2001; Zeidel et al., 2002; Cozen et al., 2004].

## 1.5 Possible mechanisms by which *H. pylori* infection induces Th1 skew

Although a Th1 skew in H. pylori-infected patients is suggested by the vast majority of research conducted on this subject, the precise mechanism by which Th1 differentiation is induced has yet to be elucidated. However, some investigators have conducted crucial studies that may explain this phenomenon: Eaton et al. reported CD4+ T cells to be essential for the development of H. pylori-induced gastritis [Eaton et al., 2001], and Nagai et al. showed the coccoid form of H. pylori to reach to Peyer's patches and then be phagocytosed by dendritic cells thereby sensitizing CD4+ T cells, and that these sensitized CD4+ T cells homed to the lamina propria of the gastric mucosa [Nagai et al., 2007]. Finally, such dendritic cells produce IL-12 which promotes Th1 differentiation after phagocytosis of H. pylori [Codolo et al., 2008].

In addition to mentioned above, a number of investigators have demonstrated a Th1 skew in patients with peptic ulcers, as compared to those with gastritis or gastric cancer [Hida et al., 1999; D'Elios et al., 2007; Goll et al., 2008; Codolo et al., 2008; Del Prete et al., 2008; Shimada et al., 2008; Hosseini et al., 2010; Watanabe et al., 2010].

We therefore conducted the current study to assess the influence of both *H. pylori* and smoking on serum immunoglobulin levels for the purpose of evaluating the presence of Th1 skew in patients with peptic ulcers.

## 2. Patients and method

### 2.1 Study design
**Study 1.** Effects of current smoking on levels of serum immunoglobulins
To evaluate the influences of smoking on serum immunoglobulin levels, serum IgG, IgA, and IgM levels were measured in both peptic ulcer and non-ulcer gastritis patients with and without *H. pylori* infection.
**Study 2.** Effects of *H. pylori* infection on levels of serum immunoglobulins in peptic ulcer patients
To evaluate the influences of *H. pylori* infection on serum immunoglobulin levels, serum IgG, IgA, and IgM were measured in peptic ulcer patients, both current smokers and non-smokers.
**Study 3.** As a control for study 2, serum IgG, IgA, and IgM levels were measured in non-ulcer gastritis patients with and without current smoking.

### 2.2 Patients
Dyspeptic patients and those recommended to undergo fiberscopic examination received gastroduodenoscopic examinations. Those endoscopically diagnosed as having gastric or duodenal ulcers were included in the current study. Following informed consent to check *H. pylori* status and immunohematologic parameters, dyspeptic patients underwent gastrofiberscopic examination. Patients with hematologic, immunologic, rheumatic, malignant, and infectious diseases were excluded. Those taking corticosteroids, antibiotics, and/or immunosuppressive drugs were also excluded. Because non-steroidal anti-inflammatory drugs (NSAIDs) [Franch *et al*, 1994; Mazzeo *et al.*, 1998; Yamaki *et al.*, 2003, 2005; Andreone *et al.*, 2004; Mored *et al.*, 2004] and proton-pump inhibitors (PPIs) [Tsutsumi *et al.*, 2005; Matsukawa *et al.*, 2007] have increasingly been reported to skew the T helper response toward type 2, patients taking these drugs were also excluded. Both smokers and non-smokers with endoscopically diagnosed non-ulcer gastritis were also evaluated as control groups.

### 2.3 Methods
Following informed consents to measure titers of serum anti-*H. pylori* IgG antibody, serum immunoglobulins and complete blood cell counts, patients with gastric or duodenal ulcer was diagnosed according to the classification of Sakita and Miwa [Matsukawa *et al.*, 1997], and those with non-ulcer gastritis did according to the updated Sydney System [Dixon *et al.*, 1996] under gastrofiberscopic observation. To evaluate *H. pylori* status, biopsy specimens were obtained from the antrum and lower body of the greater curvature in the stomach and from the major lesions. The samples from the antrum and lower body were placed in rapid urease test (RUT) kits, and the results were evaluated 24 hr later. These samples were also prepared for pathologic evaluation. Immediately after completion of the procedure, blood samples were collected to measure IgG, IgA, IgM, and anti-*H. pylori* IgG antibodies. Serum levels of IgG, IgA, and IgM were measured by an automated turbidimetric immunoprecipitation method [Matsukawa *et al.*, 1997], and the anti-*H. pylori* antibody was measured by a commercially available ELISA kit. Confirmed *H. pylori* infection required

both RUT and anti-*H. pylori* IgG antibody to be positive. Smoking status was ascertained on the day of the endoscopic examination.

### 2.3.1 Statistical analysis

Data were expressed as means+/-SD. The statistical significance of differences was anlyzed employing the Student unpaired *t-test* and the $\chi$-square test. We evaluated statistical differences using Macintosh StatView version 4, and p values less than 0.05 were accepted as statistically significant.

## 3. Results

### 3.1 Recruited patients and controls

Table 2. Profiles of patients and controlls

| Sex | Female | Male |
|---|---|---|
| Number | 90 | 146 |
| Age (years)** | 60.0+/-11.5 | 53.4+/-13.6 |
| H. pylori* | 66 (73.3%) | 127 (87.0%) |
| Smokers* | 24 (37.5%) | 82 (56.2%) |

Table 2a. Profiles of patients with peptic ulcer

| Sex | Female | Male |
|---|---|---|
| Number | 408 | 312 |
| Age (years) | 56.6+/-14.3 | 55.8+/-13.3 |
| H. pylori* | 229 (56.1%) | 192 (61.1%) |
| Smokers* | 44 (10.8%) | 106 (34.0%) |

Smokers: peptic ulcer>non-ulcer gastritis (female.=0001 and male <.0001)
*H. pylori* prevalence: peptic ulcer>non-ulcer gastritis (<.0001 for females and males)
*P<.0001 **P=.0001

Table 2b. Profiles of patients with non-ulcer gastritis

There were 146 patients with gastric ulcer, 58 with duodenal ulcer, and 32 with both types (Table 3). There were no differences in these lesions between smokers and non-smokers.

| Smokers (F:M) | | | |
|---|---|---|---|
| Body | Angle/Antrum | Duodenum | Multiple |
| 33 (7:26) | 30(10:20) | 28 (2:26) | 15 (5:10) |
| Non-smokers (F:M) | | | |
| Body | Angle/Antrum | Duodenum | Multiple |
| 51 (32:19) | 32(15:17) | 30 (15:15) | 17 (5:12) |
| Total | | | |
| Body | Angle/Antrum | Duodenum | Multiple |
| 84 (39:45) | 62(25:37) | 58 (17:41) | 32 (10:22) |

Table 3. Ulcer location (F:M)

Table 2 presents the profiles of both patients with peptic ulcer and those with non-ulcer gastritis serving as controls. In total, 236 patients (F:M=90:146) were diagnosed as having gastric and/or duodenal ulcers and were enrolled in this study. There was an age difference between female and male patients (F:M=60.0+/-11.5 vs. 53.4+/-13.6 years, p=.0001) (Table 2a). Patients with non-ulcer gastritis consisted of 408 females and 312 males, and there was no difference in age between genders (56.6+/-14.3 vs. 55.8+/-13.3 years) (Table 2b).

Patients with peptic ulcer had higher prevalences of both *H. pylori* infection and smoking, as compared to those with non-ulcer gastritis: p=.0001 for smoking in females and <.0001 for smoking in males, while p<.0001 for *H. pylori* infection in both females and males (Tables 2a and 2b).

### 3.2 Serum levels of IgG, IgA, and IgM in the current study
### 3.2.1 The results of study 1

Tables 4 and 5 show the results of study 1, examining the effects of current smoking on serum immunoglobulin levels in patients with petic ulcer and non-ulcer gastritis. There was age difference between smokers and non-smokers with *H. pylori* infection among ulcer patients (p=.0019). Smoking was associated with definite suppressions of serum IgG, IgA, and IgM levels in *H. pylori*-infected patients with peptic ulcer (p<.0001, .0006, and .0009, respectively), whereas ulcer patients without *H. pylori* infection showed no such tendency. Table 5 presents the effects of current smoking on serum immunoglobulin levels in non-ulcer patients with gastritis. There was an age difference between smokers and non-smokers (p<.0001). Among patients with non-ulcer gastritis, smokers had suppressed serum IgG (p<.0001), IgA (p<.05), and IgM levels, although the reduction of IgM in patients with *H. pylori* infection failed to reach statistical significance. Like those with *H. pylori* infection, non-ulcer patients without *H. pylori* infection also showed suppression of both IgG and IgM (p<.05, respectively).

Table 4. Influence of smoking on serum immunoglobulin levels in peptic ulcer patients

|     | Smokers | Non-smokers | P |
|-----|---------|-------------|---|
| N   | 92      | 101         |   |
| Age | 52.2+/-12.2 | 58.0+/-13.2 | .0019 |
| IgG | 1178.0+/-250.3 | 1376.6+/-343.2 | <.0001 |
| IgA | 218.4+/-98.2 | 271.4+/-109.1 | .0006 |
| IgM | 93.8+/-41.9 | 123.1/71.1 | .0009 |

Table 4a. Serum immunoglobulin levels in *H. pylori*-infected patients

|     | Smokers | Non-smokers | P |
|-----|---------|-------------|---|
| N   | 14      | 29          |   |
| Age | 56.0+/-13.7 | 60.7+/-13.7 | NS |
| IgG | 1348.6+/-254.7 | 1463.7+/-286.3 | NS |
| IgA | 295.1+/-113.2 | 253.2/-99.3 | NS |
| IgM | 105.8+/-49.8 | 123.5+/47.9 | NS |

IgG: Immunoglobulin G (mg/dl)
IgA: Immunoglobulin A (mg/dl)
IgM: Immunoglobulin M (mg/dl)
N: Number of patients
NS: Not significant
P: Probability

Table 4b. Serum immunoglobulin levels in patients without *H. pylori* infection

Table 5. Effects of smoking on serum immunoglobulin levels in non-ulcer gastritis patients

|  | Smokers | Non-smokers | P |
|---|---|---|---|
| N | 93 | 325 |  |
| Age | 53.5+/-11.6 | 60.0+/-11.4 | <.0001 |
| IgG | 1224.1+/-264.3 | 1392.1+/-278.6 | <.0001 |
| IgA | 236.6+/-97.0 | 264.0+/-112.7 | .0384 |
| IgM | 104.7+/-58.6 | 112.4+/63.5 | NS |

Table 5a. Serum immunoglobulin levels in *H. pylori*-infected patients

|  | Smokers | Non-smokers | P |
|---|---|---|---|
| N | 57 | 247 |  |
| Age | 51.9+/-13.4 | 57.8+/-13.9 | .0071 |
| IgG | 1205.5+/-278.6 | 1295.0+/-237.7 | .0228 |
| IgA | 254.7+/-118.3 | 251.0+/-89.7 | NS |
| IgM | 83.4+/-42.9 | 104.8+/69.0 | .0408 |

IgG: Immunoglobulin G (mg/dl)
IgA: Immunoglobulin A (mg/dl)
IgM: Immunoglobulin M (mg/dl)
N: Number of patients
NS: Not significant
P: Probability

Table 5b. Serum immunoglobulin levels in patients without *H.* pylori infection

### 3.2.2 The results of study 2

Table 6. Effects of *H. pylori* infection on serum immunoglobulin levels in peptic ulcer patients

| *H. pylori* | Positive | Negative | P |
|---|---|---|---|
| N | 92 | 14 |  |
| Age | 52.6+/-12.2 | 56.0+/-13.7 | NS |
| IgG | 1177.9+/-250.3 | 1348.6+/-254.7 | .0197 |
| IgA | 218.4+/-98.2 | 295.1+/-113.2 | .0092 |
| IgM | 93.8+/-41.9 | 105.8+/-49.8 | NS |

Table 6a. Serum immunoglobulin levels in smokers

| *H. pylori* | Positive | Negative | P |
|---|---|---|---|
| N | 101 | 29 |  |
| Age | 58.0+/-13.2 | 60.7+/-13.7 | NS |
| IgG | 1376.6+/-343.3 | 1463.7+/-286.3 | NS |
| IgA | 271.4+/-109.1 | 253.2+/-99.3 | NS |
| IgM | 123.1+/-71.1 | 123.5+/-47.9 | NS |

IgG: Immunoglobulin G (mg/dl)
IgA: Immunoglobulin A (mg/dl)
IgM: Immunoglobulin M (mg/dl)
N: Number of patients
NS: Not significant
P: Probability

Table 6b. Serum immunoglobulin levels in non-smokers

Table 6 presents the results of study 2, examining the effects of *H. pylori* infection on serum levels of immunoglobulins in peptic ulcer patients. As a whole, patients with peptic ulcer showed decreases in serum IgG, IgA, and IgM levels, although only the decrease in IgG reached statistical significance (data not shown). Among those with peptic ulcer, smokers with *H. pylori* infection showed decreases in both IgG and IgA (p<.0197 and .0092, respectively), whereas the difference in IgM did not reach statistical significance (Table 6a). In contrast to smokers, among patients with peptic ulcers, non-smokers with *H. pylori* infection showed no difference in IgG, IgA, or IgM levels.

### 3.2.3 The results of study 3

Table 7 presents the results of study 3, the control for study 2, examining the effects of *H. pylori* infection on serum levels of immunoglobulins in non-ulcer gastritis patients. As to the effect of *H. pylori* infection, patients with non-ulcer gastritis showed a phenomenon opposite to that in peptic ulcer patients, except for IgA in smokers. Patients with *H. pylori* infection had increased serum IgG, IgA, and IgM levels regardless of smoking status, although only the IgG difference in non-smokers (p<.0001) and the IgM difference in smokers (p=.0288) were statistically significant. Compared to patients with peptic ulcer, *H. pylori* infection, at minimum, did not suppress serum immunoglobulin levels regatdless of smoking status. *H. pylori* infection appeared to up-regulate serum immunoglobulin levels in non-ulcer patients with gastritis.

Table 7. Effect of *H. pylori* infection on serum immunoglobulin levels in patients with non-ulcer gastritis

| *H. pylori* | Positive | Negative | P |
|---|---|---|---|
| N | 93 | 57 | |
| IgG | 1234.5+/-264.3 | 1205.5+/-278.6 | NS |
| IgA | 236.6+/-97.0 | 254.7+/-111.8 | NS |
| IgM | 104.7+/-58.6 | 83.4+/42.9 | .0288 |

Table 7a. Serum immunoglobulin levels in smokers

| *H. pylori* | Positive | Negative | P |
|---|---|---|---|
| N | 325 | 247 | |
| IgG | 1392.1+/-288.7 | 1295.0+/-237.7 | <.0001 |
| IgA | 264.0+/-112.7 | 251.0+/-89.7 | NS |
| IgM | 112.4+/-63.5 | 104.8+/69.0 | NS |

IgG: Immunoglobulin G (mg/dl)
IgA: Immunoglobulin A (mg/dl)
IgM: Immunoglobulin M (mg/dl)
N: Number of patients
NS: Not significant
P: Probability

Table 7b. Serum immunoglobulin levels in non-smokers

## 4. Discussion

We initially showed definite suppression of serum immunoglobulin levels in current smokers with *H. pylori*-associated peptic ulcer (Tables 4a), and this suppression was observed even in patients without *H. pylori* infection, although the difference did not reach statistical significance possibly due to our small sample size (Table 4b). In contrast to patients with peptic ulcer, those with non-ulcer gastritis showed suppressed levels of serum immunoglobulins, regardless of *H. pylori* status. These observations support the notion that smoking causes a skewed Th1 response in current smokers, regardless of whether or not *H. pylori* infection or peptic ulceration is present. As to the Th skew in smokers, there are conflicting reports, with some reporting a Th2 skew in smokers [Hagiwara *et al.*, 2001; Zeidel *et al.*, 2002; Cozen *et al.*, 2004]. However, two noteworthy studies conducted recently have challenged this concept. Whetzel *et al.* reported elevated peripheral IFN-$\gamma$ levels, especially in female smokers, and in surgically resected specimens from the colon of smokers [Whetzel *et al.*, 2007], and Kikuchi *et al.* showed that nicotine exerted a Th1-dominant effect via nicotinic acetylcholine receptors in the intestine [Kikuchi *et al.*, 2008].

As stated in the introduction, *H. pylori* infection is known to skew T helper differentiation toward type 1 (Th1) properties (production of IL-2, IFN-$\gamma$, and TNF)- thereby counteracting Th2-dependent processes. Th1 differentiation may reduce humoral immunity by down-regulating immunoglobulin production resulting in suppressions of serum IgG, IgA, and IgM levels. *H. pylori*, therefore, is presumed to down-regulate serum immunoglobulin levels in infected individuals. On the contrary, extracellular bacterial infections usually up-regulate IgM initially, and then IgG. Because *H. pylori* extracellularly colonizes the gastric mucosa, it should induce a Th2 response because such ubiquitous bacterium would be expected to colonize the mucosa (Table 1b). In accordance with this theory, Mohammadi *et al.* reported the presence of a Th2 response to effectively reduce the  bacterial load in a mouse model of *H. pylori* infection: Th1 cells enhance gastritis and Th2 cells reduce bacterial load [Mohammadi *et al.*, 1997]. The current data from the control group in study 3 are also in accordance with this theory, i.e., *H. pylori* infection raises levels of serum immunoglobulins in both smokers (IgM) and non-smokers (IgG) with non-ulcer gastritis. This differs from the situation in patients with peptic ulcer, in whom *H. pylori* infection did not suppress serum immunoglobulin levels, of non-ulcer patients suggesting the unique phenomenon of Th1 skew seen only in patients with peptic ulcer (Table 7). Taking our current observations together, suppression, i.e., a lack of upregulation of serum immunoglobulins appears to be a unique feature of smokers with both peptic ulcer and *H. pylori* infection. Th1 skew observed in *H. pylori*-infected patients with peptic ulcer appeared to exceed the expected Th2 skew in patients infected with extracellular bacteria such as *H. pylori* itself, especially in smokers. In addition, vast majority of gastric T cells may be already polarized to produce Th1 cytokine even in the absence of *H. pylori* infection [Itoh, et al., 1999]. We therefore stress that the Th1 skew induced by *H. pylori*, smoking, and the presence of peptic ulceration may synergistically exert a Th1 response which prevails over the expected Th2 skew, i.e., up-regulation of serum immunoglobulin levels induced by the presence of extracellular bacterial infection by *H. pylori* itself.

The Th1 skew observed in patients with *H. pylori* infection indicated a Th1-polarized response to be associated with mucosal damage that can induce peptic ulcer, while a mixed Th1 and IL-4-drived Th2 polarized response appeared to be associated with a low degree of gastric inflammation and reduced bacterial load resulting in the prevention of ulcer formation [D'Elios *et al.*, 1997, 2003, 2005; Mohammadi *et al.*, 1997; Holck *et al.*, 2003]. Th2 drive therefore may be preferable to hasten ulcer healing in such patients. However, mixed or dysregulated Th responses may trigger T cell-dependent B cell activation involved in the development of low grade B cell lymphoma associated with *H. pylori* [D'Elios *et al.*, 2003, 2005].

## 5. Conclusion

As shown herein, current smoking is consitently associated with suppressed serum immunoglobulin levels (study 1), and *H. pylori* infection definitely reduced these levels in smokers with peptic ulcer (study 2). Furthermore *H. pylori* infection up-regulated IgG, IgA, and IgM in the absence of peptic ulcer. Current smoking, *H. pylori* infection, and the presence of peptic ulceration may interact to suppress the levels of serum immunoglobulins as a result of a Th1 shift which overwhelms the Th2 shift expected with extracellular bacterial infection.

## 6. References

[1] Fundamental Immunology. 6th ed., 2008 pp411-412, 742-744, 1147  Paul WE ed, Wolters Kluwer/Lppincott Williams&Wilkins, Philadelphia PA 191 USA

[2] Mosmann, T.R.& Coffman, R.I. (1989). TH1 and Th2 cells: different patterns of lymphokine secretion lead in different functional properties. *Annual Review of Immunology*, vol.7, pp145-173

[3] Steinman, L. (2007). A brief history of T(H) 17, the first major revision in the T(H)1/T(H)2 hypothesis of cell mediated tissue damage. *Nature Medicine* vol.13, pp139-145

[4] Sakaguchi, S., Sakaguchi, N., Asano, M., Itoh, M. & Toda, M. (1995). Immunologic self-tolerance maintained by activated T cells expressing IL-2 receptor alpha-chains (CD25). Breakdown of a single mechanism of self-tolerance causes various autoimmune diseases. *Journal of Immunology* vol.155, pp1151-1164

[5] Sakaguchi, S., Yamaguchi, T., Nomura, T. & Ono, M. (2008). Regulatory T cells and immune tolerance. *Cell* vol.133, pp775-787

[6] Hida, N., Shimoyama, T. Jr., Neville, P., Dixon, M.F., Axon, A.T.R., Shimoyama, T., Sir. & Crabtree, J.E. (1999). Increased expression of IL-10 and IL-12 (p40) mRNA in *Helicobacter pylori* infected gastric mucosa: relation to bacterial cag status and peptic ulceration. *Journal of Clinical Pathology* vol.52, pp658-664

[7] Holck, S., Norgaard, A., Bennedsen, M., Permin, H., Norn, S. & Andersen, L.P. (2003). Gastric mucosal cytokine responses in *Helicobacter pylori*-infected patients with gastritis and peptic ulcers. Association with inflammatory parameters and bacterial load. *FEMS Immunology and Medical Microbiolology* vol.36, pp175-180

[8] D'Elios, M.M., Amedei, A. & Del Prete, G. (2003). *Helicobacter pylori* antigen-specific-cell responses at gastric levels in chronic gastritis, peptic ulcer, gastric ulcer, gastric cancer and low-grade mucosa-associated lymphoid tissue (MALT) lymphoma. *Microbes and Infection* vol.5, pp723-730

[9] Itoh. T., Seno. H., Kita. T., Chiba. T. & Wakatsuki, Y. (2005). The response to *Helicobacter pylori* differs between patients with gastric ulcer and duodenal ulcer. *Scandinavian Journal of Gastroenterology* vol.40, pp641-647

[10] D'Elios, M.M., Amedei, A., Benagiano, M., Azzurri, A. & Del Prete, G. (2005). *Helicobcter pylori*, T cells and cytokines: "dangerous liaisons". *FEMS Immunology and Medical Microbiology* vol.44, pp113-119

[11] Goll, R., Cui, G., Olsen, T., Isaksen, V., Gruber, F. Husebekk, A. & Florholmen, J. (2007). Alterations in antral cytokine gene expression in peptic ulcer patients during ulcer healing and after *Helicobacter pylori* eradication. *Scandinavian Journal of Immunology* vol. 67, pp57-62

[12] Ayada, K., Yokota, K., Kawahara, Y., Yamamoto, Y., Hirai, K., Inaba, T., Kita, M., Okada, H., Yamamoto, K. & Oguma, K. (2009). Immune reactions against elongation factor 2 kinase: specific pathogenesis for gastric ulcer from *Helicobacter pylori* infection. *Clinical and Developmental Immunology* 2009;Article ID850623,10pages.

[13] Mohammadi, M., Czinn, S., Redline, R. & Nedrud, J. (1996). *Helicobacter*-specific cell-mediated responses display a predominant Th1 phenotype and promote a delayed-type hypersensitivity response in the stomach of mice. *Journal of Immunology* vol.156, pp4729-4738

[14] D'Elios, M.M., Manghetti, M., De Carli, M., Costa, F., Baldari, C.T., Burroni, D., Telford, J.L., Romagnani, S. & Del Prete, G. (1997). T helper 1 effector cells specific for *Helicobacter pylori* in the gastric antrum of patients with peptic ulcer disease. *Journal of Immunology* vol.158, pp962-967

[15] D'Elios, M.M., Manghetti, M., Almerigogna, F., Amedei, A., Costa, F., Burroni, D., Baldari, C.T., Romagnani, S., Telford, J.L. & Del Prete, G. (1997). Different cytokine profile and antigen-specificity repertoire in *Helicobacter pylori*-specific T cell clones from the antrum of chronic gastritis patients with or without peptic ulcer. *European Journal of Immunology* vol.27, pp1751-1755

[16] Fan, X., Crowe, S.E., Behar, S., Gunasena, H., Ye, G., Haeberle, H., Van Houten, N., Gourley, W.K. Ernst, P.B. & Reyes, V.E (1998). The effect of class II major histocompatibility complex expression on adherence of *Helicobacter pylori* and induction of apoptosis in gastric epithelial cells: a mechanism for T helper cell type 1 mediated damage. *Journal of Experimental Medicine* vol.187, pp1659-1669

[17] Bamford, K.B., Fan, X., Crowe, S.E., Leary, J.F., Gourley, W.K., Luthra, G.K., Brooks, E.G., Graham, D.Y., Reyes, V.E. & Ernst, P.B. (1998). Lymphocytes in the human gastric mucosa during *Helicobacter pylori* infection have a T helper cell 1 phenotype. *Gastroenterology* vol.114, pp482-492

[18] Sommer, F., Faller, G., Konturek, P., Kirchner, T., Hahn, E.G., Zeus, J., Rollinghoff, M. & Lohof, M. (1998). Antrum- and corpus mucosa-infiltrating CD4(+) lymphocytes in *Helicobacter pylori* gastritis display a Th1 phenotype. *Infection and Immunity* vol.66, pp5543-5546

[19] Lindholm, C., Quiding-Jarbrink, M., Lonroth, H., Hamlet, A. & Svennerholm, A.M. (1998). Local cytokine response in *Helicobacter pylori*-infected subjects. *Infection and Immunity* vol.66, pp5964-5971

[20] Ihan, A., Tepes, B. & Gubina, M. (2000). Diminished Th1-type cytokine production in gastric mucosa T lymphocytes after *H. pylori* eradication in duodenal ulcer patients. *Pflugers Archives-European Journal of Physiology* vol.440, pp[Suppl]:R89-R90

[21] Smythies, L.E., Waites, K.B., Lindsey, J.R., Harris, P.R., Ghiara, P. & Smith, P.D. (2000). *Helicobacter pylori*-induced mucosal inflammation is Th1 mediated and exacerbated in IL-4, but not IFN-gamma, gene-deficient mice. *Journal of Immunology* vol.165, pp1022-1029,

[22] Akhiani, A.A., Pappo, J., Kabok, Z., Schon, K., Gao, W., Franzen, L.E. & Lycke N. (2002). Protection against *Helicobacter pylori* infection following immunization is IL-12 dependent and mediated by Th1 cells. *Journal of Immunology* vol.169, pp6977-6984

[23] Guiney, D.G., Hasegawa, P. & Cole, S.P. (2003). *Helicobacter pylori* preferentially induces interleukin 12 (IL-12) rather than IL-6 or IL-10 in human dendritic cells. *Infection and Immunity* vol.71, pp4163-4166

[24] Amedei, A., Cappon, A., Codolo, G., Cabrelle, A., Polenghi, A., Benagiano, M., Tasca, E., Azzurri, A., D'Elios, M.M., Del Prete, G. & de Bernard, M. (2006). The neutrophil-activating protein of *Helicobacter pylori* promotes Th1 immune responses. *Journal of Clinical Investigation* vol.116, pp1092-1101

[25] Taylor, J.M., Ziman, M.E., Huff, J.L., Moroski, N.M., Vajdy, M. & Solnick, J.V. (2006). *Helicobacter pylori* lipopolysaccharide promotes a Th1 type immune response in immunized mice. *Vaccine* vol.24, pp4987-4994

[26] D'Elios, M.M., Amedei, A., Cappon, A., Del Prete, G. & de Bernard, M. (2007). The neutrophil-activating protein of *Helicobacter pylori* (HP-NAP) as an immune modulating agent. FEMS *Immunology and Medical Microbiology* vol.50, pp157-164

[27] Goll, R., Cui, G., Olsen, T., Isaksen, V., Gruber, F., Husebekk, A. & Florholmen, J. (2008). Alteration in antral cytokine gene expression in peptic ulcer patients during ulcer healing and after *Helicobacter pylori* eradication. *Scandinavian Journal of Immunology* vol.67, pp57-62

[28] Codolo, G., Mazzi, P., Amedei, A., Del Prete, G.D., Berton, G., D'Elios, M.M. & Bernard, M. (2008). The neutrophil-activating protein of *Helicobacter pylori* down-modulates Th2 inflammation in ovalbumin-induced allergic asthma. *Cellular Microbiology* vol.10, pp2355-2363

[29] Del Prete, G., Chiumiento, L., Amedei, A., Piazza, M., D'Elios, M.M., Codolo, G., Bernard, M., Masetti, M. & Bruschi, F. (2008). Immunosuppression of Th2 responses in Trichinella spiralis infection by *Helicobacter pylori* neutrophil-activating protein. *Journal of Allergy and Clinical Immunology* vol.122, pp908-913

[30] Shimada, M., Ando, T., Peek, R.M., Watanabe, O., Ishiguro, K., Maeda, O., Ishikawa, D., Hasegawa, M., Ina, K., Ohmiya, N., Niwa, Y. & Goto, H. (2008). *Helicobacter pylori* infection upregulates interleukin-18 production from gastric epithelial cells. *European Journal of Gastroenterology* vol.20, 1144-1150

[31] Watanabe, T., Asano, N., Kitani, A., Fuss, I.J., Chiba, T. & Strober, W. (2010). NOD1-mediated mucosal host defense against *Helicobacter pylori*. *International Journal of Inflammation* Article ID476482,6 pages.

[32] Hosseini, M.E., Oghalaie, A., Habibi, G., Nahvijoo, A., Hosseini, Z.M., Tashakoripoor, M. & Mohammadi, N.M. (2010). Molecular detection of host cytokine expression in *Helicobacter pylori* infected patients via semi-quantitative RT-PCR. *Indian Journal of Medical Microbiology* vol.28, pp40-44

[33] Itoh, T., Wakatsuki, Y., Yoshida, M., Usui, T., Matsunaga, Y., Kaneko, S., Chiba, T. &Kita, T. (1999). The vast majority of gastric T cells are polarized to produce T helper 1 type cytokines upon antigenic stimulation despite the absence of *Helicobacter pylori* infection. *Journal of Gastroenterology* vol.34, pp560-570

[34] Campbell, D.I., Pearce, M.S., Parker, L. & Thomas, J.E. (2004). IgG subclass responses in childhood *Helicobacter pylori* duodenal ulcer: evidence of T-helper cell type 2 responses. *Helicobacter* vol.9, pp289-292

[35] Kido, M., Tanaka, J., Aoki, N., Iwamoto, S., Nishiura, H., Chiba, T. & Watanabe, N. (2010). *Helicobacter pylori* promotes the production of thymic stromal lymphopoietin by

gastric epithelial cells and induces dendritic cell-mediated inflammatory Th2 responses. *Infection and Immunity* vol.78, pp108-114

[36] Kayhan, B., Arasli, M., Eren, H., Aydemir, S., Kayhan, B., Aklas, E. & Tekin, I. (2008). Analysis of peripheral blood lymphocyte phenotypes and Th1/Th2 cytokines prophile in the systemic immune responses of *Helicobacter pylori* infected individulas. *Microbiology and Immunology* vol.52, pp531-538

[37] Bergman, M.P., Engering, A., Smits, H.H., van Vliet, S.J., van Bodegraven, A.A., Wirth, H., Kapsenberg, M.L., Vandenbroucke-Grauls, C.M.J.E., van Kooyk, Y. & Applemelk, B.J. (2004). *Helicobacter pylori* modulates the T helper cell 1/T helper cell 2 balance through phase-variable interaction between lipopolysaccharide and DC-SIGN. *Journal of Experimental Medicine* vol.200, pp979-990

[38] Andersen, P., Pedersen, O.F., Bach, B. & Bonde, G.J. (1982). Serum antibodies and immunoglobulins in smokers and non-smokers. *Clinical and Experimental Immunology* vol.47, pp467-473

[39] Tollerud, D.J., Brown, L.M., Blattner, W.A., Weiss, S.T., Maloney, E.M., Kurman, C.C., Nelson, D.L. & Hoover, R.N. (1995). Racial difference in serum immunoglobulin levels: relationship to cigarette smoking, T-cell subsets, and soluble interleukin-2 receptors. *Journal of Clinical and Laboratory Analysis* vol.9, pp37-41

[40] Barbour, S.E., Nakashima, K., Zhang, J., Tangada, S., Hahn, C., Schenkein, H.A. & Tew, J.G. (1997). Tobacco and smoking: environmental factors that modify the host response (Immune system) and have an impact on periodontal health. *Critical Review in Oral Biology and Medicine* vol.8, pp437-460

[41] Gonzalez-Quintela, A., Alende, R., Gude, F., Campos, J., Rey, J., Meijide, L.M., Fernandez-Merino, C. & Vidal, C. (2008). Serum levels of immunoglobulins (IgG, IgA, IgM) in a general adult population and their relationship with alcohol consumption, smoking and common metabolic abnormalities. *Clinical and Experimental Immunology* vol.151, pp42-50

[42] Hallquist, N., Hakki, A., Wecker, L., Friedman, H. & Pross, S. (2000). Differential effects of nicotine and aging on splenocyte proliferation and the promotion of Th1-vs. Th2-type cytokines. *Proceedings of Society for Experimental Biology and Medicine* vol.224, pp141-146

[43] Whetzel, C.A., Corwin, E.J. & Klein, L.C. (2007). Disruption in Th1/Th2 response in young adult smokers. *Addictive Behaviors* vol.32, pp1-8

[44] Kikuchi, H., Itoh, J. & Fukuda, S. (2008). Chronic nicotine stimulation modulates the immune response of mucosal T cells to Th1-dominant pattern via nAChR by upregulation of Th1-specific transcriptional factor. *Neuroscience Letter* vol.432, pp217-221,

[45] Hagiwara, F., Takahashi, K., Okubo, T., Ohno, S., Ueda, A., Aoki, A., Odagiri, S. & Ishigatsubo Y. (2001). Cigarette smoking depletes cells spontaneously secreting Th1 cytokines in the human airway. Cytokines vol.14, pp121-126,

[46] Cozen, W., Diaz-Sanchez, D., Gauderman, W.J., Zadnik, J., Cockburn, M.G., Gill, P.S., Masood, R., Hamilton, A.S., Jyrala, M. & Mack, T.M. (2004). Th1 and Th2 cytokines and IgE levels in identical twins with varying levels of cigarette consumption. *Journal of Clinical Immunology* vol.24, pp617-22

[47] Zeidel, A., Beilin, B., Yardeni, I., Mayburg, E., Smirnov, G. & Bessler, H. (2002). Immune response in asymptomatic smokers. *Acta Anaesthesiologica Scandinavica* vol.46, pp959-964,

[48] Eaton, K.A. & Mefford, M.E. (2001). Cure of *Helicobacter pylori* infection and resolution of gastritis by adoptive transfer of splenocytes in mice. *Infection and Immunity* vol.69, pp1025-1031

[49] Nagai, S., Mimuro, H., Yamada, T., Baba, Y., Moro, K., Nochi, T., Kiyono, H., Suzuki, T Sasakawa, C. & Koyasu, S. (2007). Role of Peyer's patches in the induction of *Helicobacter pylori*-induced gastritis. *Proceedings of the National Academy of Sciences of the United States of America* vol.104, pp8971-8976

[50] Franch, A., Castellote, M. & Castell, M. (1994). Effect of acetylsalicylic acid and dexamethasone on antibody production in adjuvant arthritis. *Rheumatology International* vol.14, pp27-31

[51] Mazzeo, D., Panina-Bordignon, P., Recalde, H., Sinigaglia, F. & D'Ambrosio, D. (1998). Decreased IL-12 production and Th1 cell development by acetyl salcilic acid-mediated inhibition of NF-kappa B. *European Journal of Immunology* vol.28, pp3205-3213

[52] Yamaki, K., Uchida, H., Harada, R., Yanagisawa, R., Takano, H., Hayashi, H., Mori, Y. & Yoshino, S. (2003). Effect of nonsteroidal anti-inflammatory drug indomethacin on Th1 and Th2 immune response in mice. *Journal of Pharmaceutical Sciences* vol.92:1723

[53] Andreone, P., Gramenzi, A., Loggi, E., Faverelli, L., Cursaro, C., Margotti, M., Biselli, M., Lorenzini, S. & Bernardi, M. (2004). In vivo effect of indomethacin and interferon on Th1 and Th2 cytokine synthesis in patients with chronic hepatitis C. *Cytokine* vol.26, pp95-101

[54] Mored, H., Stoof, T.J., Boorsma, D.M., von Blomberg, B.M., Gibbs, S., Bruynzeel, D.P, Scheper, R.J. & Rustemeyer, T. (2004). Identification of anti-inflammatory drugs according to their capacity to suppress type-1 and type-2 cell profiles. *Clinical and Experimental Allergy* vol.34, pp1868-1875

[55] Yamaki, K., Uchida, H., Mori, Y. & Yoshino, S. (2005). Effect of varying types of anti-arthritic drugs on Th1 and Th2 immune responses in mice. *International Journal of Immunopathology and Pharmacology* vol.18,pp133-144

[56] Tsutsumi, Y., Kanamori, H., Yamato, H., Ehira, N., Kawamura, T., Umehara, S., Mori, A., Obara, S., Ogura, N., Tanaka, J., Asaka, M., Imamura, M. & Msauzi, N. (2005). Randomized study of *Helicobacter pylori* eradication therapy and proton pump inhibitor monotherapy for idiopathic thrombocytopenic purpura. *Annals of Hematology* vol.84, pp807-811,

[57] Matsukawa, Y., Kurosaka, H., Kato, K., Hayashi, I., Minekawa, K., Arakawa, Y. & Sawada, S. (2007). Lansoprazole increases serum IgG and IgM in *H. pylori*-infected patients. *International Journal of Immunopathology and Pharmacology* vol.20, pp173-179

[58] Matsukawa, Y., Tomita, Y., Nishinarita, S., Horie, T., Kato, K., Arakawa, Y., Ko, K., Shimada, H., Nakano, M., Kitami, Y. & Kurosaka, H. (1997). Efficacy of lansoprazole against peptic ulcers induced by non-steroidal anti-inflammatory drugs: endoscopic evaluation of ulcer healing. *Journal of International Medical Research* vol.25, pp190-195,

[59] Dixon, M., Genta, R.M, Yardley, J.H. & Correa, P. (1996). Classification and grading gastritis: The updated Sydney system. *American Journal of Surgical Pathology* vol.20, pp1161-1181

[60] Mohammadi, M., Nedrud, J., Redline, R., Lycke, N. & Czinn, S. (1997). Murine, CD4 T-cell response to *Helicobacter* infection:Th1 cells enhence gastritis and Th2 cells reduce bacterial load. *Gastroenterology* vol.113, pp1848-1857

# 12

# Activation of the Hypothalamic-Pituitary-Adrenocortical Axis as a Gastroprotective Component of Stress Response

Ludmila Filaretova
*Laboratory of Experimental Endocrinology*
*Pavlov Institute of Physiology*
*Russia*

## 1. Introduction

Gastric ulcer disease remains widespread; a stressful lifestyle and non-steroidal anti-inflammatory drugs (NSAIDs) make significant contributions to this pathological situation (Glavin et al., 1991; Hawkey, 2000; Laine et al., 2008). Despite indubitable advances in elucidation of the pathogenesis of gastric ulceration, there are gaps in our understanding of ulcerogenesis, particularly the role of key hormonal system of adaptation: the hypothalamic-pituitary-adrenocortical (HPA) axis.

## 2. Glucocorticoid hormones and gastric ulceration

Glucocorticoid hormones and gastric ulceration have been discussed in many contexts. The action of acute and chronic treatment of patients or experimental animals with glucocorticoids as well as the effects of basal and stress-induced glucocorticoid production on the gastric mucosa has been considered. Although there is a long-standing debate over whether glucocorticoid therapy by itself leads to peptic ulcer disease in human (Luo et al., 2009; Olsen et al., 2010), it is established that administration of glucocorticoids to experimental animals can result in an acute gastric erosion (Bandyopadhyay et al., 1999, as cited in Filaretova et al., 2009b; Black, 1988, as cited in Filaretova et al., 1998; Takeuchi et al., 2008). In the same time, in some cases administration of glucocorticoids to animals can attenuate gastric erosion (Derelanko & Long 1982; Filaretova et al., 2009b; McCafferty et al., 1995). It is also known that basal glucocorticoid production contribute to the maintenance of the gastric mucosal integrity (Takeuchi et al., 1989). The glucocorticoids may modulate the cytoprotective effect of adrenal catecholamines (Hernandez et al., 1984). They may have a permissive role in allowing gastroprotective mechanisms to exert their full potential. A permissive role was suggested in gastric mucosal protection induced by prostaglandins (PGs), sulfhydryls, cimetidine (Szabo et al., 1983) or interleukin-1 (Perretti et al., 1992).

The most controversial question is the question about the action of stress-produced glucocorticoids. Based on the notion that exogenous glucocorticoids used at pharmacological doses have ulcerogenic properties, the increase of glucocorticoids during stress was also considered to be an ulcerogenic factor. In the same time, it is known that glucocorticoid hormones released during acute stress-induced activation of the HPA axis help the body overcome negative effects of stress stimuli (Munk et al., 1984, as cited in Filaretova et al., 1998). Despite this knowledge, it has been generally accepted for several decades that stress-produced glucocorticoids cause an ulcerogenic response in the stomach, and stress-induced activation of the HPA axis is considered a pathogenic component of this response.

As the widely held view about the ulcerogenic role of glucocorticoids released during stress is difficult to reconcile with the adaptive role of the HPA axis hormones, we designed experiments in rats to clarify the validity of this view. The results obtained do not support the traditional paradigm and suggest that glucocorticoids released during acute activation of the HPA axis are important gastroprotective factors. In the chapter, we review our results on the role of glucocorticoids in gastroprotection.

## 2.1 Gastroprotective action of stress-produced glucocorticoids

Various stressful stimuli activate the HPA axis, and consequently, the production of glucocorticoids, and severe stress stimuli may also induce gastric erosion, called "stress ulcers". Hans Selye, the "Father" of the field of research into stress, attracted attention to these signs of stress. His greatest contributions were the demonstration of the stress triad (gastrointestinal ulceration, thymico-lymphatic atrophy, and adrenal hypertrophy) and of the role of the hypothalamus in activating the hypophysis, which, in turn, stimulates the adrenals to produce corticoids (Selye, 1967). From the very outset, researchers have focused on the idea that stress-generated glucocorticoids are causally related with gastric ulcerogenesis. This possibility was also investigated in hypophysectomized and adrenalectomized animals by Selye himself, who observed that although stress-induced thymico-lymphatic atrophy was inhibited in these animals, "stress ulcers" were not prevented, and concluded that the formation of "stress ulcers" depends on not only the pituitary-adrenal axis but other factors as well. He also proposed that neurostimulators play a major role in stress-induced ulcerogenesis, although high levels of corticoids in blood could be a sensitizing factor (Selye, 1967). Weiss (Weiss, 1971, as cited in Filaretova et al., 1998) found in rats that the severity of stress-induced ulceration is positively correlated with the level of corticosterone in plasma and proposed that "steroids, in quantities that the animal is capable of secreting, may contribute to the production of ulcers". Further support for this idea came from the observation that animals with hippocampal lesions had increased levels of plasma corticosterone and developed more gastric ulcers during stress (Murphy et al., 1979, as cited in Filaretova et al., 1998). One approach used to support the view that stress-generated glucocorticoids are ulcerogenic was a groundless extrapolation of the ulcerogenic properties of exogenous glucocorticoids observed at high pharmacological doses to the properties of endogenous glucocorticoids released during stress.

From the beginning (Filaretova, 1990), we have focused on the idea that glucocorticoids released during acute stress also have an adaptive effect on the stomach and, therefore, are gastroprotective rather than ulcerogenic. To test this hypothesis, we examined the effect of glucocorticoid deficiency or the glucocorticoid receptor antagonist RU-38486 on water and immersion-restraint-induced or cold-restraint-induced gastric erosion in rats (Filaretova, 1990, 2006; Filaretova et al., 1998). Different approaches were used to inhibit the stress-induced release of corticosterone: the inhibition of corticotropin-releasing hormone synthesis in the hypothalamic paraventricular nucleus by intrahypothalamic implantation of dexamethasone, the immunoneutralization of ACTH by pretreatment with ACTH antiserum, and the inhibition of the HPA axis at the hypothalamic and the pituitary levels by pretreatment with a pharmacological dose of cortisol one week before stress. Corticosterone replacement, that is, the injection of corticosterone at a dose mimicking the stress-induced rise in corticosterone (4 mg/kg) 15 min before stress, was used in our experiments.

Intrahypothalamic dexamethasone implantation significantly decreased the stress-induced increase in corticosterone and markedly provoked the gastric erosion caused by stress. Corticosterone replacement prevented the aggravating effect of dexamethasone on the ulceration. ACTH antiserum administered shortly before cold-restraint stress decreased the release of corticosterone in response to stress and enhanced the severity of the gastric erosion (Filaretova et al., 1998). Pretreatment with glucocorticoid (cortisol) at a pharmacological dose caused an inhibition of the HPA axis at the hypothalamic and pituitary levels via a negative feedback mechanism and resulted in a long-lasting decrease in the stress-induced rise in corticosterone levels (Filaretova, 2006; Filaretova et al., 2001a). It is important to emphasize that animals were stressed one week after the treatment with cortisol when the exogenous hormone had already been eliminated but the corticosterone response to stress was still inhibited. The cortisol pretreatment increased the ulcerogenic action in both models of stress, and acute corticosterone replacement that mimicked the stress-induced corticosterone response reduced gastric erosion in rats with an inhibited HPA axis (Filaretova, 1990, 2006). These results support the idea that the gastric ulcerogenic response to stress is potentiated by a reduction of stress-induced glucocorticoid production.

Glucocorticoid antagonists offer another way to demonstrate the role of the stress-induced rise in corticosterone in the gastric ulcerogenic response to stress. The specific progesterone/glucocorticoid receptor antagonist RU-38486 is known to bind with a high affinity to type II glucocorticoid receptors and may influence peripheral as well as central glucocorticoid receptors (Moguilewski & Philibert, 1984, as cited in Filaretova et al., 1998). In the simultaneous presence of glucocorticoids and the antagonist in vivo, glucocorticoid receptors are predominantly occupied by the antagonist (Alexandrova, 1994). The RU-38486-glucocorticoid receptor complex is incapable of nuclear translocation and does not produce a biological effect (Moguilewski & Philibert, 1984, as cited in Filaretova et al., 1998). For this reason the glucocorticoid receptor antagonist RU-38486 can be a tool for investigating modes of glucocorticoid action. It was found that the occupation by RU-38486 of glucocorticoid receptors during cold-restraint stress aggravates the stress-induced gastric erosion (Filaretova et al., 1998). We believe these results support the gastroprotective role of glucocorticoids released during stress. These data also suggest that gastroprotective action of glucocorticoids may occur, at least partly, through the classical genomic mechanism. There is also evidence that glucocorticoids can act through nongenomic pathways (Whitehouse, 2011). We do not rule out that nongenomic mechanisms may also be involved in gastroprotective action of glucocorticoids.

To investigate contribution of glucocorticoids to the maintenance of gastric mucosal integrity during stress we predominantly used ulcerogenic stress models, although in some cases we also used non-ulcerogenic stress models. Using the ulcerogenic models we demonstrated that glucocorticoids released in response to the ulcerogenic stimuli attenuated their harmful action on the gastric mucosa. Our data obtained from the non-ulcerogenic models suggests that mild stress stimuli don't damage the gastric mucosa due to physiologic gastroprotective action of glucocorticoids released in response to these stimuli (Filaretova, 1990; Filaretova et al., 2001a). Indeed, we showed that in rats with glucocorticoid deficiency normally non-ulcerogenic stress stimulus turns into an ulcerogenic one (Filaretova, 1990). Another striking demonstration of the physiological gastroprotective role of glucocorticoids is the participation of glucocorticoids in gastroprotective effects of preconditioning stress (Filaretova et al., 2008). Preconditioning mild stress may attenuate gastric injury caused by severe stress and this effect is known to be mediated by PGs (Tanaka et al., 2007). It is known that mild stressors induce an increase in glucocorticoid production, however, it remained unknown whether glucocorticoids released during preconditioning mild stress contribute to the gasroprotective effect of mild stress against severe stressors. The contribution of glucocorticoids to the protective effect of preconditioning mild stress on gastric mucosa has not been investigated previously, apparently due to the prevailing traditional point of view on ulcerogenic action of glucocorticoids released during stress. Our findings about gastroprotective role of glucocorticoids produced during ulcerogenic stress allowed us to hypothesize that glucocorticoids contribute to gastroprotective effect of preconditioning non-ulcerogenic stress. To verify the hypothesis we compared the effects of mild stress on gastric erosion caused by severe stress in rats with normal and deficient corticosterone response to preconditioning mild stress. To inhibit glucocorticoid synthesis during mild stress metyrapone was injected shortly before the onset of mild stress. Metyrapone pretreatment caused a fast inhibition of corticosterone response to mild stress and prevented its protective effect on gastric ulceration induced by severe stress. The results obtained argue for a participation of glucocorticoids in the protective influence of preconditioning mild stress on gastric mucosa (Filaretova et al., 2008). We consider this fact as a further support for the point of view that glucocorticoids released during an acute stress are naturally occurring gastroprotective factors.

Therefore, our data allows us to conclude that an acute stress-induced increase of glucocorticoids has gastroprotective action against stress-induced gastric damage. It should be emphasized that our studies on the mode of gastroprotection by glucocorticoids have been performed on animals during acute ulceration. The effects of glucocorticoids on the gastric mucosa during chronic stress conditions may be different from those observed in acute experiments.

## 2.2 Gastroprotective action of glucocorticoids during treatment with non-steroidal anti-inflammotary drugs

According to our results (Filaretova et al., 2001b, 2002a), NSAID treatment, similar to stress, may activate the HPA axis. Administration of both indomethacin and aspirin induced a release of corticosterone, which in turn may help to protect the gastric mucosa against NSAIDs. Indeed, adrenalectomy prevented NSAID-induced corticosterone release and markedly worsened the gastric erosion caused by NSAIDs. Acute corticosterone replacement, mimicking the indomethacin- and aspirin-induced rise in corticosterone, also prevented the aggravation of gastric ulcers generated by adrenalectomy (Filaretova et al., 2002a). The aggravation of NSAID-induced gastric erosion was also demonstrated in another model of glucocorticoid deficiency where the NSAID-induced corticosterone rise was prevented by pharmacological blockade of the HPA axis (Filaretova et al., 2001b, 2005).

Likewise, pretreatment of the animals with RU-38486, the glucocorticoid receptor antagonist, significantly aggravated the severity of gastric erosion induced by indomethacin as well as aspirin (Filaretova et al., 2002a). It is thus assumed that endogenous glucocorticoids released during NSAID treatment increase the resistance of the gastric mucosa to NSAID-induced injury.

The gastric ulcerogenic properties of NSAIDs limit the use of these drugs for the treatment of chronic inflammatory disorders, and it has been considered that combined treatment with therapeutic doses of glucocorticoid increases the risk of gastric ulceration (Hawkey, 2000). The results obtained in our studies (Filaretova et al., 2001b, 2002a, 2005) suggest that the increased risk of adverse gastric reactions should be considered when NSAIDs are used in patients with impaired glucocorticoid production.

Endogenous glucocorticoids may have a permissive role in allowing gastroprotective mechanisms against NSAID-induced injury to exert their full beneficial potential. This action was suggested in gastric mucosal protection against aspirin-induced erosion induced by cimetidine (Szabo et al., 1983) or interleukin-1 (Perretti et al., 1992). Likewise, a normal basal production of glucocorticoids is also important for the gastric mucosa to resist indomethacin- (Takeuchi et al., 1989) or aspirin-induced damage (Perretti et al., 1992). Furthermore, both aspirin and indomethacin at ulcerogenic doses stimulate glucocorticoid production to cause an acute elevation of glucocorticoid content in the physiological range, which in turn protects against gastric damage induced by these NSAIDs.

These data together with our previous findings support the point of view that glucocorticoids released during acute activation of the HPA axis caused by stress or NSAIDs as well as other ulcerogenic stimuli (Filaretova et al., 2001a) act as gastroprotective hormones. From the beginning (Filaretova, 1990), we have focused on the hypothesis that glucocorticoids released during stress also have an adaptive effect on the stomach. The results obtained in our studies confirm this hypothesis and furthermore demonstrate that glucocorticoids released in response to NSAIDs or other ulcerogenic stimuli also have an adaptive effect on the stomach. In turn, it means that an acute HPA axis activation is a physiologic gastroprotective component of acute stress response.

It is known that both humoral and neuronal factors, such as PGs, nitric oxide (NO), and capsaicin-sensitive afferent neurons, play a pivotal role in the defense against gastric mucosal injury (Holzer, 1998; Wallace, 1997). They contribute to gastroprotection by modulating mucosal blood flow, mucus secretion, and repair of injured gastric mucosa. We showed that glucocorticoids released in response to ulcerogenic stimuli are naturally occurring gastroprotective factors and exert many of the same actions in the stomach as PGs, NO, and capsaicin-sensitive afferent neurons. This has prompted us to consider the interaction between glucocorticoid hormones and other protective factors in the maintenance of gastric mucosal integrity.

We compared the effects of the drug-induced inhibition of PG or NO production or the desensitization of capsaicin-sensitive sensory neurons on the gastric mucosa in rats with deficient or with normal glucocorticoid production, under normal or ulcerogenic conditions. Indomethacin at 35 mg/kg (s.c.) was used as an ulcerogenic stimulus. The glucocorticoid deficiency was caused by adrenalectomy one week before the experiment. Two kinds of corticosterone replacement were used in adrenalectomized rats. Indomethacin at a nonulcerogenic dose (5 mg/kg i.p.) or L-NAME (50 mg/kg s.c.) was acutely given to inhibit PG and NO production, respectively. For the desensitization (functional ablation) of capsaicin-sensitive afferent neurons, rats were given subcutaneous injections of capsaicin in 3 consecutive doses of 20, 30, and 50 mg/kg (Bobryshev et al., 2005; Filaretova et al., 2007). Adrenalectomy by itself did not cause damage in the stomach. Neither inhibition of PG or NO, nor sensory deafferentation by itself provoked any damage in the gastric mucosa of sham-operated rats. However, each of these treatments damaged the gastric mucosa in adrenalectomized rats, and all of these responses were prevented by corticosterone in drinking water at a concentration mimicking the basal corticosterone level in normal rats (Bobryshev et a., 2005; Filaretova et al., 2007).

Indomethacin-induced gastric erosion was aggravated to a similar extent by adrenalectomy, inhibition of NO production, or desensitization of capsaicin-sensitive afferent neurons. These data suggest that the role of glucocorticoid hormones in protection of the gastric mucosa against indomethacin is no less significant than that of NO or capsaicin-sensitive afferent neurons. The combination of adrenalectomy with inhibition of NO production or sensory deafferentation markedly potentiated the aggravating effect of these treatments by themselves on indomethacin-induced gastric erosions: the mean erosion area was increased approximately 5 or 10 times, respectively. Corticosterone at a dose mimicking the indomethacin-induced corticosterone rise totally prevented the aggravating effect of adrenalectomy in these experiments (Bobryshev et al., 2005; Filaretova et al., 2007). These results demonstrate that the effect of inhibition of NO production or sensory deafferentation on indomethacin-induced gastric erosion is significantly modified by glucocorticoid deficiency. This, in turn, suggests the important role of glucocorticoid hormones in the maintenance of gastric mucosal integrity under adverse conditions when the gastroprotective action of NO or capsaicin-sensitive neurons is impaired.

Thus, our data demonstrates a pivotal compensatory role of glucocorticoids in the maintenance of gastric mucosal integrity in the case of impaired gastroprotective mechanisms provided by PGs, NO and capsaicin-sensitive afferent neurons. The compensatory gastroprotective role of glucocorticoids during PG deficiency (Filaretova et al., 2002a) or desensitization of capsaicin-sensitive afferents (Bobryshev et al., 2005) may be provided through enhancement of their production in these situations. We also showed that glucocorticoid deficiency, in turn, induces a compensatory enhancement in PG production in the stomach through COX-2 expression, which contributes to maintain the gastric mucosal integrity (Filaretova et al., 2002b). These date allowed us to conclude that there is some cooperative interaction between glucocorticoids and PGs in gastroprotection, in a way that a deficiency of one protective factor can lead to an apparently compensatory increase of the other. The gastric mucosa becomes more susceptible to injury during deficiency of both glucocorticoids and PGs (Filaretova et al., 2002b). This finding is important for clinical practice, especially for NSAID users. This further supports a warning that the increased risk of adverse gastric reactions should be considered when NSAIDs are used in patients with impaired glucocorticoid production.

It has been suggested that "PGs, NO, and sensory neuropeptides act in concert in the maintenance of mucosal viability" (Whittle et al., 1990). The suggestion was confirmed and reinforced by other investigations. Our data adds new information to such a "concerted" modulation of the gastric mucosal integrity and suggests that glucocorticoids are also important participants in this modulation. According to the data the ability of glucocorticoids protect the gastric mucosa seems especially important for the maintenance of gastric mucosa when the protective mechanism provided by PGs or NO or capsaicin-sensitive afferent neurons is impared. We consider this fact as a striking manifestation of adaptive role of glucocorticoids.

## 2.3 Mechanisms of gastroprotective action of glucocorticoids: the maintenance of gastric mucosal integrity through the maintenance of general body homeostasis

There may be multiple targets for glucocorticoids to exert their beneficial influence on the gastric mucosa. We demonstrated that the gastroprotective action of glucocorticoids is provided by the maintenance of gastric mucosal blood flow, mucus secretion and repair processes as well as the attenuation of pathogenic elements such as the enhanced gastric motility (Filaretova et al., 1999, 2001b, 2002b,c, 2004). Anti-inflammatory properties of glucocorticoids may also contribute to their gastroprotective action. Glucocorticoids as anti-inflammatory hormones may contribute to gastroprotection by inhibition of neutrophil adherence (Wallace, 1997) and attenuation of microvascular permeability (Filaretova et al., 2002c).

Because the glucocorticoid receptors are expressed ubiquitously it is possible that glucocorticoids may act directly on local gastric targets as well as using a more general mechanism. The contribution of glucocorticoids to the maintenance of gastric mucosal integrity may be closely related with their contribution to general body homeostasis (Filaretova et al., 2006). General homeostasis's various links can be primary targets of glucocorticoid action and, therefore, the maintenance of general body homeostasis by glucocorticoids may be the base for their action on the maintenance of gastric mucosal integrity. The following facts support this statement.

Glucocorticoids participate in maintaining normal blood glucose level that is especially important for the brain. There is a close relationship between HPA axis activity and blood glucose regulation. Hypoglycemia is the major trigger that activates the HPA axis and leads to enhancement of glucocorticoid production (Erturk et al., 1998, as cited in Filaretova et al., 2006). Glucocorticoids increase hepatic gluconeogenesis, inhibit glucose uptake in adipocytes and fibroblasts, sensitize the liver to glucagon and epinephrine, decrease the hepatic sensitivity to insulin and, as a result, they increase blood glucose level (Chan et al., 2002). In turn, maintaining the normal blood glucose level is important for the maintenance of gastric mucosal integrity. Insufficient supply of glucose may stimulate hypothalamic glucose-sensitive neurons (Mobbs et al., 2001, as cited in Filaretova et al., 2002c), resulting in a vagally-mediated increase in gastric motility and secretion (Shiraishi, 1988, as cited in Filaretova et al., 2002c) that are well-known pathogenic elements in various gastric ulcerogenic models. Exogenous glucose reverses the hypoglycemia-induced stimulation of hypothalamic glucose-sensitive neurons (Oomura et al., 1974, as cited in Filaretova et al., 2002c), inhibits vagally-mediated gastric hypermotility (Barnett & Owyang, 1988, as cited in Filaretova et al., 2002c) and attenuates gastric ulceration (Takeuchi et al., 1990, as cited in Filaretova et al., 2002c). It was reasonable to assume that the maintenance of glucose homeostasis by glucocorticoid hormones could be fundamental to their beneficial actions on local gastric targets.

The data obtained from the model of indomethacin-induced ulceration demonstrates that the maintenance of glucose homeostasis by glucocorticoids is responsible for their beneficial actions on gastric motility. Although the mechanisms by which indomethacin induces gastric injury involves multiple, closely interacting elements such as depletion of PGs, gastric hypermotility, microcirculatory disturbances, neutrophil-endothelial cell interactions and superoxide radicals (Takeuchi et al., 1991; Wallace, 1997), gastric hypermotility may be a key element in the pathogenesis of indomethacin-induced gastric damage (Takeuchi et al., 1989). The glycoprivic response is involved in the mechanism of gastric hypermotility induced by NSAIDs (Mersereau & Hinchey, 1982, as cited in Filaretova et al., 2002c). To understand the mechanisms underlying glucocorticoids' gastroprotective actions against indomethacin-induced injury, we investigated the effect of adrenalectomy, with or without corticosterone replacement, on gastric motility and blood glucose level 4 hours after administration of indomethacin at the ulcerogenic dose. We confirmed (Filaretova et al., 2002c) that indomethacin significantly enhanced gastric motility in sham-operated rats, and this hypermotility response was significantly aggravated in adrenalectomized rats, in parallel with an increase in gastric lesion score (Takeuchi et al., 1989). These results support a causal relationship between gastric hypermotility and lesion formation following administration of indomethacin. Blood glucose levels were low in adrenalectomized rats and decreased further after administration of indomethacin. This suggests a relation between low blood glucose levels, enhanced gastric motility and ulcerogenic responses to indomethacin. Indeed, adrenalectomized rats (with deficiency of corticosterone) given indomethacin showed minimum blood glucose levels, maximum gastric motility index values and maximum gastric lesion score when compared to sham-operated indomethacin-treated group (Filaretova et al., 2002c). A single injection of corticosterone to adrenalectomized animals, at the dose imitating the indomethacin-induced rise in corticosterone, restored blood glucose levels and significantly reduced gastric hypermotility and ulcerogenic responses to indomethacin, whereas these beneficial effects of corticosterone was attenuated by a glucocorticoid receptor antagonist RU-38486 (Filaretova et al., 2002a,c). The findings suggest that there is close relationship between the gastroprotective action of glucocorticoids and their attenuation of gastric hypermotility through maintaining blood glucose level.

The contribution of glucocorticoids to general body homeostasis involves their beneficial influences on cardiovascular system. The major actions of glucocorticoids on cardiovascular system are to enhance vascular reactivity to other vasoactive substances and to maintain systemic blood pressure (Darlington et al., 1989, as cited in Filaretova et al., 2006; Grunfeld & Eloy, 1987). Glucocorticoid deficiency is associated with reduced response to vasoconstrictors such as norepinephrine and angiotensin II. The latter stage of glucocorticoid deficiency is associated with cardiovascular collapse and heart failure in mammals after various stressors (Cleghorn, 1983, as cited in Filaretova et al., 2006). Glucocorticoid replacement is crucial in the treatment of patients with adrenal crisis, including the patients with Addison's disease (Darlington et al., 1989, as cited in Filaretova et al., 2006). On the contrary, glucocorticoid excess induces hypertension in human and rats. Hypertension is seen in patients with excessive glucocorticoid secretion, occurring in most patients with Cushing's syndrome and in patients with glucocorticoid treatment (Nieman et al., 1985, as cited in Filaretova et al., 2006). It was reported that a patient with Cushing's syndrome was treated successfully with glucocorticoid receptor antagonist RU-38486 at high dose (Nieman et al., 1985, as cited in Filaretova et al., 2006). Experimental data obtained in adrenalectomized animals with or without glucocorticoid replacement (Darlington et al., 1989; Darlington & Tehrani, 1997, as cited in Filaretova et al., 2006) as well as in rats with occupation of glucocorticoids receptors by RU-38486 (Grunfeld & Eloy, 1987, as cited in Filaretova et al., 2006) confirm and further develop clinical observations about the important contribution of glucocorticoid hormones to the regulation of blood pressure.

Under certain conditions, maintaining blood pressure is especially important for the maintenance of gastric mucosal integrity. There is evidence showing the linear correlation between the graded systemic hypotension and the mucosal blood flow as an important defensive factor (Guth, 1992). It was hypothesized that the blood flow to the stomach, a nonessential organ, decreases more rapidly and at an early stage of graded hypotension, in order to maintain blood flow to the essential organs such as the brain and kidney. The decrease in submucosal and mucosal blood flow during stress is an important factor, leading to mucosal ischemia, impairment in tissue resistance, and subsequent ulceration in stressed animals (Guth, 1992; Tarnasky et al., 1990). These facts allow us to assume that maintaining systemic blood pressure by glucocorticoids may be fundamental to their beneficial action on gastric blood flow and, consequently, on gastric mucosal integrity.

Utilizing an in vivo microscopy technique for the direct visualization of the gastric microcirculation (Filaretova et al., 1999) as well as methods creating the alterations in glucocorticoid supply, we examined whether gastric microcirculation and arterial blood pressure are involved in the mechanism of gastroprotective action of glucocorticoids during 3 hour water immersion-restraint stress. To this end the effects of deficiency of glucocorticoid production followed by corticosterone replacement on the stress-induced gastric microcirculation, systemic arterial pressure and gastric erosion were investigated. The stress-induced glucocorticoid production was inhibited by a single high dose of cortisol injected one week before stress. Gastric microcirculation was evaluated by measurement of the blood flow velocity in submucosal and mucosal microvessels (Filaretova et al., 1999).

Water immersion-restraint stress caused decrease in blood flow velocity in submucosal and mucosal gastric microvessels. The deficiency of glucocorticoids during water immersion-restraint stress promoted the stress-induced decrease of blood flow velocity in submucosal and mucosal microvessels, and corticosterone replacement prevented this effect (Filaretova et al. 1999, 2004). The results suggest that glucocorticoids released during water immersion-restraint stress maintain gastric blood flow during the stress. Our data also confirms that the decrease in gastric blood flow is associated with the reduction in systemic blood pressure. Mean systemic blood pressure in stressed rats with glucocorticoid deficiency was about 60 mm Hg, and these animals had a very low gastric blood flow velocity and large erosion area. Corticosterone replacement increased both systemic blood pressure and gastric blood flow and, as a result, improved the resistance of gastric mucosa to ulcerogenic stress action. It means that the improvement of gastric blood supply by glucocorticoids is provided, at least partly, through their beneficial action on systemic blood circulation. The data suggests that the gastroprotective actions of glucocorticoids during water immersion-restraint stress may be provided by the maintenance of gastric blood flow that may be brought about by their beneficial effect on arterial blood pressure (Filaretova et al. 1999, 2004).

Thus, glucocorticoids released during activation of the HPA axis may contribute to protection of the gastric mucosa by maintaining general body homeostasis, including glucose levels and systemic blood pressure, which could be a basis for their beneficial influence on gastric mucosal integrity.

## 2.4 How gastroprotective action of glucocorticoids may be transformed to proulcerogenic one

Thus, in general glucocorticoid hormones may have dual action on the stomach: physiological gastroprotective and pathological proulcerogenic one. In al physiologic conditions, even in acute stress situations, glucocorticoids have an adaptive effect on the stomach and, therefore, are gastroprotective, while in some situations their action on the gastric mucosa may become proulcerogenic. It is important to understand how physiological gastroprotective action can be transformed to pathological proulcerogenic effect.

Because the maintenance of glucose homeostasis by glucocorticoids could be fundamental to their gastroprotective action (Filaretova et al., 2002c, 2006), it was reasonable to assume that glucocorticoid-induced disturbance of glucose regulation, observed in clinical and experimental situations (Subramanian & Trence, 2007, as cited in Filaretova et al., 2009a), may contribute to ulcerogenic action of glucocorticoids on the gastric mucosa. We supposed that short-term maintenance of blood glucose level provides the gastroprotective action of glucocorticoids, while long-lasting maintenance of blood glucose level or long-lasting hyperglycemia through a disturbance of carbohydrate regulation may account, at least partly, for the ulcerogenic action of glucocorticoids. Thus, we hypothesized that glucocorticoid-induced long-lasting maintenance of blood glucose level accompanied by their catabolic effects may be responsible for the transformation of gastroprotective action of glucocorticoids to their proulcerogenic effect.

We verified the hypothesis investigating the effects of exogenous glucocorticoid and dexamethasone was selected for this aim as synthethic long-acting glucocorticoid. Stress and indomethacin were used as ulcerogenic stimuli because both of them are considered as most significant ulcerogenic factors in human (Laine et al., 2008). It is important to note that both stimuli were applied to rats after 24 hour fasting. Taking into consideration that action of exogenous glucocorticoids on the gastric mucosa is depended on the dose (Laine et al., 2008) first, we investigated dose-dependent effects of dexamethasone. Surprisingly, dexamethasone, even at pharmacological dose 10 mg/kg protected the gastric mucosa against stress- and indomethacin-induced injury, at least, during first hour of its action (Filaretova et al., 2009a,b).

Because dexamethasone at the dose of 1 mg/kg decreased the gastric erosion area and maintained blood glucose level in fasted stressed or indomethacin-pretreated rats (in the case of its injection 1 h before the onset of cold-restraint or indomethacin administration) this dose has been selected for the next step, time-dependent study. The results obtained demonstrate that single injection of dexamethasone at a dose of 1 mg/kg may attenuate or aggravate both cold-restraint- and indomethacin-induced gastric erosion depending on the duration of its action before the onset of the stress or indomethacin, respectively. Short-lasting (1-12 hours) action of dexamethasone attenuated cold-restraint- and indomethacin-induced gastric ulceration. However long-lasting (21-24 hours) dexamethasone action resulted in an aggravation of cold-restraint- and indomethacin-induced gastric erosion (Filaretova et al., 2009a,b). The findings suggest that manifestation of gastroprotective or ulcerogenic action of glucocorticoids used at the same dose may be dependent very much on the time interval between the hormonal injection and onset of ulcerogenic stimulus. Prolongation of dexamethasone action may lead to enhancement of gastric mucosal susceptibility to ulcerogenic action of cold-restaint or indomethacin.

Both short- and long-lasting dexamethasone actions resulted in maintenance of blood glucose level in fasted stressed and indomethacin-treated rats. Dexamethasone-induced long-lasting maintenance of blood glucose level accompanied with the signs of catabolic effects. It should be note that dexamethasone-induced increase in the lost of body weight during fasting preceded the appearance of its ulcerogenic action. Thymus weight was used as another marker of dexamethasone-induced catabolic effects. It is known that glucocorticoids at pharmacological doses tend to kill off many of the thymus cells. This phenomenon is the basis for the immunosuppressive use of glucocorticoids (Young et al., 1981, as cited in Filaretova et al., 2009a). It was shown that dexamethasone accelerates the rate of apoptosis in thymocytes (de Belle et al., 1994, as cited in Filaretova et al., 2009a). According to our data in distinguish from the body weight changes the thymus weight changes started earlier. These findings are in agreement with the data of literature showed that metabolic glucocorticoid effects in thymus cells evolve more rapidly comparing those in other target cells. The most prominent effect of glucocorticoid in thymus cells is a large inhibition of glucose transport that reaches 25-30% by about 30 min after the hormone addition. The metabolic inhibitions followed by cell destruction (Young et al., 1981, as cited in Filaretova et al., 2009a).

Dexamethasone treatment inhibited cold-restaint- and indomethacin-induced corticosterone production. Because according to our data deficiency of corticosterone aggravates cold-restaint- and indomethacin-induced gastric erosion, it is quite possible that simultaneous corticosterone deficiency and consequences of disturbances of carbohydrate regulation contributed together to proulcerogenic effect of long-lasting dexamethasone treatment.

We prolonged our study till the 7th day to clarify the questions how long dexamethasone effects may be continued and whether they are reversible. It was found that the dexamethasone-induced proulcerogenic action was continued till the 5th day and then, on the 7th day was disappeared. The restoration of stress- or indomethacin-induced corticosterone production, which preceded the restoration of normal susceptibility of the gastric mucosa to ulcerogenic action of cold-restraint, may contribute to this event. The gradual restoration of normal body and spleen weight is a good symptom of reversibility dexamethasone-induced catabolic effects. Disappearance of dexamethasone-induced maintenance of blood glucose level preceded the restoration of normal body and spleen weight.

In our experimental situations the transformation of gastroprotective action of dexamethasone to proulcerogenic one occurred 18 h after its administration, but it is clear that in general this time interval depends on many factors, including a kind of glucocorticoid and its dose, a specificity of situation. As far back as 1950 it was noted on the base of clinical observations that it needs at least 5-7 days of corticosteroids use before appearance of ulcer symptoms (Sandweiss, 1954, as cited in Filaretova et al., 2009a). One of the principles for minimizing undesirable side effects of glucocorticoid therapy is "keep treatment as short as possible, since treatment lasting 5 to 7 days shows fewer side effects" (Longui, 2007, as cited in Filaretova et al., 2009a). It is more often glucocorticoid-induced ulcer symptoms appeared after much more long hormonal treatment. Our results allow us to speculate that glucocorticoid-induced disturbance of carbohydrate regulation, which needs time for developing, contributes to appearance of ulcer symptoms after long-lasting hormonal therapy. It means that control of glucose regulation and its correction in case of need may be considered as useful approach minimizing ulcerogenic side effect of glucocorticoid therapy.

In conclusion, the data obtained so far suggest that short-lasting maintenance of blood glucose levels may be responsible for the gastroprotective action of glucocorticoids, while glucocorticoid-induced long-lasting maintenance of blood glucose levels accompanied with the signs of their catabolic effect and glucocorticoid-induced corticosterone deficiency may be responsible, at least partly, for the transformation of gastroprotective action of glucocorticoids to their proulcerogenic effect (Filaretova et al. 2009a, 2009b). Further investigation of detailed mechanisms underlying proulcerogenic glucocorticoid action is the task of our future studies. We take into consideration other, additional, possibilities for explanation the question how physiological gastroprotective action can be transformed to pathological proulcerogenic effect.

## 3. Conclusion

According to our data an acute stress-induced increase of glucocorticoids has a gastroprotective action against stress-induced gastric injury but is not ulcerogenic, as it has generally been considered for some decades. Beneficial action of high levels of endogenous glucocorticoids released during acute stress on the stomach is opposite to the harmful actions of exogenous glucocorticoids at pharmacological doses used as a hormonal therapy. NSAIDs as well as other ulcerogenic stimuli, similar to stress, induce an increase in glucocorticoid production that in turn helps the gastric mucosa to resist the harmful actions of these stimuli. It is assumed that the adaptive action of glucocorticoids released during acute activation of the HPA axis may be applied to the gastric mucosa. Glucocorticoids exert gastroprotective actions in co-operation with PGs, NO and capsaicin-sensitive sensory neurons: their compensatory gastroprotective action is observed when the protective mechanism provided by either of these factors is impared. Gastroprotective effects of glucocorticoids may be mediated by multiple actions, including maintenance of gastric mucosal blood flow, mucus production, and attenuation of enhanced gastric motility and microvascular permeability. The contribution of glucocorticoids to gastroprotection is tightly related with their contribution to general body homeostasis. Glucocorticoids released during activation of the HPA axis may contribute to protection of the gastric mucosa by maintaining general body homeostasis, including glucose levels and systemic blood pressure, which could be a basis for their beneficial influence on gastric mucosal integrity. These findings further support idea that gastroprotective action of glucocorticoids is an essential element of their general adaptive action. In conclusion, the results obtained in our studies suggest that glucocorticoids released during acute activation of the HPA axis are naturally occurring protective factors that play an important role in maintenance of the gastric mucosal integrity. In turn, it means that acute activation of the HPA axis is a gastroprotective component of stress response.

## 4. Acknowledgment

I would like to show my thanks to Professor A. Filaretov for supporting this field of research in the very beginning; to my colleagues Dr. T. Podvigina, Dr. P. Bobryshev, Dr. T. Bagaeva, Dr. O. Morozova and my long-standing assistance Mrs. T. Kolbasova for their active participation in developing this research study; to Professor G. Makara from the Institute of Experimental Medicine (Budapest) and Professor K. Takeuchi from the Kyoto Pharmaceutical University for making it possible to continue this research in their laboratories and for their kind support. This study was supported by grants of RFBR-10-04-00605; FNM RAS-2009-2011; DBS RAS-2009-2011.

## 5. References

Alexandrova, M. (1994). Stress induced tyrosine aminotransferase activity via glucocorticoid receptor. *Horm Metab Res*, Vol.26, No.2, (February 1994), pp. 97–99, ISSN 0170-5903

Bobryshev, P.Yu., Bagaeva, T.R., Podvigina, T.T. & Filaretova, L. (2005). Gastroprotective action of glucocorticoid hormones in rats with desensitization of capsaicin-sensitive sensory neurons. *Inflammopharmacology*, Vol.13, No.1-3, (February 2005), pp. 217-228, ISSN 0925-4692

Chan, O., Chan, S., Inouye, K., Shum, K., Matthews, S.G. & Vranic, M. (2002). Diabetes impairs hypothalamo-pituitary-adrenal (HPA) responses to hypoglycemia, and insulin treatment normalizes HPA but not epinephrine responses. *Diabetes*, Vol.51, No.6, (June 2002), pp. 1681-1689, ISSN 0012-1797

Derelanko, M. J. & Long, J. F. (1982). Influence of prednisolone on ethanol-induced gastric injury in the rat. *Dig Dis Sci*, Vol.27, No.2, (February 1982), pp. 149-154, ISSN 0163-2116

Filaretova, L. (1990). The dependence of the formation of stress gastric ulcers on the function of hypothalamo-hypophyseal-adrenocortical system. *Sechenov Physiol J USSR*, Vol.76, No.11, (November 1990), pp. 1594-1600, ISSN 0015-329X

Filaretova, L.P. (2006). The hypothalamic-pituitary-adrenocortical system: hormonal brain-gut interaction and gastroprotection. *Autonomic Neurosci: Basic and Clinical*, Vol.125, No.1-2, (April 2006), pp. 86-93, ISSN 1566-0702

Filaretova, L.P., Bagaeva, T.R. & Makara, G.B. (2002a). Aggravation of nonsteroidal antiinflammatory drug gastropathy by glucocorticoid deficiency or blockade of glucocorticoid receptor in rats. *Life Sci*, Vol.71, No.21, (October 2002), pp. 2457-2468, ISSN 0024-3205

Filaretova, L.P., Filaretov, A. & Makara, G.B. (1998). Corticosterone increase inhibits stress-induced gastric erosions in rats. *Am J Physiol*, Vol.274, No.6, (June 1998), pp. G1024-G1030, ISSN 0193-1857

Filaretova, L., Bagaeva, T., Amagase, K. & Takeuchi, K. (2008). Contribution of glucocorticoids to protective influence of preconditioning mild stress against stress-induced gastric erosions. *Ann N Y Acad Sci*, Vol.1148, (December 2008), pp. 209-212, ISSN 0077-8923

Filaretova, L., Bagaeva, T., Podvigina, T. & Makara, G. (2001a). Various ulcerogenic stimuli are potentiated by glucocorticoid deficiency in rats. *J Physiol Paris*, Vol.95, No.1-6, (January-December 2001), pp. 59-65, ISSN 0928-4257

Filaretova, L.P., Maltcev, A.N., Bogdanov, A.I. & Levkovich, Yu.I. (1999). Role of gastric microcirculation in the gastroprotection by glucocorticoids released during water-restraint stress in rats. *Chin J Physiol*, Vol.42, No.3, (September 1999), pp. 145-152, ISSN 0304-4920

Filaretova, L., Morozova, O., Bagaeva, T. & Podvigina T. (2009a). From gastroprotective to proulcerogenic action of glucocorticoids on the gastric mucosa. *J Physiol Pharmacol*, Vol.60, Supp.l 7, (December 2009), pp. 79-86, ISSN 0867-5910

Filaretova, L., Podvigina, T., Bagaeva, T. & Makara G. (2001b). Gastroprotective action of glucocorticoids during the formation and the healing of indomethacin-induced gastric erosions in rats. *J Physiol Paris*, Vol.95, No.1-6, (January-December 2001), pp. 201-208, ISSN 0928-4257

Filaretova, L., Podvigina, T., Bagaeva, T. & Morozova, O. (2009b). Dual action of glucocorticoid hormones on the gastric mucosa: how the gastroprotective action can be transformed to the ulcerogenic one. *Inflammopharmacology*, Vol.17, No.1, (February 2009), pp. 15-22, ISSN 0925-4692

Filaretova, L., Tanaka A., Komoike, Y. & Takeuchi, K. (2002b). Selective cyclooxygenase-2 inhibitor induces gastric mucosal damage in adrenalectomized rats. *Inflammopharmacology*, Vol.10, No.4-6, pp. 413-422, ISSN 0925-4692

Filaretova, L., Bobryshev, P., Bagaeva, T., Podvigina, T. & Takeuchi K. (2007). Compensatory gastroprotective role of glucocorticoid hormones during inhibition of prostaglandin and nitric oxide production and desensitization of capsaicin-sensitive sensory neurons. *Inflammopharmacology*, Vol.15, No.4, (August 2007), pp. 146-153, ISSN 0925-4692

Filaretova, L.P., Podvigina, T.T., Bagaeva, T.R., Tanaka, A. & Takeuchi, K. (2005). Gastroprotective action of glucocorticoid hormones during NSAID treatment. *Inflammopharmacology*, Vol.13, No.1-3, (February 2005), pp. 27-43, ISSN 0925-4692

Filaretova, L.P., Podvigina, T.T., Bagaeva, T.R., Tanaka A. & Takeuchi K. (2004). Mechanisms underlying gastroprotective action of glucocorticoids released in response to ulcerogenic stress factors. *Ann NY Acad Sci*, Vol.1018, (June 2004), pp. 288-293, ISSN 0077-8923

Filaretova, L., Podvigina, T., Bobryshev, P., Bagaeva, T., Tanaka, A. & Takeuchi K. (2006). Hypothalamic-pituitary-adrenocortical axis: the hidden gold in gastric mucosal homeostasis. *Inflammopharmacology*, Vol. 14, No.5-6, (December 2006), pp. 207-213, ISSN 0925-4692

Filaretova, L., Tanaka, A., Miyazawa, T., Kato, S. & Takeuchi K. (2002c). Mechanisms by which endogenous glucocorticoids protects against indomethacin-induced gastric injury in rats. *Am J Physiol*, Vol.283, No.5, (November 2002), pp. G1082-G1089, ISSN 0193-1857

Glavin, G.B., Murison, R., Overmier, J.B., Pare, W.P., Bakke, H.K., Henke, P.G. & Hernandez, D.E. (1991). The neurobiology of stress ulcers. *Brain Res Brain Res Rev*, Vol.16, No.3, (September-December 1991), pp. 301-343.

Guth, P.H. (1992). Current concept in gastric microcirculatory pathophysiology. *Yale J Biol Med*, Vol.65, No.6, (November-December 1992), pp. 677-688, ISSN 0044-0086

Hawkey, C.J. (2000). Nonsteroidal anti-inflammatory drug gastropathy. *Gastroenterology*, Vol.119, No.2, (August 2000), pp. 521-535, ISSN 0016-5085

Hernandez, D.E., Adcock, J.W., Nemeroff, C.B., Prange & A.J. Jr. (1984). The role of the adrenal gland in cytoprotection against stress-induced gastric ulcers in rats. *J Neurosci Res*, Vol.11, No. 2, pp. 193-201, ISSN 0360-4012

Holzer, P. (1998). Neural emergency system in the stomach. *Gastroenterology*, Vol.114, No.4, (April 1998), pp. 823-839, ISSN 0016-5085

Laine, L., Takeuchi, K. & Tarnawski, A. (2008). Gastric mucosal defense and cytoprotection: bench to bedside. *Gastroenterology*, Vol.135, No.1, (July 2008), pp. 41-60, ISSN 0016-5085

Luo, J.C., Chang, .F.Y., Chen, T.S., Ng, Y.Y., Lin, H.C., Lu, C.L., Chen, C.Y., Lin, H.Y. & Lee S.D. (2009). Gastric mucosal injury in systemic lupus erythematosus patients receiving pulse methylprednisolone therapy. *Br J Clin Pharmacol*, Vol.68, No.2, (August 2009), pp. 252-259, ISSN 0306-5251

McCafferty, D.M., Granger, D.N. & Wallace, J.L. (1995). Indomethacin-induced gastric injury and leukocyte adherence in arthritic versus healthy rats. *Gastroenterology*, Vol.109, No.4, (October 2005), pp. 1173-1180, ISSN 0016-5085

Olsen, M., Christensen, S., Riis, A. & Thomsen, R.W. (2010). Preadmission use of systemic glucocorticoids and 30-day mortality following bleeding peptic ulcer: a population-based cohort study. *Am J Ther*, Vol.17, No.1, (January-February 2010), pp. 23-29, ISSN 1075-2765

Perretti, M., Mugridge, K.G., Wallace, J.L. & Parénte, L. (1992). Reduction of aspirin-induced gastric damage in rats by interleukin-1 beta: possible involvement of endogenous corticosteroids. *J Pharmacol Exp Ther* , Vol.61, No.3, (June 1992), pp. 1238-1247, ISSN 0022-3565

Selye, H. (1967) *In Vivo. The case for supramolecular biology presented in six informal, illustrated lectures*. Liveright, New York, US

Szabo, S., Callagher, G.T., Horner, H.C., Frankel, P.W., Underwood, R.H., Konturek, S.J., Brzozowski T. & Trier JS. (1983). Role of the adrenal cortex in gastric mucosal protection by prostaglandins, sulfhydryls, and cimetidine in the rat. *Gastroenterology*, Vol.85, No.6, (December 1983), pp. 1384-1390, ISSN 0016-5085

Takeuchi, Y., Takahashi, M. & Fuchikami, J. (2008) Vulnerability of gastric mucosa to prednisolone in rats chronically exposed to cigarette smoke. *J Pharmacol Sci*, Vol.106, No.4, (April 2008), pp. 585-592, ISSN 1347-8613

Takeuchi, K., Nishiwaki, H., Okada, M., Niida, H. & Okabe, S. (1989). Bilateral adrenalectomy worsens gastric mucosal lesions induced by indomethacin in the rat. Role of enhanced gastric motility. *Gastroenterology*, Vol.97, No.2, (August 1989), pp. 284-293, ISSN 0016-5085

Takeuchi, K., Ueshima, K., Hironaka, Y., Fujioka, Y., Matsumoto, J. & Okabe S. (1991). Oxygen free radicals and lipid peroxidation in the pathogenesis of gastric mucosal lesions induced by indomethacin in rats. *Digestion*, Vol.49, No.3, pp. 175-184, ISSN 0012-2823

Tanaka, A., Hatazawa, R., Takahira, Y., Izumi, N., Filaretova, L. & Takeuchi, K. (2007) Preconditioning stress prevents cold restraint stress-induced gastric lesions in rats: roles of COX-1, COX-2, and PLA2. *Dig Dis Sci*, Vol.52, No.2, (February 2007), pp. 478-487, ISSN 0163-2116

Tarnasky, P.R., Livingston, E.H., Jacobs, K.M., Zimmerman, B.J., Guth, P.H. & Garrick, T.R. (1990). Role of oxyradicals in cold water immersion restraint-induced gastric mucosal injury in the rat. *Dig Dis Sci*, Vol.35, No.2, (February 1990), pp. 173-177, ISSN 0163-2116

Wallace, J.L. (1997). Nonsteroidal anti-inflammatory drugs and gastroenteropathy: the second hundred years. *Gastroenterology*, Vol.112, No.3, (March 1997), pp. 1000-1016, ISSN 0016-5085

Whitehouse, M.W. (2011). Anti-inflammatory glucocorticoid drugs: reflections after 60 years. *Inflammopharmacology*, Vol.19, No.1, (February 2011), pp. 1-19, ISSN 0925-4692

Whittle, B.J.R., Lopez-Belmonte, J. & Moncada, S. (1990). Regulation of gastric mucosal integrity by endogenous nitric oxide: interactions with prostanoids and sensory neuropeptides in the rats. *Br J Pharmacol*, Vol.99, No.3, (March 1990), pp. 606-611, ISSN 0007-1188

# 13

# *Helicobacter pylori* and Host Response

Mario M. D'Elios[1] and Marina de Bernard[2]
*[1]Department of Internal Medicine, University of Florence*
*[2]Venetian Institute of Molecular Medicine, University of Padua*
*Italy*

## 1. Introduction

*Helicobacter pylori*, a pathogen infecting the gastric antrum of half of the adult population worldwide, is thought to be the major cause of acute and chronic gastroduodenal pathologies, including gastric and duodenal ulcer, gastric cancer and gastric B-cell lymphoma of mucosa-associated lymphoid tissue (MALT) (Marshall et al., 1994; Parsonnet et al., 1991; Wotherspoon et al., 1991). Despite a vigorous humoral response against *H. pylori* antigens, most of infected subjects fails to eliminate the pathogen spontaneously. As in other infectious diseases, besides the virulence of the pathogen, both the natural and the specific immune responses of the host are crucial for determining the outcome of the infection. The immune system has evolved different defence mechanisms against pathogens. The first defensive line is provided by 'natural' immunity, including phagocytes, T cell receptor (TCR) $\gamma\delta$+ T cells, natural killer (NK) cells, mast cells, neutrophils and eosinophils, as well as complement components and pro-inflammatory cytokines, such as interferons (IFNs), interleukin (IL)-1, IL-6, IL-12, IL-18 and tumor necrosis factor (TNF)-$\alpha$. The more specialized TCR $\alpha\beta$+ T lymphocytes provide the second defence wall. These cells account for the specific immunity, which results in specialized types of immune responses which allow vertebrates to recognize and clear (or at least control) infectious agents in different body compartments. Viruses growing within infected cells, are faced through the killing of their host cells by CD8+ cytotoxic T lymphocytes (CTL). Most of microbial components are endocytosed by antigen-presenting cells (APC), processed and presented preferentially to CD4+ T helper (Th) cells. Th cells co-operate with B cells for the production of antibodies which opsonize extracellular microbes and neutralize their exotoxins. This branch of the specific Th cell-mediated immune response is known as humoral immunity. Other microbes, however, survive within macrophages in spite of the unfavorable microenvironment and antigen-activated CD4+ Th cells are required to activate macrophages, whose reactive metabolites and TNF-$\alpha$ finally lead to the destruction of the pathogens. This branch of the specific Th cell-mediated response is known as cell-mediated immunity (CMI).

Most of successful immune responses involve both humoral and cell-mediated immunity. CD4+ Th cells can develop different polarized patterns of cytokine production, such as type-1 or Th1, type-2 or Th2, type-17 or Th17 (Mosmann et al., 1986; Del Prete et al., 1991; Korn et al., 2009).

Th1 cells produce IFN-γ, IL-2 and TNF-β, elicit macrophage activation and delayed-type hypersensitivity (DTH) reactions, whereas Th2 cells produce IL-4, IL-5, IL-10 and IL-13, which act as growth/differentiation factors for B cells, eosinophils and mast cells and inhibit several macrophage functions (Del Prete, 1998). A new subset of Th cells, named Th17 cells, producing IL-17 alone or in combination with IFN-γ, has been identified recently (Weaver et al., 2006). Th17 cells play a critical role in protection against microbial challenges, particularly extracellular bacteria and fungi (Bettelli et al., 2007).

However, most of T cells do not express a polarized cytokine profile; such T cells (coded as Th0) represent a heterogenous population of partially differentiated effector cells consisting of multiple subsets which secrete different combinations of both Th1 and Th2 cytokines. The cytokine response at effector level can remain mixed or further differentiate into the Th1 or the Th2 pathway under the influence of polarizing signals from the microenvironment. Human Th1 and Th2 cells e.g. also differ for their responsiveness to cytokines. Both Th1 and Th2 cells proliferate in response to IL-2, but Th2 are more responsive to IL-4 than Th1; on the other hand IFN-γ tend to inhibit the proliferative response of Th2 cells (Del Prete et al., 1993). Th1 and Th2 cells substantially differ for their cytolytic potential and mode of help for B-cell antibody synthesis. Th2 clones, usually devoid of cytolytic activity, induce IgM, IgG, IgA, and IgE synthesis by autologous B cells in the presence of the specific antigen, with a response which is proportional to the number of Th2 cells added to B cells. In contrast, Th1 clones, most of which are cytolytic, provide B-cell help for IgM, IgG, IgA (but not IgE) synthesis at low T-cell/B-cell ratios. At high T-cell/B-cell ratios there is a decline in B-cell help related to the Th1-mediated lytic activity against antigen-presenting autologous B-cells (Del Prete et al., 1991b). Th1 and Th2 cells exhibit different ability to activate cells of the monocyte-macrophage lineage. Th1, but not Th2, help monocytes to express tissue factor (TF) production and procoagulant activity (PCA). In this type of Th cell-monocyte cooperation, both cell-to-cell contact and Th1 cytokines (namely IFN-γ), are required for optimal TF synthesis and PCA, whereas Th2-derived IL-4, IL-10 and IL-13 are strongly inhibitory (Del Prete et al., 1995a).

The factors responsible for the Th cell polarization into a predominant Th profile have extensively been investigated. Current evidence suggests that Th1, Th2 and Th17 cells develop from the same Th-cell precursor under the influence of mechanisms associated with antigen presentation (Kamogawa et al., 1993; Korn et al. 2009). Both environmental and genetic factors influence the Th1 or Th2 differentiation mainly by determining the 'leader cytokine' in the microenvironment of the responding Th-cell. IL-4 is the most powerful stimulus for Th2 differentiation, whereas IL-12, IL-18 and IFNs favor Th1 development (D'Elios et al., 1999). A role has been demonstrated for the site of antigen presentation, the physical form of the immunogen, the type of adjuvant, and the dose of antigen (Constant et al., 1997). Several microbial products (particularly from intracellular bacteria) induce Th1-dominated responses because they stimulate IL-12 production. IFN-γ and IFN-α favor the Th1 development by enhancing IL-12 secretion by macrophages and maintaining the expression of functional IL-12 receptors on Th cells (Szabo et al., 1995). IL-18 sustains the expression of IL-12Rβ, indicating that IL-12 and IL-18 synergize in inducing and maintaining Th1 development (Xu et al., 1998). On the other hand, IL-11 and PGE2 would promote Th2 cell polarization (D'Elios et al., 1999). Other microbial products and stimuli induce a preferential activation of Th17 responses (Codolo et al., 2008a; Korn et al., 2009).

## 2. Immune responses in *H. pylori* infection

### 2.1 Innate reponses in *H. pylori* infection

Most of *H. pylori*-infected patients are unable to clear the pathogen, leading to postulate that *H. pylori* might somehow hamper the host immune response. It has been shown that *H. pylori* may interfere with protective immunity by acting on professional APC through the release of its vacuolating cytotoxin (VacA), which impairs antigen processing and the subsequent priming of efficient immune response (Molinari et al., 1998). The failure of clearing *H. pylori* from the gastric environment almost invariably leads to chronic antral gastritis. Colonization of the stomach by *H. pylori* is consistently accompanied by inflammation of the gastric mucosa, which varies according to the host immune reaction against the pathogen. Once in the stomach, *H. pylori* first activates the natural immunity cellular compartment, represented by macrophages and neutrophils. IL-8 expression by gastric epithelium following contact with *H. pylori* plays a major role in the initial host response to the bacterium, since this chemokine acts as a strong chemotactic and activating factor for neutrophils, which in turn contribute to initiate and expand the inflammatory cascade (Crabtree et al., 1993). Furthermore, certain *H. pylori* components, such as HP-NAP, the lipopolysaccharide, VacA or the cytotoxin-associated protein CagA, as well as the urease or the heat shock proteins (HSP) are allowed to cross the damaged layer of gastric cells and to come in contact with macrophages. Activation of macrophages, mainly exerted by HP-NAP, results in the release of several cytokines, including IL-12, IL-1, IL-6, TNF-α, IFN-α and chemokines, such as IL-8. Moreover, also neutrophils are able to produce IL-12 and IL-23 in response to HP-NAP (Amedei et al, 2006). This is an important step of the natural history of *H. pylori* infection, because the local cytokine "milieu", particularly the IL-12 and IL-23 produced by cells of the natural immunity is crucial in driving the subsequent specific T-cell response into a more or less polarized Th1 pattern. Furthermore *H. pylori* may results in activation not only of TLR receptor (e.g. by HP-NAP) but also of the cytoplasmic nucleotide-binding oligomerization domain (NOD)1, member of the NOD-like receptors (NLR) family. In particular, *H. pylori* peptidoglycan, acting in concert with the bacterial type IV "syringe", encoded by the cag PAI, following the engagement of NOD1 in gastric epithelial cells, leads to the generation of protective Th1 responses (Kaparakis et al., 2007; Pritz et al., 2007; Watanabe et al., 2010).

### 2.2 Th response in *H. pylori* infection

The The pattern of cytokines produced by the immunological active cells recruited in the antral mucosa of *H. pylori* -infected patients with peptic ulcer were analyzed by RT-PCR. Antral biopsies from patients with ulcer showed IL-12, IFN-γ, and TNF-α but not IL-4, mRNA expression, whereas virtually no mRNA encoding for cytokines was found in the mucosa of *H. pylori* -negative controls (D'Elios *et al.*, 1997b). In the same biopsies, immunohistochemistry showed remarkable in vivo activation of IFN-γ, but not IL-4, producing T cells (D'Elios *et al.*, 1997c).

Several studies have examined the antigen specificity and the cytokines produced by the *H. pylori*-specific Th cells derived from the antral mucosa of *H. pylori* -infected patients. Gastric biopsies were pre-cultured in IL-2-conditioned medium in order to preferentially expand T cells activated in vivo, and T-cell blasts were cloned according to a high efficiency technique allowing the growth of virtually every single T cell (D'Elios *et al.*, 1997).

In *H. pylori* infected patients the proportion of *H. pylori* -reactive gastric T-cells in each patient was variable, ranging from 2 to 33% of CD4+ clones. The majority of gastric-derived T cells were specific for CagA or for HP-NAP, whereas a minority were specific for VacA, for urease, or for HSP (D'Elios *et al.*, 1997b; Amedei *et al.*, 2006). Among the *H. pylori* - reactive clones from low grade gastric B-cell lymphoma (MALToma), 25% were specific for urease, 4% for VacA, and 71% proliferated only to *H. pylori* lysate (D'Elios *et al.*, 1999). These data suggest that in MALToma urease is an important target of the gastric T-cell response and that some other still undefined antigens of *H. pylori* may be relevant in driving Th and B-cell activation and proliferation.

In peptic ulcer patients, in vitro stimulation with the appropriate *H. pylori* antigens induced the great majority of *H. pylori*-reactive Th clones to produce IFN-γ but not IL-4 (expressing thus a polarized Th1 profile). Under the same experimental conditions, most of *H. pylori*-specific T-cell clones derived from uncomplicated chronic gastritis showed a Th0 phenotype, producing IL-4 and/or IL-5 together with IFN-γ, whereas only one third of *H. pylori*-specific gastric T cells was polarized towards the Th1 effectors (D'Elios et al., 1997d). Also in MALToma patients most of *H. pylori*-specific T cell clones derived from the gastric mucosa were able to produce both Th1 and Th2 cytokines (D'Elios et al., 1999).

Detailed analysis of the antigen-induced B-cell help exerted in vitro by *H. pylori*-reactive gastric T-cell clones provided new information on the mechanisms possibly associated with the onset of low-grade B-cell lymphoma of the gastric MALT, rare complication of chronic *H. pylori* infection. Functional analysis of *H. pylori*-specific Th clones derived from the gastric antrum of infected patients showed that *in vitro* stimulation with the appropriate *H. pylori* antigen resulted in the expression of their helper function for B-cell proliferation and Ig production (D'Elios et al., 1997b). This can provide convincing explanation for the intense B-cell activation in the lymphoid tissue associated with, or newly generated in, the antral mucosa during chronic *H. pylori* infection. Such a sustained *H. pylori* -induced T cell-dependent B-cell activation is responsible for the high levels of specific antibodies found in the serum of *H. pylori* -infected patients (Rathbone et al., 1986; Crabtree et al., 1995). In chronic gastritis patients either with or without ulcer, the helper function to B cells exerted by *H. pylori* antigen-stimulated gastric T-cell clones was negatively regulated by the concomitant cytolytic killing of B cells (D'Elios et al., 1997b). In contrast, gastric T-cell clones from MALToma patients were surprisingly unable to down-modulate their antigen-induced help for B cell proliferation (D'Elios et al., 1999). Indeed, none of the gastric *H. pylori*-specific T-cell clones from MALToma was able to express perforin-mediated cytotoxicity against autologous B cells. Moreover, most Th clones from uncomplicated chronic gastritis induced Fas-Fas ligand-mediated apoptosis in target cells, whereas only a minority of *H. pylori* - specific gastric clones from MALToma patients were able to induce apoptosis in target cells, including autologous B cells (D'Elios et al., 1999).

There are a number of postulated mechanisms whereby *H. pylori* can induce mucosal injury, and some are certainly related to many of the *H. pylori* pathogenic products described (Telford et al., 1994; Tomb et al., 1997). Indeed in many infectious (and non-infectious) diseases, the type of immune response elicited is important for protection, but, under certain circumstances, it may also contribute to the pathogenesis of disease. A number of studies from different research groups seem to agree on that Th1 polarization of immune response to *H. pylori* is associated with more severe disease (D'Elios et al., 1997b; Hauer et al., 1997; Bamford et al., 1998; Sommer et al., 1998). Preferential activation of Th1 cells and the subsequent production of their cytokines, namely IFN-$\gamma$ and TNF-$\alpha$, in the absence of Th2 cytokines can potentiate gastrin secretion and pepsinogen release, as observed in vitro in animal models (Weigert et al., 1996). Data from our laboratory indicate that also in humans TNF-$\alpha$ and IFN-$\gamma$ are able to dose-dependently stimulate pepsinogen release from isolated gastric chief cells. In this model, simultaneous addition of IL-4 was not synergic, rather inhibitory, on the IFN-$\gamma$-induced pepsinogen release by chief cells, whereas it had no effect on the pepsinogen release induced by TNF-$\alpha$ (D'Elios et al., 1998). Moreover Th1 cells are able to induce both tissue factor production by monocytes (Del Prete et al., 1995a) and the activation of coagulation cascade, followed by microvascular thrombosis and consequent alteration of epithelial cell integrity. A number of studies suggest that chronic inflammation (e.g. triggered by infectious agents like *H. pylori*) may be important in the pathogenesis of atherothrombosis (Elizalde et al., 1997; Danesh et al., 1997). Indirect support to the hypothesis that the Th1-type of gastric immune response against *H. pylori* contributes to the pathogenesis of peptic ulcer comes from the observation that in kidney graft recipients (undergoing strong immunosuppression) peptic ulcer and active inflammatory lesions were virtually absent, in spite of a higher prevalence of *H. pylori* colonization (Hruby et al., 1997). The results obtained so far clearly demonstrated that gastric T-cell response to *H. pylori* antigens characterized by a mixed Th1-Th2 cytokine profile is apparently associated with low rate of ulcer complication. The concept that Th2 cytokines, particularly IL-4 and IL-10, are important in balancing and quenching some immunopathological effects of polarized Th1 responses is supported by other clinical and experimental observations. Holding in mind the concept of Th1/Th2 balance, one may reconsider what clinicians know from a long time, that, during pregnancy, patients suffering of peptic ulcer significantly reduce their dyspeptic symptoms and tend to undergo remission for the time of pregnancy (Cappell et al., 2003). This might be an indirect effect of the preferential Th2 "switch" occurring in pregnancy, which makes the mother able to "tolerate" her offspring by inhibiting Th1 responses, which would otherwise promote "graft" (fetus) rejection.

In favor of a role for the immune system in influencing gastric acid secretion and the onset of peptic ulcer disease is the interesting observation in rats that immune cells of gastric mucosa, but not epithelial cells, expressed in vivo detectable mRNA for gastrin, muscarine and histamine receptors. Such information supports the hypothesis that the primary target of antiulcer drugs may primarily be the immune cells in the gastric environment (Mezey et al., 1992). Many studies performed in mice demonstrated that T-cell dependent immune response are needed for protection against *H. pylori* whereas antibody response is not strictly required for protective immunity (Ermak et al., 1998). However if the T-cell response induced against *H. pylori* is not appropriate it may even result in a damage for the host, as demonstrated by several reports also in animal models. Transferring T cells derived from *H. pylori* infected patients into SCID mice has proven to be effective in inducing gastric ulcer in those mice, thus demonstrating that host immunity is involved in the development of peptic ulcers (Yokota et al., 1999). In *H. felis* -infected mice, neutralization of IFN-$\gamma$ significantly reduced the severity of gastritis, strongly supporting the concept that preferential activation of a Th1-type response, far from being protective, rather contributes to the development and maintenance of gastric immunopathology. The magnitude of *H. felis* -induced inflammation in IL-4-deficient mice was higher than in their wild-type counterparts. Moreover, infection with *H. felis* induced minimal inflammation in BALB/c mice, whose genetic background is prone to high IL-4 production in response to different antigens. The results of these studies provide further evidence that a polarized Th1 response is associated with gastric inflammation and disease whereas, when a mixed Th1/Th2 response is raised, it is able to reduce the unbalanced proinflammatory Th1 response (Mohamadi et al., 1996). If the hypothesis that some local IL-4 production may result in protection from ulcer is correct, the so-called "African enigma" (i.e. discrepancy between high rate of *H. pylori* infection and low prevalence of peptic ulcer)(Holcombe et al., 1992) may be explained, at least in part, on the basis of the acquired cytokine background of African people living in endemic areas of helminth infection, which is known to elicit strong and persistent Th2-dominated responses. Theoretically, a Th2-oriented host immunological background would be a misfortune for efficient defence against mycobacteria, but would provide at the same time an advantage for developing milder responses to a pathogen like *H. pylori,* so widespread even in infancy. Thus, peptic ulcer may be regarded as the immunopathological outcome of a chronic inflammatory process induced by some *H. pylori* strains in subjects genetically and/or environmentally biased to develop strong Th1-polarized responses.

Although related to *H. pylori* infection, low-grade gastric MALT lymphoma is a very rare complication and represents a model to study the interplay between chronic infection, immune response and lymphomagenesis. This type of lymphoma represents the first described neoplasia susceptible to regression following antibiotic therapy resulting in *H. pylori* eradication (Wotherspoon et al., 1993). A prerequisite for lymphomagenesis is the development of secondary inflammatory MALT induced by chronic *H. pylori* challenge (Isaacson, 1994). The tumor cells of low-grade gastric MALT lymphoma are memory B cells still responsive to differentiation signals, such as CD40 costimulation and cytokines produced by antigen-stimulated T helper cells, and dependent for their growth on the stimulation by *H. pylori* -specific T cells (Hussel et al., 1996; Greiner et al., 1997). In early phases, this tumor is sensitive to withdrawal of *H. pylori* -induced T-cell help, providing an explanation for both the tumor tendency to remain localized to the primary site and its regression after *H. pylori* eradication with antibiotics (Wotherspoon et al., 1993; Bayerdoffer et al., 1995). The growth of neoplastic B cells may depend on evasion from T cell-mediated cytotoxicity. In this regard, gastric T cells from MALT lymphoma showed both defective perforin-mediated cytotoxicity and poor ability to induce Fas-Fas ligand-mediated apoptosis, thus providing a possible explanation for their enhanced helper activity on B-cell proliferation. Both defects were restricted to MALT lymphoma-infiltrating T cells, since specific T helper cells from peripheral blood of the same patients expressed the same degree of either cytolytic potential or pro-apoptotic activity as T cells from chronic gastritis patients (D'Elios et al., 1999). The reason why gastric T cells of MALT lymphoma, while delivering full help to B cells, are apparently deficient in mechanisms involved in the concomitant control of B-cell growth, remains unclear. It has been shown that VacA toxin inhibits antigen processing in APC, but not the exocytosis of perforin-containing granules of NK cells (Molinari et al., 1998). It is possible that, in some *H. pylori* -infected individuals, other bacterial components affect the development or the expression in gastric T cells of regulatory cytotoxic mechanisms on B-cell proliferation, allowing exhaustive and inbalanced B-cell help and lymphomagenesis to occur.

### 2.3 *H. pylori*, asthma and allergy
The severity and incidence of asthma have increased drastically in the developed nations of the world over the last decades. Although the underlying reason is still unknown, clinical,

epidemiological and experimental evidence indicate that infectious diseases can influence the development of allergic disorders (Strachan et al., 1989; Roumier et al., 2008). Accordingly, an inverse correlation has been demonstrated between the onset of allergic disorders and the incidence of infections. This may be the result of an inhibition of allergic Th2 inflammation exerted by Th1 responses; the latter are elicited by infectious agents and are able to induce the production of IFN-g, IL-12, IL-18 and IL-23 (Herz et al, 2000). This view is supported by studies showing that development of asthma can be prevented in animals by administering live or killed bacteria or their components, which induce Th1 responses (Wohlleben et al., 2006). We demonstrated that *H. pylori* inhibited Th2 responses in asthmatic patients (Amedei et al., 2006). Interestingly, on the basis of large epidemiological studies, a consistent negative association between *H. pylori* infection and the presence of allergic disorders, such as asthma and rhinitis, has recently been proposed (Chen et al., 2007). Although it is an undoubtedly interesting theory, no convincing molecular mechanism has been suggested to support it.

Our studies carried out with *H. pylori* may help in the understanding of this complex issue. We have shown that the addition of the *H. pylori* protein HP-NAP to allergen-induced T-cell lines derived from allergic asthmatic patients led to a drastic increase in IFN-γ-producing T cells and to a decrease in IL-4-secreting cells, thus resulting in a redirection of the immune response from a Th2 to a Th1 phenotype (Amedei et al., 2006). These results suggest that HP-NAP might be the key element responsible for the decrement of allergy frequency in *H. pylori*-infected patients. Several studies were devoted to the definition of new immune-modulating factors able to inhibit Th2 responses and consequently, different compounds have been proposed for the treatment and prevention of asthma, including several TLR ligands mimicking the effects of microbial components, such as dsRNA, CpG-oligodeoxynucleotides and imidazoquinolines (Hirota et al., 2002; Trujillo-Vargas et al., 2005).

We demonstrated that in allergic asthmatic patients, the typical Th2 responses can be redirected toward Th1 by HP-NAP and that the activity of HP-NAP required the engagement of TLR2 (Amedei et al., 2006; Codolo et al., 2008b). To address whether HP-NAP, on the basis of its immune-modulating activity, could be beneficial for the prevention and treatment of bronchial asthma, it was administered via the intraperitoneal or the intranasal route using a mouse model of allergic asthma induced by inhaled ovalbumin (OVA). Groups of nine C57BL/6j, wild-type or *tlr2-/-* mice were treated with OVA alone, or with OVA plus HP-NAP administered intraperitoneally or mucosally. In both systemic and mucosal protocols, mice were treated with OVA according to a standardized procedure consisting of a first phase of sensitization with intraperitoneal OVA and a second phase of induction of the allergic response with aerosolized OVA on day 8, followed by repeated aerosol challenge with the allergen on days 15–18. Control animals were injected with phosphate-buffered saline (PBS) alone and then exposed to aerosolized PBS. In the systemic protocol, mice were treated with intraperitoneal HP-NAP on day 1, whereas in the mucosal protocol mice received intranasal HP-NAP on days 7 and 8 (Codolo et al., 2008b).

After priming and repeated aerosol challenge with OVA, Th2 responses were induced in the mouse lung. Accordingly, following OVA treatment, eosinophils were recruited and activated in bronchial airways, and serum IgE levels increased. Both systemic and mucosal administration of HP-NAP strongly inhibited the development of airway eosinophilia and bronchial inflammation. Likewise, HP-NAP treatment strongly affected the cytokine release in the lung, reducing the production of IL-4, IL-5 and GM-CSF. Systemic HP-NAP also significantly resulted in both the reduction of total serum IgE and an increase in IL-12 plasma levels. However, no suppression of lung eosinophilia and bronchial Th2 cytokines was observed in *tlr2-/-* mice following HP-NAP treatment (Codolo et al., 2008b). This phenomenon can be explained by the inhibition of the allergic Th2 inflammation seen when Th1 responses are elicited by infectious agents able to induce the production of IFN-γ, IL-12 and IL-23. HP-NAP, by acting on innate immune cells via TLR2 agonistic interaction, induces an IL-12- and IL-23-enriched milieu, and in such a way it represents a key factor able to induce a Th2-Th1 redirection. Furthermore, HP-NAP administration *in vivo* resulted in inhibition of the typical Th2-mediated bronchial inflammation of allergic bronchial asthma. Thus, combined, these results support the view that the increased prevalence and severity of asthma and allergy in Western countries may be related, at least in part, to the decline of *H. pylori* infection, which is able to induce a long-lasting Th1 background, and suggest that the use of a microbial product derived from *H. pylori*, such as as HP-NAP, may help the prevention and treatment of bronchial asthma and allergic diseases. At the same time, we do not suggest infecting people with *H. pylori* or leaving a *H. pylori* infection without antibiotic treatment to treat asthma and allergy.

## 3. Conclusion

*Helicobacter pylori* infects almost half of the population worldwide and represents the major cause of gastroduodenal diseases, such as duodenal and gastric ulcer, gastric adenocarcinoma, autoimmune gastritis, and B-cell lymphoma of mucosa-associated lymphoid tissue. Different bacterial and environmental factors, other concomitant infections, and host genetics may influence the balance between mucosal tolerance and inflammation in the course of *H. pylori* infection. *Helicobacter pylori* induces the activation of a complex and fascinating cytokine and chemokine network in the gastric mucosa. The type of innate and acquired immune responses provides an useful model for explaining both different types of protection and the pathogenetic mechanisms of several disorders elicited by *H. pylori*. A predominant *H. pylori*-specific Th1 response, characterized by high IFN-γ, TNF-α, and IL-12 production associates with peptic ulcer, whereas combined secretion of both Th1 and Th2 cytokines are present in uncomplicated gastritis. Gastric T cells from MALT lymphoma exhibit abnormal help for autologous B-cell proliferation and reduced perforin- and Fas-Fas ligand-mediated killing of B cells. In *H. pylori*-infected patients with autoimmune gastritis cytolytic T cells infiltrating the gastric mucosa cross-recognize different epitopes of *H. pylori* proteins and $H^+K^+$ ATPase autoantigen. An inverse association between *H. pylori* prevalence and the frequencies of asthma and allergies was demonstrated, and the Neutrophil Activating Protein of *H. pylori*, according to its ability in inhibiting allergic inflammation of bronchial asthma, could be the factor responsible for this negative relationship. Given that resistance to antibiotic is increasing and the effectiveness of current therapeutic regimens is decreasing the design of an efficient vaccine for *H. pylori* will represent a novel and very important tool against both infection, peptic ulcer and gastric cancer.

## 4. Acknowledgment

This work was supported in part by MIUR PRIN 2008 to M.M.D.E., and by MIUR PRIN 2006 and Research Grant by University of Padova (CPDA074121/07) to M.d.B.

# 5. References

Amedei, A., Cappon, A., Codolo, G., Cabrelle, A., Polenghi, A.,Benagiano, M., Tasca, E., Azzurri, A., D'Elios, M.M., Del Prete, G. & De Bernard, M. (2006). The neutrophil-activating protein of *Helicobacter pylori* promotes Th1 immune responses. *The Journal of Clinical Investigation*, Vol.116, No.4, (April 2006), pp. 1092–1101, ISSN 0021-9738

Bacon, C.M., Petricoin, E.F., Ortaldo, J.E., Rees, R.C., Larner, A.C., Johnston, J.A., & O'Shea, J.J. (1995). Interleukin 12 induces tyrosine phosphorylation and activation of STAT4 in human lymphocytes. *Proceedings of the National Academy of Sciences of the United States of America*, Vol.92, No.16, (August 1995), pp. 7307-7311

Bamford, K.B., Fan, X., Crowe, S.E., Leary, J.F., Gourley, W.K., Luthra, G.K., Brooks, E.G., Graham, D.Y., Reyes, V.E., & Ernst, P.B. (1998). Lymphocytes in the human gastric mucosa during Helicobacter pylori have a T helper cell 1 phenotype. *Gastroenterology*, Vol.114, No.3, (March 1998), pp. 482-492, ISSN 0016-5085

Bayerdoffer, E., Neubauer, A., Rudolph, B., Thiede, C., Lehn, N., Eidt, S., & Stolte, M. (1995). Regression of primary gastric lymphoma of mucosa-associated lymphoid tissue after cure of *Helicobacter pylori* infection. *Lancet*, Vol.345, No.8965, (June 1995), pp. 1591-1594, ISSN 0140-6736

Bettelli, E., Oukka, M. & Kuchroo, V.K. (2007) Th-17 cells in the circle of immunity and autoimmunity. *Nature Immunology*, Vol.8, No.4, (April 2007), pp. 345–350, ISSN 1529-2908

Cappell, M.S. (2003) Gastric and duodenal ulcers during pregnancy. *Gastroenterology Clinics of North America*, Vol.27, No.1, (March 2003), pp. 263–308, ISSN 0889-8553

Chen, Y., Blaser, M.J. (2007). Inverse associations of *Helicobacter pylori* with asthma and allergy. *Archives of Internal Medicine*, Vol.167, No.8, (April 2007), pp. 821–827, ISSN 0003-9926

Codolo, G., Amedei, A., Steere, A.C,. Papinutto, E., Cappon, A., Polenghi, A., Benagiano, M., Paccani, S.R., Sambri, V., Del Prete, G., Baldari, C.T., Zanotti, G., Montecucco, C., D'Elios, M.M. & de Bernard, M. (2008). Borrelia burgdorferi-NapA driven Th17 cell inflammation in Lyme arthritis. *Arthritis and Rheumatism*, Vol.58, No.11, (November 2008), pp. 3609–3617, ISSN 0004-3591

Codolo, G., Mazzi, P., Amedei, A., Del Prete, G., Berton, G., D'Elios, M.M. & de Bernard, M. (2008). The neutrophil-activating protein of *Helicobacter pylori* down-modulates Th2 inflammation in ovalbumin-induced allergic asthma. *Cellular Microbiology*, Vol.10, No.11, (November 2008), pp. 2355–2363, ISSN 1462-5814

Constant, S.L. & Bottomly, K. (1997). Induction of Th1 and Th2 CD4+ T cell responses: The alternative approaches. *Annual Review of Immunology*, Vol.15, (1997), pp. 297-322, ISSN 0732-0582

Cover, T.L. & Blaser, M.J. (1996). *Helicobacter pylori* infection, a paradigm for chronic mucosal inflammation: pathogenesis and implications for eradication and prevention. *Advances in Internal Medicine*, Vol.41, (1996), pp. 85-117

Crabtree, J.E., Peichl, P., Wyatt, J.I., Stachl, U. & Lindley, I.J. (1993). Gastric interleukin-8 and IgA IL-8 autoantibodies in *Helicobacter pylori* infection. *Scandinavian Journal of Immunology*, Vol.37, No.1, (January 1993), pp. 65-70, ISSN 0300-9475

Crabtree, J.E., Eyre, D., Levy, L., Covacci, A., Rappuoli, R. & Morgan, A.G. (1995). Serological evaluation of *Helicobacter pylori* eradication using recombinant CagA protein. *Gut.* 36:A46, ISSN 0017-5749

Dallman, M.J. (1995). Cytokines and transplantation: Th1/Th2 regulation of the immune response to solid organ transplants in the adult. *Current Opinion in Immunology*, Vol. 7, No.5, (October 1995), pp. 632-638, ISSN 0952-7915

Danesh, J., Collins, R., & Peto, R. (1997). Chronic infections and coronary heart disease: is there a link? *Lancet*, Vol.350, No.9075, (August 1997), pp. 430-436, ISSN 0140-6736

D'Elios, M.M., Josien, R., Manghetti, M., Amedei, A., De Carli, M., Cuturi, M.C., Blancho, G., Buzelin, F., Del Prete, G. & Soulillou, J.P. (1997). Predominant Th1 infiltration in acute rejection episodes of human kidney grafts. *Kidney International*, Vol.51, No.6, (June 1997), pp. 1876-1884, ISSN 0085-2538

D'Elios, M.M., Manghetti, M., De Carli, M., Costa, F., Baldari, C.T., Burroni, D., Telford, J.L., Romagnani, S. & Del Prete, G. (1997). Th1 effector cells specific for *Helicobacter pylori* in the gastric antrum of patients with peptic ulcer disease. *Journal of Immunology*, Vol.158, No.2, (January 1997), pp. 962-967, ISSN 0022-1767

D'Elios, M.M., Romagnani, P., Scaletti, C., Annunziato, F., Manghetti, M., Mavilia, C., Parronchi, P., Pupilli, C., Pizzolo, G., Maggi, E., Del Prete, G. & Romagnani S. (1997). In vivo CD30 expression in human diseases with predominant activation of Th2-like T cells. *Journal of Leukocyte Biology*, Vol.61, No.5, (May 1997), pp. 539- 544, ISSN 0741-5400

D'Elios, M.M., Manghetti, M., Almerigogna, F., Amedei, A., Costa, F., Burroni, D., Baldari, C.T., Romagnani, S., Telford, J.L. & Del Prete, G. (1997). Different cytokine profile and antigen-specificity repertoire in *Helicobacter pylori*-specific T cell clones from the antrum of chronic gastritis patients with or without peptic ulcer. *European Journal of Immunoogy*, Vol.27, No.7, (july 1997), pp. 1751-1755, ISSN 0014-2980

D'Elios, M.M., Andersen, L.P., & Del Prete, G. (1998). Inflammation and host response. The year in *Helicobacter pylori. Current Opinion in Gastroenterology*, Vol.14, (1998), pp. 15-19, ISSN 0267-1379 D'Elios, M.M., Amedei, A., Manghetti, M., Costa, F., Baldari, C.T., Quazi A.S., Telford, J.L., Romagnani, S. & Del Prete, G. (1999). Impaired T-cell regulation of B-cell growth in Helicobacter pylori-related gastric low-grade MALT lymphoma. *Gastroenterology*, Vol.117, No.5, (November 1999), pp. 1105-1112, ISSN 0016-5085

D'Elios, M.M. & Del Prete, G. (1999). Th1/Th2 cytokine network. *Topics in Neuroscience*, Martino, G. & Adorini, L., eds. Springer-Verlag, Berlin, pp. 68-82 Del Prete, G., De Carli, M., Mastromauro, C., Macchia, D., Biagiotti, R., Ricci, M. & Romagnani, S. (1991). Purified protein derivative of *Mycobacterium tuberculosis* and excretory-secretory antigen(s) of *Toxocara canis* expand in vitro human T cells with stable and opposite (type 1 T helper or type 2 T helper) profile of cytokine production. *The Journal of Clinical Investigation*, Vol.88, No.1, (July 1991), pp. 346-351, ISSN 0021-9738

Del Prete, G.F., De Carli, M., Ricci, M., & Romagnani, S. (1991). Helper activity for immunoglobulin synthesis of T helper type 1 (Th1) and Th2 human T cell clones: the help of Th1 clones is limited by their cytolytic capacity. *The Journal of Experimental Medicine*, Vol.174, No.4, (October 1991), pp. 809-813, ISSN 0022-1007

Del Prete, G., De Carli, M., Almerigogna, F., Giudizi, M.G., Biagiotti, R. & Romagnani, S. (1993). Human IL-10 is produced by both type 1 helper (Th1) and type 2 helper (Th2) T cell clones and inhibits their antigen-specific proliferation and cytokine production. *Journal of Immunology*, Vol.150, No.2, (January 1993), pp. 353-360, ISSN 0022-1767

Del Prete, G., De Carli, M., Lammel, R.M., D'Elios, M.M., Daniel, K.C., Giusti, B., Abbate, R. & Romagnani S. (1995). Th1 and Th2 T-helper cells exert opposite regulatory effects on procoagulant activity and tissue factor production by human monocytes. *Blood*, Vol.86, No.1, (July 1995), pp. 250-257, ISSN 0006-4971

Del Prete, G. (1998). The concept of Type-1 and Type-2 helper T cells and their cytokines in humans. *International Reviews of Immunology*, Vol.16, No.3-4, (1998), pp. 427-455

Elizalde, J.L., Gomez, J., Panes, J., Lozano, M., Casadevall, M., Ramirez, J., Pizcueta, P., Marco, F., Rojas, F.D., Granger, D.N. & Pique, J.M. (1997). Platelet activation in mice and human *Helicobacter pylori* infection. *The Journal of Clinical Investigation*, Vol.100, No.5, (September 1997), pp. 996-1005, ISSN 0021-9738

Ermak, T.H., Giannasca, P.J., Nichols, R., Myers, G.A., Nedrud, J., Weltzin, R., Lee, C.K., Kleanthous, H. & Monath, T.P. (1998) Immunization of mice with urease vaccine affords protection against Helicobacter pylori infection in the absence of *The Journal of Experimental Medicine*, Vol.188, No.12, (December 1998), pp. 2277-2288, ISSN 0022-1007

Ferrick, D.A., Schrenzel, M.D. & Mulvania T. (1995). Differential production of IFN-γ and IL-4 in response to Th1- and Th2-stimulating pathogens by gamma delta T cells in vivo. *Nature*, Vol.373, No.6511, (January 1995), pp. 255-258, ISSN 0028-0836

Fiorucci, S., Santucci, L., Migliorati, G., Riccardi, C., Amorosi, A., Mancini, A., Roberti, R. & Morelli, A. (1996). Isolated guinea pig gastric chief cells express tumor necrosis factor receptors coupled with the sphingomyelin pathway. *Gut.*, Vol.38, No.2, (February 1996), pp. 182-189, ISSN 0017-5749

Fritz, J.H., Le Bourhis, L., Sellge, G., Magalhaes, J.G., Fsihi, H.,Kufer, T.A., Collins, C., Viala, J., Ferrero, R.L., Girardin, S.E. & Philpott, D.J.(2007). Nod1-mediated innate immune recognition of peptidoglycan contributes to the onset of adaptive immunity. *Immunity*, Vol.26, No.4, (April 2006), pp.445–59, ISSN 1074-7613

Greiner, A., Knorr, C., Qin, Y., Sebald, W., Schimpl, A., Banchereau, J. & Muller-Hermelink, H.K. (1997). Low-grade B cell lymphomas of mucosa-associated lymphoid tissue (MALT-type) require CD40-mediated signaling and Th2-type cytokines for in vitro growth and differentiation. *The American Journal of Pathology*, Vol.150, No.5, (May 1997), pp. 1583-1593, ISSN 0002-9440

Hauer, A.C., Finn, T.M., MacDonald, T.T., Spencer, J. & Isaacson, P.G. (1997). Analysis of TH1 and TH2 cytokine production in low grade B cell gastric MALT-type lymphomas stimulated in vitro with *Helicobacter pylori*. *The Journal of Clinical Pathology*, Vol.50, No.11, (November 1997), pp. 957-959, ISSN 0021-9746

Herz, U., Lacy, P., Renz, H. & Erb, K. (2000). The influence of infections on the development and severity of allergic disorders. *Current Opinion in Immunology*, Vol.12, No.6, (December 2000), pp. 632–640, ISSN 0952-7915

Hirota, K., Kazaoka, K., Niimoto, I., Kumihara, H., Sajiki, H., Isobe, Y., Takaku, H., Tobe, M., Ogita, H., Ogino, T., Ichii, S., Kurimoto, A. & Kawakami, H. (2002). Discovery of 8-hydroxyadenines as a novel type of interferon inducer. *Journal of Medicinal Chemistry*, Vol.45, No.25, (December 2002), pp. 5419–5422, ISSN 0022-2623

Holcombe, C. (1992). *Helicobacter pylori* : the African enigma. 1992. *Gut*. Vol.33, No.4, (April 1992), pp. 429-431, ISSN 0017-5749

Hruby, Z., Myszka-Bijak, K., Gosciniak, G., Blaszczuk, J., Czyz, W., Kowalski, P., Falkiewicz, K., Szymanska, G. & Przondo-Mordarska, A. (1997). *Helicobacter pylori* in kidney allograft recipients: high prevalence of colonization and low incidence of active inflammatory lesions. *Nephron*, Vol.75, No.1, (1997), pp. 25-29 Hussell, T., Isaacson, P.G., Crabtree, J.E. & Spencer, J. (1996). *Helicobacter pylori* -specific tumour-infiltrating T cells provide contact dependent help for the growth of malignant B cells in low-grade gastric lymphoma of mucosa-associated lymphoid tissue. *The Journal of Pathology*, Vol.178, No.2 (February 1996), pp. 122-127, ISSN 0022-3417

Isaacson, P.G. (1994). Gastrointestinal lymphoma. *Human Pathology*, Vol.25, No.10, (October 1994), pp. 1020-1029, ISSN 0046-8177

Kamogawa, Y., Minasi, L.E., Carding, S.R., Bottomly, K. & Flavell, R.A. (1993). The relationship of IL-4- and IFN-γ-producing T cells studied by lineage ablation of IL-4-producing cells. *Cell*, Vol.75, No.5, (December 1993), pp. 985-995, ISSN 0092-8674 Kaparakis, M., Philpott, D.J., Ferrero, R.L. (2007). Mammalian NLR proteins; discriminating foe from friend. *Immunology and Cell Biology*, Vol.85, No.6, (August-September 2007), pp. 495–502, ISSN 0818-9641

Korn, T., Bettelli, E., Oukka, M., Kuchroo, V.K. (2009). IL-17 and Th17 Cells. *Annual Review of Immunology*, Vol.27, (2009), pp.485-517 Marshall, B.J. (1994). *Helicobacter pylori*. *Am. J. Gastroenterol*. 89: 116-128, ISSN 0002-9270

Mezey, E. & Palkovits, S. (1992). Localization of targets for anti-ulcer drugs in cells of the immune system. *Science*, Vol.258, No.5088, (December 1992), pp. 1662-1665, ISSN 0036-8075

Mohammadi, M., Czinn, S., Redline, R. & Nedrud, J. (1996). *Helicobacter*-specific cell-mediated immune response display a predominant Th1 phenotype and promote a delayed-type hypersensitivity response in the stomachs of mice. *Journal of Immunology*, Vol.156, No.12, (June 1996), pp. 4729-4738, ISSN 0022-1767

Molinari, M., Salio, M., Galli, C., Norais, N., Rappuoli, R., Lanzavecchia, A. & Montecucco, C. (1998). Selective inhibition of Ii-dependent antigen presentation by *Helicobacter pylori* toxin VacA. *The Journal of Experimental Medicine*, Vol.187, No.1, (January 1998), pp. 135-140, ISSN 0022-1007

Mosmann, T.R., Cherwinski, H., Bond, M.W., Giedlin, M.A. & Coffman, R.L. (1986). Two types of murine T cell clone. I. Definition according to profiles of lymphokine activities and secreted proteins. *Journal of immunology*, Vol.136, No.7, (April 1986), pp. 2348-2357, ISSN 0022-1767 Mosmann, T.R. & Sad, S. (1996). The expanding universe of T-cell subsets: Th1, Th2 and more. *Immunology Today*, Vol.17, No.3, (March 1996), pp. 138-146

Niessner, M. & Volk, B.A. (1995). Altered Th1/Th2 cytokine profiles in the intestinal mucosa of patients with inflammatory bowel disease as assessed by quantitative transcribed polymerase chain reaction (RT-PCR). *Clinical and Experimental Immunology*, Vol.101, No.3, (September 1995), pp. 428-435, ISSN 0009-9104

Parronchi, P., Romagnani, P., Annunziato, F., Sampognaro, S., Becchio, A., Giannarini, L., Maggi, E., Pupilli, C., Tonelli, F. & Romagnani, S. (1997). Type 1 T-helper cells predominance and interleukin-12 expression in the gut of patients with Crohn's disease. *The American Journal of Pathol*ogy, Vol.150, No.3, (March 1997), pp. 823-831, ISSN 0002-9440

Parsonnet, J., Friedman, G.D., Vandersteen, D.P., Chang, Y., Vogelman, J.H., Orentreich, N. & Sibley, R.K. (1991). *Helicobacter pylori* infection and the risk of gastric cancer. *The New England Journal of Med*icine, Vol. 325, No.16, (October 1991), pp. 1127-1131, ISSN 0028-4793

Piccinni, M.P., Beloni, L., Livi, C., Maggi, E., Scarselli, G. & Romagnani, S. (1998). Role of type 2 T helper (Th2) cytokines and leukemia inhibitory factor (LIF) produced by decidual T cells in unexplained recurrent abortions. *Nature Medicine*, Vol.4, No.9, (September 1998), pp. 1020-1024

Rathbone, B.J., Wyatt, J.I., Worsley, B.W., Shires, S.E., Trejdosiewicz, L.K. & Heatley, R.V. (1986). Systemic and local antibody responses to gastric *Campylobacter pyloridis* in non-ulcer dyspepsia. *Gut*, Vol.27, No.6, (June 1986), pp. 642-647, ISSN 0017-5749

Rincon, M. & Flavell, R.A. (1997). T cell subsets: transcriptional control in the Th1/Th2 decision. *Current Biology*, Vol.7, No.11, (November 1997), pp. 729-732, ISSN 0960-9822 Roumier, T., Capron, M., Dombrowicz, D. & Faveeuw, C. (2008). Pathogen induce regulatory cell populations preventing allergy through the Th1/Th2 paradigm point of view. *Immunologic research*, Vol.40, No.1, (2008), pp. 1-17, ISSN 0257-277X

Sommer, F., Faller, G., Konturek, P., Kirchner, T., Hahn, E.G., Zeus, J., Röllinghoff, M. & Lohoff, M. (1998). Antrum- and corpus mucosa-infiltrating CD4(+) lymphocytes in *Helicobacter pylori* gastritis display a Th1 phenotype. *Infection and Immunity*, Vol.66, No.11, (November 1998), pp. 5543-5546, ISSN 0019-9567

Strachan, D.P. (1989). Hay fever, hygiene and household size. *BMJ* Vol.299, No.6710, (November 1989), pp. 1259–1260 Szabo, S., Jacobson, N.G., Dighe, A.S., Gubler, U. & Murphy, K.M. (1995). Developmental committment to the Th2 lineage by extinction of IL-12 signaling. *Immunity*, Vol.2, No.6, (June 1995), pp. 665-675, ISSN 1074-7613

Szabo, S.J., Glimcher, L.H. & Ho, I.C. (1997). Genes that regulate interleukin-4 expression in T cells. *Current Opinion in Immunology*, Vol.9, No.6, (december 1997), pp. 775-781, ISSN 0952-7915

Telford, J.L., Ghiara, P., Dell'Orco, M., Comanducci, M., Burroni, D., Bugnoli, M., Tecce, M.F., Censini, S., Covacci, A., Xiang, Z., Papini, E., Montecucco, C., Parente, L. & Rappuoli, R. (1994). Gene structure of the *Helicobacter pylori* cytotoxin and evidence of its key role in gastric disease. *The Journal of Experimental Medicine*, Vol.179, No.5, (May 1994), pp. 1653-1670, ISSN 0022-1007

Tomb, J.F., White, O., Kerlavage, A.R., Clayton, R.A., Sutton, G.G., Fleischmann, R.D., Ketchum, K.A., Klenk, H.P., Gill, S., Dougherty, B.A., Nelson, K., Quackenbush, J., Zhou, L., Kirkness, E.F., Peterson, S, Loftus B., Richardson, D., Dodson, R., Khalak, H.G., Glodek, A., McKenney, K., Fitzegerald, L.M., Lee, N., Adams, M.D., Hickey, E.K., Berg, D.E., Gocayne, J.D., Utterback, T.R., Peterson, J.D., Kelley, J.M., Cotton, M.D., Weidman, J.M., Fujii, C., Bowman, C., Watthey, L., Wallin, E., Hayes, W.S., Borodovsky, M., Karp, P.D., Smith, H.O., Fraser, C.M., Venter, J.C. (1997). The complete genome sequence of the gastric pathogen *Helicobacter pylori. Nature*, Vol.388, No.6642, (August 1997), pp. 539-547, ISSN 0028-0836

Trinchieri, G. (1995). Interleukin-12: a proinflammatory cytokine with immunoregulatory functions that bridge innate resistance and antigen-specific adaptive immunity. *Annual Review of Immunology*, Vol.13, (1995), pp. 251-276, ISSN 0732-0582

Trujillo-Vargas, C.M., Mayer, K.D., Bickert, T., Palmetshofer, A., Grunewald, S., Ramirez-Pineda, J.R., Polte, T., Hansen, G., Wohlleben G. & Erb KJ. (2005). Vaccinations with T-helper type 1 directing adjuvants havedifferent suppressive effects on the development of allergen-induced T-helper type 2 responses. *Clinical and Experimental Allergy*, Vol. 35, No.8, (August 2005), pp. 1003–1013, ISSN 0954-7894

Weaver, C.T., Harrington, L.E-, Mangan, P.R., Gavriel,i M. & Murphy, K.M. (2006). Th17: an effector CD4 T cell lineage with regulatory T cell ties. *Immunity*, Vol.24, No.6, (June 2006), pp. 677–688, ISSN 1074-7613

Weigert, N., Schaffer, K., Schusdziarra, V., Classen, M. & Schepp, W. (1996). Gastrin secretion from primary cultures of rabbit antral G cells: stimulation by inflammatory cytokines. *Gastroenterology*, Vol.110, No.1, (January 1996), pp. 147-154, ISSN 0016-5085

Wohlleben, G. & Erb, K.J. (2006). Immune stimulatory strategies for the prevention and treatment of asthma. *Current Pharmaceutical Design*, Vol.12, No.25, (2006), pp. 3281–3292 , ISSN 1381-6128

Wotherspoon, A.C., Ortiz-Hidalgo, C., Falzon, M.F. & Isaacson, P.G. (1991). *Helicobacter pylori* associated gastritis and primary B-cell lymphoma. *Lancet*, Vol.338, No.8776, (November 1991), pp. 1175-1176, ISSN 0140-6736

Wotherspoon, A.C., Doglioni, C., Diss, T.C., Pan, L., Moschini, A., De Boni, M. & Isaacson, P.G. (1993). Regression of primary low grade B cell gastric lymphoma of mucosa-associated lymphoid tissue type after eradication of *Helicobacter pylori*. *Lancet*, Vol.342, No.8871, (September 1993), pp. 575-577, ISSN 0140-6736

Yokota, K., Kobayashi, K., Kahawara, Y., Hayashi, S., Hirai, Y., Mizuno, M., Okada, H., Akagi, T., Tsuji, T. & Oguma, K. (1999). Gastric ulcers in SCID mice induced by *Helicobacter pylori* infection after transplanting lymphocytes from patients with gastric lymphoma. *Gastroenterology*, Vol.117, No.4, (October 1999), pp. 893-899, ISSN 0016-5085

# Permissions

The contributors of this book come from diverse backgrounds, making this book a truly international effort. This book will bring forth new frontiers with its revolutionizing research information and detailed analysis of the nascent developments around the world.

We would like to thank Jianyuan Chai, Ph.D, for lending his expertise to make the book truly unique. He has played a crucial role in the development of this book. Without his invaluable contribution this book wouldn't have been possible. He has made vital efforts to compile up to date information on the varied aspects of this subject to make this book a valuable addition to the collection of many professionals and students.

This book was conceptualized with the vision of imparting up-to-date information and advanced data in this field. To ensure the same, a matchless editorial board was set up. Every individual on the board went through rigorous rounds of assessment to prove their worth. After which they invested a large part of their time researching and compiling the most relevant data for our readers. Conferences and sessions were held from time to time between the editorial board and the contributing authors to present the data in the most comprehensible form. The editorial team has worked tirelessly to provide valuable and valid information to help people across the globe.

Every chapter published in this book has been scrutinized by our experts. Their significance has been extensively debated. The topics covered herein carry significant findings which will fuel the growth of the discipline. They may even be implemented as practical applications or may be referred to as a beginning point for another development. Chapters in this book were first published by InTech; hereby published with permission under the Creative Commons Attribution License or equivalent.

The editorial board has been involved in producing this book since its inception. They have spent rigorous hours researching and exploring the diverse topics which have resulted in the successful publishing of this book. They have passed on their knowledge of decades through this book. To expedite this challenging task, the publisher supported the team at every step. A small team of assistant editors was also appointed to further simplify the editing procedure and attain best results for the readers.

Our editorial team has been hand-picked from every corner of the world. Their multi-ethnicity adds dynamic inputs to the discussions which result in innovative outcomes. These outcomes are then further discussed with the researchers and contributors who give their valuable feedback and opinion regarding the same. The feedback is then collaborated with the researches and they are edited in a comprehensive manner to aid the understanding of the subject.

Apart from the editorial board, the designing team has also invested a significant amount of their time in understanding the subject and creating the most relevant covers. They scrutinized every image to scout for the most suitable representation of the subject and create an appropriate cover for the book.

The publishing team has been involved in this book since its early stages. They were actively engaged in every process, be it collecting the data, connecting with the contributors or procuring relevant information. The team has been an ardent support to the editorial, designing and production team. Their endless efforts to recruit the best for this project, has resulted in the accomplishment of this book. They are a veteran in the field of academics and their pool of knowledge is as vast as their experience in printing. Their expertise and guidance has proved useful at every step. Their uncompromising quality standards have made this book an exceptional effort. Their encouragement from time to time has been an inspiration for everyone.

The publisher and the editorial board hope that this book will prove to be a valuable piece of knowledge for researchers, students, practitioners and scholars across the globe.

# List of Contributors

**Maria Izabel Gomes Silva and Francisca Cléa Florenço de Sousa**
Federal University of Ceará, Brazil

**Tat-Kin Tsang**
University of Chicago, USA

**Manish Prasad Shrestha**
Saint Francis Hospital, University of Illinois, USA

**Iván Ferraz-Amaro and Federico Díaz-González**
Rheumatology Service, Hospital Universitario de Canarias, Santa Cruz de Tenerife, Spain

**Wang G.Z**
College of Life Science, Zhejiang University, P.R. China
Institute of Medicine, Qiqihaer Medical College, P. R. China

**Wang J.F**
College of Life Science, Zhejiang University, P.R. China

**Ahmet Uyanıkoğlu, Ahmet Danalıoğlu, Filiz Akyüz, Binnur Pınarbaşı, Kadir Demir, Sadakat Özdil, Fatih Beşışık, Güngör Boztaş, Zeynel Mungan and Sabahattin Kaymakoğlu**
İstanbul University, Faculty of Medicine, Department of Gastroenterohepatology, Turkey

**Mine Güllüoğlu and Yersu Kapran**
İstanbul University, Faculty of Medicine, Department of Pathology, Turkey

**Petr Lukes, Jaromir Astl and Jan Betka**
Charles University in Prague, 1st Faculty of Medicine, Department of Otorhinolaryngology and Head and Neck Surgery, Faculty Hospital Motol, Prague, Czech Republic

**Emil Pavlik and Bela Potuznikova**
Charles University in Prague, 1st Faculty of Medicine, Institute of Immunology and Microbiology, Prague, Czech Republic

**Jan Plzak and Martin Chovane**
Charles University in Prague, 1st Faculty of Medicine, Department of Otorhinolaryngology and Head and Neck Surgery, Faculty Hospital Motol, Prague, Czech Republic
Charles University in Prague, 1st Faculty of Medicine, Institute of Anatomy, Prague, Czech Republic

**Matteo Fornai, Luca Antonioli, Rocchina Colucci, Marco Tuccori and Corrado Blandizzi**
Department of Internal Medicine, University of Pisa, Pisa, Italy

**Jianyuan Chai**
VA Long Beach Healthcare System, Long Beach and the University of California, Irvine, USA

**Thomas Brzozowski Aleksandra Szlachcic, Robert Pajdo, Zbigniew Sliwowski, Danuta Drozdowicz, Jolanta Majka, Wladyslaw Bielanski, Stanislaw J. Konturek and Wieslaw W. Pawlik**
Department of Physiology, Jagiellonian University Medical College, Cracow, Poland

**Peter. C. Konturek**
Thuringia-Clinic Saalfeld Georgiou's Agricola GmbH Teaching Hospital of the University of Jena, Germany

**Trinidad Parra-Cid and Miryam Calvino-Fernández**
Unidad de Investigación. Hospital Universitario de Guadalajara, Spain
CIBERehd (Centro de Investigación Biomédica en Red, Enfermedades Hepáticas y Digestivas), Spain

**Javier P. Gisbert**
Servicio de Aparato Digestivo. Hospital Universitario de La Princesa e Instituto de Investigación Sanitaria Princesa (IP)(Madrid), Spain
CIBERehd (Centro de Investigación Biomédica en Red, Enfermedades Hepáticas y Digestivas), Spain

**Yoshihiro Matsukawa**
Division of Hematology and Rheumatology, Department of Medicine, Nihon University School of Medicine, Japan

**Kimitoshi Kato**
Division of Gastroenterology and Hematology, Department of Medicine, Nihon University School of Medicine, Japan

**Ludmila Filaretova**
Laboratory of Experimental Endocrinology, Pavlov Institute of Physiology, Russia

**Mario M. D'Elios**
Department of Internal Medicine, University of Florence, Italy

**Marina de Bernard**
Venetian Institute of Molecular Medicine, University of Padua, Italy